Autism and Child Psychopathology Series

Series Editor
Johnny L. Matson
Baton Rouge, Louisiana, USA

More information about this series at http://www.springer.com/series/8665

Peter Sturmey

Reducing Restraint and Restrictive Behavior Management Practices

Springer

Peter Sturmey
Department of Psychology
Queens College
City University of New York
Flushing
New York
USA

ISSN 2192-922X ISSN 2192-9238 (electronic)
Autism and Child Psychopathology Series
ISBN 978-3-319-17568-3 ISBN 978-3-319-17569-0 (eBook)
DOI 10.1007/978-3-319-17569-0

Library of Congress Control Number: 2015937493

Springer Cham Heidelberg New York Dordrecht London

Printed on acid-free paper

Springer International Publishing AG Switzerland is part of Springer Science+Business Media (www.springer.com)

To Raul Antonio Gordillo

Preface

Restrictive behavioral practices include physical and personal restraints, seclusion and time-out rooms, emergency "prn" medication, movement restrictions through environmental modification, such as barriers and loss of property. This issue has garnered attention due to restraint-related deaths and repeated calls for elimination of restrictive behavioral practices. Such calls for action tend to be emotional and ideological appeals to solve the problem, often in response to restraint-related deaths or media exposes of abusive practices. Unfortunately, exactly how to reduce restrictive behavioral practices is often unclear.

This volume will address this issue in two parts. The first part of this book will define clearly what constitutes restrictive behavioral practices, survey the extent of the problem and highlight both historical and contemporary descriptions of restrictive behavioral practices. It will demonstrate that restrictive behavioral practices continue to be used, commonly in contemporary services, including community services, and perhaps are commonly also used in families. The second part of the volume will review the outcome research literature. This will include a review applied behavior analysis, mostly, but not exclusively for children and adults with Intellectual Disabilities, other interventions, such as mindfulness and staff education programs in nursing homes, and interventions for large-scale organizations, such as entire mental health services. The final chapter will identify future direction for research and practice.

There are a number of published books in this area. One group of books includes reprints of historical books which described medieval restraint and torture devices (Santini and Ness 2011), early programs to eliminate restraint (Conolly 1856/1973; Jarvis and Clark 1869/2013; Tuke 1813/2009), and reviews of the history of restraint use primarily in psychiatric settings (Deutch 1946). A second group related to restraint use and reduction with specific populations and/or settings. These include books on restraint in seniors and nursing home (Hughes 2010; Stumpf et al. 1998), nursing (Lipson and Braun 1993; Kumar 2007) and how to meet restraint-related regulations for medical facilities and some nursing home regulations (Joint Commission on Accreditation of Healthcare 2002; Zusman 1997; Zusman 1999); books on restraint in psychiatric services (Beer et al. 2001; Deutch 1946; Tardiff 1984), including a description of an evaluation of a course to reduce restraint in psychiatric settings (Ryan 2009) and a book on reducing seclusion in mental health settings (Alty and Mason 1994); books on restraint in services for people with developmental disabilities (Allen 2002; Allen 2009), including legal aspects of physical interventions (Karim 2014; Lyon and Imor 2004), codes of practice, (British Institute for Learning Disabilities 2014. Several books have addressed the use of restraints with children including use of restraint in schools (Johnson undated; Peterson 2013) and youth services (Kupfersmid and Monkman 1988). One volume addressed the use of restraints in a variety of social care settings (Hughes 2009). Finally, one illustrative manual described how to use painful join locking, joint hyperextension and limb-breaking personal restraints on the streets (Christensen 2006). Most contemporary books review limited literature focusing on specific populations, settings or contexts, and/or report outcome for specific programs. Some are highly practitioner-oriented, but do not support their interventions with research and others merely document and lament the excessive use of restraint without offering specific solutions as how to reduce restraint use safely. Therefore, the aims of this book are: (a) to review the research literature broadly across different populations, settings and contexts, and, based on this review, (b) identify the interventions methods most likely to result in safe reduction of restraint and other restrictive behavior management practices, such as seclusion, locked room time out; and (c) illustrate the application of effective, evidence-based interventions for safe reductions in restraint use.

"No form of strait-waistcoat, no leg-locks, no any contrivance confining the trunk or limbs, or any muscles, is now in use. The coercion chairs, about forty in number, have been altogether removed from the wards."

John Connolly, 1856

Contents

About the Author

Peter Sturmey Ph.D. is Professor of Psychology at The Graduate Center and Queens College, City University of New York and a member of the doctoral program in behavior analysis. He has published widely on intellectual and other developmental disabilities and made many national and international presentations for more than 30 years. His main focus of research is training staff and parents and evidence-based practice and Intellectual Disabilities.

Part I
Foundational Issues

The first six chapters of this volume focus on the nature of restrictive behavior management practices, such as restraint, seclusion, PRN medication, and other restrictive procedures. These six chapters discuss the definition of restrictive behavior management practices, document the extent of their use, their correlates and at-risk populations, and settings. Restrictive behavior management practices have an extensive history, which, this book argues, sadly repeats itself again and again. Thus, the chapters on history cover the use of elimination of restraint in the nineteenth century, and charts the continued use of restrictive behavior management practices through to the time when this volume was written.

Chapter 1
Definitions and Rationales

Restraint and restrictive behavioral practices (RRBPs) have always been controversial. They often appear demeaning and stressful to the person restrained and the person implementing the procedure. They may be dangerous to both parties; restraint-related deaths have been reported for over 200 years and continue to be reported. When there are alternate, effective methods of managing undesirable behavior, few would advocate for the use of RRBPs. Many human service policies, laws, and codes of professional conduct call for the use of RRBPs to be highly circumscribed, to be limited to only emergency situations, or to be completely eliminated. The need to safely reduce or eliminate RRBPs has been recognized since the late eighteenth century, yet services and families continue to use RRBPs and, if they are interested in reducing or eliminating their use, often continue to struggle to do so. Yet, RRBPs remain widespread and are sometimes even seen as desirable. This chapter has two aims. The first is to attempt to define RRBPs in different populations and contexts. The second is to identify the rationale for their use.

1.1 Restrictive Behavior Management Practices: Some Examples

Consider first some examples of RRBPs:

- A nurse places an agitated medical patient in a bed and prevents them from tearing an intravenous drip by placing mittens on their hands, tying their wrists to bed rails, and securing the bedrails so the person cannot get out of bed. The patient and their family are grateful that the patient's safety is assured and admire the nursing and medical staff's professionalism and calm in dealing with a dangerous situation.

P. Sturmey, *Reducing Restraint and Restrictive Behavior Management Practices*,
Autism and Child Psychopathology Series, DOI 10.1007/978-3-319-17569-0_1

- A teacher of children aged 7–8 years is fired when parents find out that she taped children's mouths shut to stop them talking in class. The parents go to the media and sue the school for emotional damages to the children and family members.
- While waiting for their car to be worked on, two parents, irritated by their 2-year-old daughter's annoying behavior, repeatedly reprimand her. After they both return to their cell phones, she continues to try to pound the table and walk round the room and talk to strangers. As their irritation increases, they place her in her stroller and tie her in using the safety harnesses that come with the stroller. After she continues to try to walk while attached to the stroller, they finally place the locks on the stroller and place a table in front of her so that she cannot move. Other members of the public scowl disapprovingly, but say nothing.
- An 85-year-old woman in a nursing home with dementia repeatedly wanders using her walking frame and sometimes staggers, bangs her legs, and looks like she might fall. Direct carestaff send much time redirecting her back from the nursing home lobby where she repeatedly demands candy bars and coffee. Her treatment team decides to deny her access to her walking frame to prevent falls and to obtain a medical order to do so.
- A 3-year-old girl with severe Intellectual Disabilities (ID) and autism comes into a preschool program with arm splints to prevent head banging. Whenever the restraints are removed, she bangs her head approximately 100 times per minute, resulting in bruising and sometimes bleeding. Her mother and father made the arm splints themselves. The school staff continue to use the restraints because the parents asked them to do so and because they do not know of anything else to do. At the end 2 years in preschool, the girl continues to be restraints continuously and self-injures just frequently and intensely. She graduates on to another school program where they continue to use restraints for many years.
- In an inpatient program for adolescents with emotional disorders, a teenage girl becomes upset and threatens to cut herself because another girl on the unit flirted with her boyfriend repeatedly. Staff warn her to calm down, but she threatens and attacks them. They use physical restraint methods, which the program trained them to use, to take her down. During the takedown, both she and the staff are bruised. This happens repeatedly over several months, and the staff use combinations of physical takedowns, pro re nata (PRN; "as needed"), medication to sedate her, and seclusion. Injuries continue to occur to her, other residents, and staff.
- In a special treatment unit for adults with Prader–Willi syndrome (a rare genetic syndrome characterized by frequent ID, overeating, life-threatening obesity, self-injury in the form of chronic skin picking) all food is locked up. Access to the kitchen, refrigerator, and pantry doors is prevented as they are locked when staff are not in the kitchen. Families are not permitted to bring high-calorie food, and residents may not use their own money to do so. Behavioral incidents related to food stealing are common and result in injuries to clients and staff.
- When teaching a 26-month-old child with autism to sit down and keep their hands down, their applied behavior analyst blocks their legs with her own legs for several minutes at a time and gradually reduces the blocking. She also briefly

holds the child's arms down for up to 5 s to help her learn to keep her hands down. The child finds this quite distressing for the first few sessions and cries and struggles a lot. After 2 weeks, the child sits for up to 2 h with his hands down and is able to begin learning. Without this procedure, it is unlikely that the child will benefit from early intervention.

- Following a stroke that paralyzes a patient's left arm, the patient agrees to receive "constraint-induced therapy" (Taub 2012) which consists of physically restraining the non-affected arm for much of the day for several weeks, shaping[1] movement in the affected arm, and a package of homework assignments to transfer treatment gains from therapy sessions to activities of daily living in the natural environment. Some weeks later, the patient has made much faster recovery than otherwise would have been expected and has functional use of their left arm.
- A driver is pulled over by the police for driving 120 miles/h. In the back of the car are two children, both of whom were not restrained in car seats, one of whom was on the car floor. The driver was jailed for several months, in part for endangering the children by failing to restrain them and thereby exposing them to potential injury and death.
- City social services entered a family home after an anonymous report to find that the family had constructed a cage in their garage to contain their aggressive and highly active child with autism. The cage did not result in physical injuries to the child. The family, who were immigrants with limited English and little knowledge of local services, had done so because they were concerned to protect their other children and did not know how to manage their child's aggressive behavior, even though local educational services had some knowledge of the child's behavioral issues at home. Social services removed all children from the home, placed them in foster care, and prosecuted the bewildered parents for child abuse. The child with autism continued not to receive effective behavioral services and was periodically physically restrained by residential staff for many months without a behavior support plan.

These examples illustrate the widespread use of restraint and other restrictive behavioral practices. Some are acceptable and even required by the law in some circumstances. Others are illegal and often considered examples of abuse.

1.2 Definitional Issues

The definition of restraint and other restrictive behavioral practices is unclear. Terms such as "restraint" are defined by different groups—laws, local services, and professional bodies—at different time and for different purposes. Sometimes the

[1] Shaping, sometimes known as the "method of successive approximations" is a behavioral procedure which involves reinforcement of better and better approximations to a final behavioral goal and extinction of previously reinforced responses. Extinction refers to no longer reinforcing responses that were previously reinforced.

authors of such definitions have implicit or explicit motivations, such as defending or propagating certain practices or commercial products, such as staff training packages. Thus, RRBPs may include physical restraint, mechanical restraint, and other restrictions to movement or access to personal properties, such as barriers. It may also refer to PRN ("as needed") medication or rapid tranquilization (Pilowsky et al. 1992), and is sometimes also used to refer to psychotropic medication more generally, especially when it is used for general sedation of reduction in all behavior. There are also gray areas, such as some medical and physical therapy procedures, and some societally sanctioned forms of restrictive behavior management practices. Sometimes people deliberately chose to manage their own behavior (Skinner 1953) using restrictive behavior management practices, such as self-restraint and use of sedating medication, including some psychiatric patients who administer or request their own PRN medication. For example, teaching to someone to fold their arms or place their hands in the pockets to reduce fidgeting or even more serious behavior problems would be seen as highly desirable by many, whereas personal or mechanical restraint imposed on the person to make them fold their arms by another would usually be seen as much less acceptable. Some teaching procedures, such as physical prompting, shadowing[2], making students sit in certain set places, and non-exclusionary time-out[3] also involve movement restriction. Such procedures, such as guiding a child's hand while learning to write is usually seen as innocuous as they are often effective in helping the child learn and appear to cause little or no distress to the child. An example of a teaching procedure that raises a little more concern is that of discrete trial teaching with children with disabilities. Early on, it is often necessary to block escape from teaching situations by placing the therapists' legs around the child's legs and/or physically holding the child's hands down briefly during early teaching sessions as these behaviors interfere with learning. Such procedures probably involve extinction of learned escape behavior and are both distressing to the child and to parents. Finally, some services and families use one-on-one or additional enhanced staffing which may also restrict movement.

Not all forms of restrictive behavior management procedures are deemed inappropriate. For example, we restrict people's movement through traffic lights, signals, barriers, and written directions. Such restraint on movement is seen as benign and nonintrusive, as it results in a more orderly society, benefits many, and is nonharmful. We often restrict children's movement in ways that are generally considered acceptable. Thus, children may be strapped into strollers, kept in play pens, walked around on reigns, or made to walk holding other people's hands. Implicitly, we may think that there are probably benefits to children in learning self-control

---

[2] Shadowing is a behavioral prompting procedure used to fade (reduce) physical prompts. In shadowing, the trainer systematically reduces physical prompts by following the trainee's movements with their hands very closely at first and gradually increasing the distance little by little, following the student's movements with her hands very near but not touching the child. The teacher then gradually increases the distance of her hands from the student.

[3] Non-exclusionary time-out refers to procedures in which the reinforcer maintaining the problem behavior is removed contingent on the behavior, but, in contrast to exclusionary time-out procedures, the person is not excluded from the setting in which the problem behavior occurred.

by eventually fading out these mechanical and personal restraints, so eventually they remain in certain areas or next to adults without requiring mechanical or personal restraints to do so. We rarely object when teachers require badly behaved children or children engaging in dangerous behavior to sit in certain places where they can be supervised more closely and kept safe, and some caregivers approve of time-outs in certain circumstances involving movement restriction as a disciplinary procedure to reduce problem behavior as popularized by TV's *Super Nanny* series. In certain circumstances, many parents and caregivers approve or request restraints for medical, dental, and other therapeutic procedures, such as splints and slings, to promote healing, pharmacological sedation, and various forms mechanical and personal restraint during dental and medical procedures where there is a risk of harm or behavioral problems that interfere with the procedures and/or pose a danger to the child. Some of these latter examples begin to shade into unacceptable practices, as when alternative behavior management practices exist that are equally or more effective and/or more safe than more restrictive alternatives. For example, if children can undergo anxiety-provoking dental and medical procedures without physical restraints or chemical sedation by using simple educational interventions, modeling, relaxation, or reinforcement procedures, then these restrictive alternatives would usually be said to be unwarranted and unethical by many parents and professionals. This is especially important as when the medical treatment is for life-threatening conditions, such as pediatric cancers, the procedures are painful and distressing, but equally effective alternate methods of behavior management are available (Jay et al. 1985). Strangely, practitioners sometimes prefer traditional restrictive and sometimes less-effective procedures to alternatives. For example, Allen et al. (1990) found that dentists preferred restrictive behavior management practices such as hand-over-mouth restraint, rather than tell–show–do[4] or modeling, perhaps because of the general professional acceptance of such restrictive practices at the time of the study, perceived excessive time needed for alternative strategies, and lack of training and behavioral skill on the part of dentists to use alternative strategies.

By law, we often require people to restrain themselves or others to reduce risk of injury to the person and avoid or reduce the cost of injury to society. Some examples of mechanical restraints here include child car seats, seat belts in cars, restraints during potentially dangerous carnival rides, and helmets while riding on bikes, motor bikes, and skate boards. Most people see these practices as innocuous, if sometimes inconvenient, although cultural standards vary from society to society and over time. Often, failure to engage in these practices results in negative punishment procedures[5] in the form of fines, loss of driving privileges, and loss or suspension of driving licenses. Some examples of personal restraints include the legal requirement to protect others from harm in certain circumstances. For example, failure to

[4] "Tell–show–do" is a behavior management strategy used in dentistry to reduce anxiety which involves instruction, modelling and use of a dental procedure.

[5] Negative punishment is a behavioral procedure in which a stimulus is removed contingent on that response that results in the future weakening of behavior.

prevent someone from harm, such as a person walking into traffic, may be criminal. Failure to pull the person back, perhaps even forcibly and resulting in harm in some circumstances may be legally required. Not to restrain the other person may result in legal punishment for failing to act resulting in harm to another person.

Many forms of legal punishment involve movement restriction. Handcuffs, ankle bracelets, court orders to not go into certain areas or near certain people, curfews, and imprisonment are all examples of this kind of movement restriction. They involve both restrictions on movement and may also involve restrictions in access to reinforcement. Sometimes, people present themselves for incarceration or other restrictive legal punishment, perhaps to avoid even greater negative consequences of their behavior, such as avoiding guilt or even greater sentences (Skinner 1953).

Certain forms of medical, dental, and various therapies involve restraint. An interesting example comes from constraint-induced movement therapy, a therapy for stroke and other neurological disorders, that includes mechanical restraint of the non-affected body part among other treatment components, to encourage movement in the affected body part (Taub 2012). People who are overweight also voluntarily have their jaws wired to make eating difficult. Dentists may use a variety of pharmacological restraints, such as valium, nitrous oxide, and general sedation; mechanical restraints, such as papoose boards for children and people with disabilities; and personal restraints, such as hand-over-mouth restriction, hand-over-mouth-with-airway restriction.

There are also cultural variations in the use of restraint. For example, different cultures use different forms of restraint to swaddle infants during sleeping and do so for different periods of time. Different cultures also use different forms of mechanical restraints to transport children (Nelson et al. 2000).

We also routinely restrain animals. We walk them and tie them up with leashes, keep them in cages, restrict their movement with electric fences and devices that administer aversive stimuli, and use mechanical devices to stop them injuring themselves after surgery or because of behavioral issues. Animals are also harnessed to make cutting their claws and coats more easy for humans. Animals are restrained in various ways to keep them safe during surgery and veterinary procedures. Humans also restraint animals when working for humans as in when we milk cows, plough fields, or drag vehicles using animal labor. Most of these practices are acceptable to many, but not all people. If these practices result in injury or distress to the animals, then these practices are often seen are cruel and may result in punishment for the humans who cased the harm.

1.2.1 Restraint

Some definitions of restraint are very broad. For example, consider this definition: "Restraint includes any action, word or deed that is used for the purpose or intent of restricting the free movement or decision-making abilities of another person" (Nurses and Midwives Board of Western Australia 2009). This definition is broad indeed and defined restraint as any action with the *purpose* or *intent* of restricting either movement or decision-making ability. It is problematic in that it requires the person doing the restraining to have a purpose or intent to restrict; it can be hard to determine a person's purpose or intent.

A more operationalized definition comes from Applied Behavior Analysis International (2010) that defined restraint as follows: "*Restraint* involves physically holding or securing the individual, either: a) for a brief period of time to interrupt and intervene with severe problem behavior, or b) for an extended period of time using mechanical devices to prevent otherwise uncontrollable problem behavior (e.g., self-injurious behavior) that has the potential to produce serious injury. When used in the context of a behavior intervention plan, restraint in some cases serves both a protective and a therapeutic function. These procedures can reduce risks of injury and can facilitate learning opportunities that support appropriate behavior." This definition distinguishes personal and mechanical restraint, brief versus extended use, two different functions of restraint—protection and treatment—and claims that restraint may reduce injuries and increase opportunities for learning. Such narrow and specific definitions of restraint are preferred over the former broad definitions because they are more precise and analytic and avoid the impossibility of divining people's intensions.

1.2.2 Acceptable and Unacceptable Restrictive Procedures

There are many forms of restrictive behavior management practices which are seen in many different contexts, populations, and settings for a wide variety of non-problematic and problematic behavior. In some contexts, such as services for vulnerable populations, prisons, detention of immigrants, and systems of staff training programs, for example, forms of acceptable and unacceptable restraints are codified. How can we make sense of these different restrictive behavior management practices and what makes them acceptable or unacceptable?

One distinction that is often made is the application of force to restrict movement. Thus, a person's movement is surely restricted when another person or a sign says, "Stop!" We rarely are concerned with such practices, even though it surely restricts our movement as much as a physical barrier or physical force; however, if there are many instructions prohibiting movement, we see such practices more negatively and call it nagging or label it disrespectful, unloving, or unprofessional. Some behavioral skills training procedures, such as prompt fading and shadowing, are similar in that, although they do not involve touch once the prompt is faded, they do exert clear and explicit control over the person's behavior in a way some find offensive until those prompts are further faded.

But once some form of force—even mere physical contact—is applied, we are much more likely to view such procedures as more undesirable than effective alternatives. Thus, even when we lightly guide someone's hand to pick up a spoon or a pencil or if we gently block a person from grabbing food with their hands, such procedures are seen as an undesirable, but perhaps necessary procedure in some cases. As more force is applied and the greater the extent of the restriction on physical movement of the person, the less acceptable the intervention is seen. Occasionally, people request physical restraint. For example, a person with severe self-injury might say, “Hold my hand. I am scared,” which might be a form of self-management to prevent engaging in self-injury (Skinner 1953), and, presumably, since the outcome is relatively good, the person does not self-injure; we might view such a restraint as more acceptable than alternatives, such as involuntary personal or mechanical restraints.

“Hold still! It will only hurt a bit!” We are often able to voluntarily immobilize ourselves as when we are given a shot or eye drops, or when we give blood. Skinner (1953) noted that one form of self-control is indeed to stiffen up our muscles to prevent ourselves from moving. We physically restraint ourselves when we fold our hands or arms to stop fidgeting or worse, bite our tongue, and clasp our hand over our mouth to stop staying something we have regretted saying in the past. We also voluntarily use mechanical restraint, for example, when we splint broken fingers or place physical therapy devices such as knee or wrist braces when injured or correcting a medical problem. Even when we have a sprained or fractured limb, we often voluntarily place our limbs in restraint, such as when we put our arms in a sling to prevent movement and promote healing. If we have an itchy rash, we jam our fingers in our pockets or wear cotton gloves to stop ourselves scratching. When we do this or see other people do it, the procedure is safe and there are benefits to the person, then we have few objections. Indeed, we might admire someone who does this as someone who is brave or who has good self-control. Often we expect parents and other caretakers to teach their children to have such self-control. If a child is harmed because they cannot do this, we might consider the parent too indulgent or negligent by placing their child at risk for preventable harm. If an adult fusses over having shots, we might think them self-indulgent and immature. Indeed, some forms of intervention to prevent the use of restrictive behavior management practices involve teaching people to engage in these forms of self-control and self-restraint as alternatives to being restrained by other people. Let us now turn to restraints that other people apply to us, either by the force of their bodies or through application of mechanical restraints and barriers.

The term “personal restraint” refers to a wide range of less and more restrictive, forceful, and sometimes potentially dangerous and unacceptable forms of movement restriction delivered by other people. Everyday examples, which are usually unremarkable and acceptable, include briefly holding someone’s hand or holding their hand down or blocking someone’s movement when it causes alarm or has the potential for danger or harm to the person blocked or someone else, such as one person holding put their hand to block someone flailing around.

Some common forms of personal restraints include methods to restrict hand and body movements, such as basket holds and personal restraints in chairs. There are also various forms of “takedowns” in which the person restraint is forced onto the floor and held there, such as two- and three-person takedowns. There are personal holds on the floor which may be in the face-up (supine) or face-down (prone) position and may involve varying number of other people. There are various escort and carrying methods to assist in moving someone away from danger, reducing harm to others, or requiring to move somewhere, such as attend a clinic or go onto a plane during deportation.

Common mechanical restraints include some treatment devices for medical, dental, nursing, physical, and occupational therapy and other professional treatments which include mechanical restraint. This refers to a very wide range of procedures which are innocuous and low risk and some that are intrusive and risky. Strait jackets are used to restrict arm and body movement. Restraint boards are used while medical and dental procedures sometimes are used in behavior management and sometimes during moving people. Bed rails are used to keep people in bed and are often used in services for seniors and in their family home to restrict movement out of bed. Various forms of ties are used to tie down arms, legs, and trunk for medical patients who are delirious or agitated, who are a danger to themselves or who may interfere with medical equipment, such as lines and catheters. Ties are also used to prevent self-injury, as when individuals with Lesch–Nyhan syndrome are tied to their wheelchair, furniture, or beds to prevent biting their fingers or other forms of self-injury. Gloves and mittens are sometimes used to prevent individuals reopening wounds or engaging in self-injury, such as chronic hand mouthing, or when individuals who exhibit pica[6] are prevented from putting some inedible objects in their mouth which pose a danger of choking. Some services develop their own mechanical devices to carry someone such as chairs bolted to wooden board. Rarely, cages are used to contain people, but occasional examples arise in certain services, and sometimes services and families devise their own cages to restrain children and sometimes individuals with disabilities. (See Chap. 6, for some examples of this.)

The use of environmental barriers to block movements is common: Our world is full of physical barriers to stop people walking in dangerous places, such as wet floor or where construction is taking place. Barriers are used sometimes in a systematic way, for example, to prevent wandering in people with dementias, both as a routine part of the environment in a nursing home, and sometimes as part of a behavior support plan. Staff and parents sometimes improvise their own devices to block movement as when teachers block a child in the corner of a classroom using desks and other furniture.

Sometimes we restrict movement through other forms of environmental modification. There is a whole industry of "child proofing" one's home to protect a child from injury by making doors difficult to open, electrical outlets and medicine containers inaccessible, and access to dangerous devises such as cookers and pools difficult. In some services, door handles are placed where clients cannot reach or use them or the handles are modified so that only staff and/or family can use them. Sometimes services such as schools lock children in classrooms, closets, or storage rooms.

[6] Pica refers to eating inedible objects.

1.2.3 Van Houten's Seven Dimensions of Restraint

It is difficult to place order on all these different restraint procedures, but van Houten (1998) made a useful contribution by distinguishing seven dimensions along which restraint procedures can vary. First, restraint may be partial in that it selectively prevents some but not all behavior, such as blocking self-injurious behavior or preventing someone leaving a teaching area, or total, as in movement suppression where almost all movements is prevented. Second, restraints vary by their duration. Some restraints are very brief, as in blocking or brief hand holding, or may be extensive in time. Third, restraints vary by the degree of resistance the person restrained makes. Fourth, restraints vary by the degree they remove the person from ongoing reinforcement. For example, blocking allows continued access to many forms of reinforcement other than those available for the blocked response, whereas preventing a child from moving in a classroom by tying them to a chair gives access to few forms of reinforcement. Fifth, restraints vary by their degree of discomfort. Some may not involve discomfort and others are specifically designed to inflict pain, as in the use of some restraint techniques used in youth services. Sixth, restraint methods differ by the amount of ongoing stimulation available. Blocking involves access to many forms of stimulation, but whole body restraint restricts access to stimulation. Finally, restraints vary by the degree to which restraints can be escaped.

These dimensions may be useful to consider when analyzing the acceptability of different forms of restraint and also when considering if and how restraint might change behavior.

1.2.4 Seclusion and Locked Room Time-Out

Sometimes people are placed in rooms designed to contain people who are violent or who may become violent. Sometimes people, including parents, do this on an occasional basis, perhaps sometimes using a child's bedroom or a closet to contain the person. Generally, this is not referred to as seclusion, although sometimes people might refer to this practice, perhaps incorrectly, as time-out. When this is done in more controlled settings, such as locked psychiatric wards or some residential programs, it may be referred to as seclusion.

Dix and Betteridge (2001) quoted the 1999 British Mental Health Act (1983) which defined seclusion as "The forcible confinement of a patient alone in a room for the protection of others from serious harm." This legal definition of seclusion features the fact that this procedure is forcible, the person is alone, and the prime reason for secluding is protection of others. Curran et al. (2005) noted that subsequently the British Court of Appeal had added that seclusion involves the use of "regular, frequent observation" and that is a medical treatment within the Mental Health Act (1983). The definition of seclusion is not consistent, and Mason (1992) noted that the term is used in widely different ways and here is little consensus about the use of the term. A more precise definition comes from Applied Behavior

Analysis International (2010) which defined seclusion as “isolating an individual from others to interrupt and intervene with problem behavior that places the individual or others at risk of harm. When used in the context of a behavior intervention plan, seclusion in some cases serves both a protective and a therapeutic function. These procedures can reduce risks of injury and can facilitate learning opportunities that support appropriate behavior....” As with Applied Behavior Analysis International’s definition of restraint, this definition is precise and delineates seclusions’ protective and potential treatment function.

In contrast, locked room time-out is a behavior modification treatment. Applied Behavior Analysis International (2010) defined time-out as “*Time-out* from reinforcement is an evidence-based treatment intervention that involves reducing or limiting the amount of reinforcement that is available to an individual for a brief period of time. It can entail removing an individual from his or her environment, or it may entail changes to the existing environment itself. When time-out involves removing an individual from the environment, it should only be used as part of an approved and planned Behavior Intervention Plan. Time-out from reinforcement is not seclusion, but it may involve seclusion if it is not safe to have others in the room. In addition, some innocuous versions of timeout from reinforcement, such as having a child take a seat away from a play area, are not deemed to be intrusive. Such procedures are commonly used and are generally safe.” This definition of time-out is functional, namely the procedure is defined by whether or not reinforcement is briefly removed, not by a specific procedure, such as locking someone in a room. Thus, it distinguishes forms of time-out that are relatively safe and acceptable from those that carry significant risks of injury and are less acceptable.

Thus, unlike seclusion, its use is a behavioral treatment to reduce specific target behaviors and it is theory-based, and time-out procedures are derived from basic learning research (Leitenberg 1965). Thus, time-out can be used for many different target behaviors, and there are many procedural variations of time-out depending upon the positive reinforcer maintaining the target behavior and it depends crucially upon two factors: (a) prior to treatment identify the positive reinforcer maintaining the target behavior, and (b) implementing a procedure that removes the contingency between the positive reinforcer and the behavior. In addition, there should be abundant positive reinforcement, including the positive reinforcer maintaining the target behavior in the time-in environment. There are numerous procedural variations in time-out. Here are four examples. First, in non-exclusionary time-out, the person wears a ribbon, badge, or other cue contingent upon a target behavior for a fixed period of time during which reinforcement is unavailable or at least minimized. The ribbon cues staff not to reinforce when the badge is worn (Foxx and Shapiro 1978). A second example is the prototypical use of time-out in child behavior management. In this variation of time-out, the person is given one firm explanation, and the parent then takes the child who sits quietly in a quiet area, such as a bedroom or the bottom of the stairs, during which no one talks to the child or person. If the child leaves, they are calmly escorted back to the area. Self-administered time-out procedures in which the person removes themselves from the reinforcer. For example, self-managed time-outs have been used in the treatment of stuttering (James 1981).

Assuming that engaging in some speech, or in vocalizations that precede speech in people who stutter, positively reinforced stuttering on an intermittent schedule of reinforcement, James (1981) taught people to stop attempting to talk and breath in slowly so they no longer engaged in these behaviors for a period of time and then restarted speaking. Finally, locked room time-out has been used as a planned behavioral intervention which assumes that placing the person in the time-out room removed the positive reinforcer maintaining that behavior. Thus, if (a) the person's target behavior is maintained by positive reinforcers such as attention, such as nagging, or tangibles, such as access to edibles, drinks, or tangible times, and (b) placing the person in the time-out room removes these positive reinforcers, then the procedure constitutes locked room time-out. If, however, the target behavior is maintained by negative reinforcement, such as escape from aversive nagging, academic, or programmatic demands, or other aversive stimuli, such as excessive noise and/or stimulation, then placing the person in a locked room will be iatrogenic since it will negatively reinforce the target behavior it is supposed to reduce. In the past, locked room time-out was used not only for aggressive and violent behavior in psychiatric in patients and adults with ID and violent behavior but also for a wide range of other populations and other target behaviors such as psychotic speech in people with schizophrenia (Travis and Sturmey 2010; Wilder et al. 2001).

Many practitioners and family members use the terms "seclusion" and "time-out" interchangeably, but this is an error. Locked room time-out and seclusion can be distinguished on the following bases. Locked room time-out is a planned treatment procedure based on a pre-treatment functional assessment or functional analysis[7] which identifies the positive reinforcer that maintains the target behavior, the procedure based on the functional assessment/functional analysis, is individualized, requires peer review and consent. Seclusion, by contrast, is not informed by a pre-intervention functional assessment or functional analysis, and is usually only implemented for the treatment of violence and aggression resulting in imminent danger; it should involve a written policy for the unit or service and is implemented in a fairly uniform manner to protect others. Although some rationales for seclusion have been offered (see below), the primary reason for seclusion is to ensure the safety of the patient or others, rather than treatment, whereas locked room time-out is a planned treatment procedure.

[7] Functional assessment and functional analysis are a set of procedures to identify the environmental variables that influence a target behavior. Functional assessment does not involve any systematic manipulation of variables whereas functional analysis does. These procedures are used before treatment and used to identify indicated and contraindicated treatments (Sturmey 1996; Sturmey 2007).

1.2.5 *PRN Medication, Psychotropic Medication and Rapid Tranquilization*

Sometimes we make moving and thinking difficult or effortful through medication through sedation and through negative side effects such as extra pyramidal symptoms. There are many culture-specific practices which are examples of this, such as giving fractious babies alcohol to calm them down, and we often manage our own behavior in a similar way (Skinner 1953). This practice is used professionally in three distinguishable ways.

First, the National Institute of Clinical Excellence (2005) defined rapid tranquilization as "the use of medication to calm/lightly sedate the service use, reduce the risk to self and/or others and achieve optimal reduction in agitation and aggression, thereby allowing psychiatric evaluation to take place and allowing comprehension and response to spoken messages through the intervention." This often involves the use and antipsychotic medication or sometimes minor tranquilizers to calm patients with psychosis. This procedure may in fact be quite restrictive as The Royal College of Psychiatrists (1998) recommended that five staff restrain the patient while the doctor injects medication, but is not involved in the restraint, and if five staff are not available, they recommended allowing the patient to leave and calling the police. Further, although the definition is using the term "light sedation," it is sometimes the case that the resulting sedation is not light.

There is an outcome literature comparing different psychotropic medications and different schedules of medication used during rapid tranquilization (see National Institute of Clinical Excellence 2014, for a systematic review). Holmes and Simmons (2008) noted that rapid tranquilization should not be confused with rapid neuroleptization, the administration of high doses of antipsychotic medication initially with the aim of achieving early remission of psychosis. Rapid tranquilization raises a number of safety and ethical issues as it comes with various risks which vary with the class of medication chosen and route of administration (e. g. oral vs. intravenous). Additionally, there are concerns over the competency and training of some physicians and the lack of policies in some services (Holmes and Simmons 2008). Ethical issues also arise relating to obtaining informed consent, patient dignity, privacy, and the extent to which other less restrictive interventions are tried first (MacPherson et al. 2005).

A second, overlapping concept is PRN ("as needed") psychotropic medication which refers to the use of psychotropic medication "as needed" for aggression, violence, or agitation. For a minority of settings and persons, PRN medication for violence and aggression is used routinely and it becomes the default method of behavior management.

A third relevant concept is routine prescribed psychotropic medication. Some view this as humane medication to treat illnesses based on diagnoses and others view it as a form of restrictive procedure, referred to as "chemical restraint," term which some practitioners regard as pejorative (Currier 2003) but is also used in some clinical guidance in some setting (Lambeth 2013). For example, in Tasmania, the law defines chemical restraint as "when medication is intentionally given to exert control over a patients' movements or behavior" (p. 1). Thus, this definition distinguishes the use of psychotropic medication to treat and the underlying mental illness from using it to control a problematic behavior. These guidelines recognize that it is a highly restrictive and potentially dangerous procedure that should be reduced by implementation of preventative and other strategies.

Sedation is also widely used in medical, dental, nursing, and other procedures in which the person's agitated behavior might pose a danger to themselves or others during the procedure or might interfere with the successful completion of the procedure. From time to time, services might use combinations of physical and/or personal restraint to allow injection of a sedative. Several studies have evaluated the acceptability of such restrictive procedures in dental treatment (Newton et al. 2003; Newton et al. 2004; Newton and Sturmey 2002), and restrictive procedures such as compulsory admission to psychiatric hospital for eating disorders (Newton et al. 2005) have found that acceptability is strongly affected by the outcome. That is, all things being equal, people prefer nonrestrictive, effective treatment; however, if restrictive procedure is effective, then people often judge it to be acceptable. Both nonrestrictive and restrictive interventions, including sedation and compulsory admission, that are ineffective are judged negatively. There is often a divergence of views on the acceptability of these procedures. Medical, nursing, and some other profession staff tend to view them much more positively than patients, who general have very negative evaluations of such procedures. (See the section on rationale for seclusion below for examples of divergence of opinions on this issue).

1.2.6 Related Concepts

Many individuals and groups have developed different definitions of restrictive behavior management practices and have done so for many different purposes. Unsurprisingly, not all such definitions and distinctions are helpful. For example, the Australian National Mental Health Consumer and Carer Forum (2009), after distinguishing physical and chemical restraint, went on to define "emotional restraint" as "when the individual consumer is conditioned to such as extent that there is a loss of confidence in being able to express their views openly and honestly to clinical staff for fear of the consequences" (p. 6) and includes threats to seclude or restrain the person. It is obviously useful to consider the effects of punishment on suppressing behavior; indeed, there are important conceptual similarities between the effects of staff and family threats on behavior since the underlying learning processes and their effects may be similar to restrictive behavior management practices. It is difficult, however, to reliably and accurately measure it (even if we are sometimes confident, we can see it). Until we can develop accurate and reliable measures of emotional restraint, it remains somewhat unhelpful.

1.3 Rationales

Several reasons have been put forward for the use of restraint and other restrictive behavior management practices. These include that restraints increase the safety of client and others, treatment of challenging behavior, and self-management through restrictive behavior management practices. The sections below review client and staff safety data and restrictive behavior management practices. Review the available data including both risks of restrictive behavior management practices and not using them and risks to clients and caregivers. In addition, a brief synopsis of the reasons for other restrictive behavior management practices, such as seclusion and PRN medication, are also given.

1.3.1 Rights and Values

Statements concerning service values often imply or explicitly state that services should not use restrictive behavior management practices. For example, the American Association on Intellectual and Developmental Disabilities Principles include "Advance the assurance of all human rights of people with intellectual and developmental disabilities, including equality, individual dignity, choice and respect. Promote…self-determination, and access to quality health, education, vocational and other human services and supports"(American Association on Intellectual and Developmental Disabilities 2014). These broad values are reflected in the American Association on Intellectual and Developmental Disabilities specific position statement on aversive procedures (American Association on Intellectual and Developmental Disabilities 2012) which condemn "inhumane forms of aversive procedures as a means of behavior support" and calls for immediate elimination of such practices. This position statement, which is designed to reflect the organization's core values, calls for interventions that do not merely reduce problem behaviors but also calls for positive behavioral supports, which "promote self-determination, productivity, independence, productivity and lifelong learning" and states that "Relationships between providers and consumers should foster empowerment of the consumer, enhance choice, and promote integration…into community settings." Hence, the American Association on Intellectual and Developmental Disabilities' specific policy on restrictive behavior management practices reflects its core values which are incompatible with the use of many restrictive behavior management practices. Likewise, in Britain, the British Institute of Learning Disabilities web page states that "We want people with learning disabilities [Intellectual Disabilities] to be valued equally, participate fully in their communities and be treated with dignity and respect" (British Institute of Learning Disabilities 2014). These value statements are generally incompatible with the use of restrictive behavior management practices and instead promote alternate forms of intervention both to promote adaptive behavior generally as well as to reduce problem behavior.

1.3.2 Safety

1.3.2.1 Client Risks

Restrictive behavior management practices are often justified in terms of preventing harm to the target person or their peers; however, there is now substantial evidence that restrictive behavior management practices, especially restraint[8], result in injuries and sometimes death. Thus, behavior management plans which incorporate restraint and prevent injuries to the client and peers and/or self-injury, presume that the programmatic restrictive behavior management practices results in less harm than otherwise would have happened. These reasons are often voiced when services used restrictive behavior management practices with children, adolescents, psychiatric inpatients and people with ID and are similarly expressed in services for seniors, related to preventing falls. (Whether or not this is true is an empirical question, which sometimes can be difficult to determine.) Some restrictive behavior management practices pose direct threats of injury to clients, including injuries during personal and restraints, such as bruising, fractures and, in some cases, even client death. Clinical teams and family members also have to weigh the evidence of short- versus long-term risks and benefits. For example, in some circumstances, brief contingent restraint might involve client discomfort and some minor injuries, such as scrapes, but might also have the long-term benefits of reduction in the target behavior and increases in adaptive behavior and personal freedom (Applied Behavior Analysis International 2010). Similarly, restraint fading for individuals with long-term restraints, such as individuals with pica or chronic self-injury, might also come with attendant risks, such and reinjuring oneself or dangerous incidents of pica.

On the other hand, restrictive behavior management practices might have short-term benefits, such as prevention of injury to the client and others. They may also, however, have long-term harms, such as reinforcing the target behavior, thereby increasing the target behavior, and medical harm, such as muscular atrophy, tendon shortening, etc. For example, in the case of seniors, restrictive behavior management practices may reduce potentially dangerous wandering, but come with long-many long-term medical risks. What is the evidence on the question of RRBPs and client harm?

There have been at several systematic reviews of restraint and seclusion most of which did not address either client or staff safety (Evans et al. 2002; Mohler et al. 2011; Salias and Fenton 2000), although two systematic reviews have addressed safety. The first comes from Day (2002) which was commissioned to conduct a review of safety of restraint following the death of Matthew Innes, a psychiatric patient, while being transported by police in a police car in New Zealand. Day conducted a systematic review of the safety of physical restraint used by law enforcement and medical staff which included both studies of personal and mechanical

[8] Restraint is also used widely in the animal literature as a procedure to study stress. For example, http://www.ncbi.nlm.nih.gov/pmc/articles/PMC3779531/.

restraints in people with behavioral problems and studies with healthy volunteers in experiments. Day retained 13 studies including 1 high-quality meta-analysis, and 12 low-quality nonexperimental studies. Based on these studies, Day concluded that there was no evidence that different forms of restraint (hog tie vs. prone (face down) restraints) were more or less dangerous than each other, but data from these studies come from healthy volunteers under very controlled conditions. He also concluded that, although the quality of evidence on safety was generally poor, restraint does contribute to death in some rare circumstances and that staff training should be undertaken to promote the use of alternatives to restraint. The second systematic review by Nelstrop et al. (2006) conducted an exhaustive search of the literature from 1985 to 2002 on the safety and effectiveness of restraints and seclusion. They found 36 studies of poor quality and were unable to make any conclusions as to the safety of restraints for either staff or clients. A third systematic review comes from Oliver et al. (2007), who reported a large systematic review and meta-analysis of strategies to prevent falls and fractures in hospitals and care homes. They found evidence that multicomponent interventions, some of which included restraint reduction, resulted in significant reduction in falls. They also meta-analyzed five restraint reduction studies of moderate quality and found that overall there was no effect on falls. (The reader should also look at treatment chapters later in this volume which include changes in injuries following individual and organizational interventions to reduce restrictive behavior management practices).

These systematic reviews concur that the overall quality of the literature at the time they were conducted was relatively low. Nevertheless, they do all concur that restraints are dangerous and potentially life threatening and that alternatives to restraint should be used in order to promote client safety. (Some exceptions to that generalization will be seen below).

1.3.2.2 People with ID

A small number of empirical studies and some intervention studies have reported data on the risks of different forms of restraint to clients. For example, Spreat et al. (1986) reported injury rates in 231 people with ID during two, 6-month periods in a long-term residential setting. They found that the overall rate of injuries was 2.9% of restraint applications and that of these injuries 91.2% were nonserious, involving scratches and abrasions, and 8.8% per "serious" involving sutures and broken teeth, etc. Interestingly, they found that injury rates were lower for planned restraint than for emergency restraints ($p<0.001$) and mechanical restraints were safer than personal restraint (15 vs. 48 injuries per 1000 restraint, $p<0.001$).

Subsequently, Williams (2009) reported safety data on 209 individuals with ID over a 12-month period. There were 349, 111, 9597, and 3276 application of planned personal, planned mechanical, emergency personal, and emergency mechanical restraints. The overall rate of injuries was 0.46% of applications. There were 60 nonserious injuries, such as scratches and abrasions, and 2 serious injuries requiring medical attention. The rate of injuries was strongly a function of the type of restraint. Namely, the rates of injuries were 5.73 % for all emergency restraints and 0.25 % for all planned restraints which was a statistically significant difference ($p<0.01$).

Some intervention studies which have reduced restraints have also reported data on client injuries. For example, Williams et al. (2009) reported multiple outcomes of a pica reduction program, which included data on both restraint and pica-related surgeries for 34 individuals with ID and life-threatening pica. The program was a comprehensive and restrictive program for pica that included environmental modifications, such as removal of all pica-related items, training in alternate behavior with pica items, and discrimination training. As well as achieving a large reduction in pica and restraints, the program eliminated pica-related surgeries. Prior to the program there were nine pica-related surgeries. These surgeries are highly risky and potentially life-threatening as many of these individuals have multiple disabilities and medical problems related to pica. After the program began there were *no* pica-related surgeries for *9* years. Thus, a carefully constructed and well-run program for severe, life-threatening pica can reduce both restraint and eliminate dangerous surgeries.

There is only limited evidence on the safety of restraint in people with ID. What there is intriguing and has important implications for services. First, two studies found that emergency restraint was more dangerous that programmatic restraint, suggesting the importance of preparing staff through effective training on the use of restraint and preventative strategies. In some services, there is pressure to remove programmatic restraint from behavior support plans. If this is done, then staff must still be well prepared in the use of restraint in order to reduce client injuries. Second, one paper showed that restraint can be greatly reduced *and* result in improved client safety. It is important to note that this was done as part of a comprehensive, well-designed, and carefully evaluated program for pica. Thus, although restraint reduction programs might also reduce client injuries, this outcome cannot be assumed, but rather must be carefully planned and evaluated.

1.3.2.3 Seniors

Restraint in the form of bed rails, chair restraint, and staff and family members denying seniors access to walking prostheses are commonly used to restrict both purposeful walking that is judged to be dangerous due to the potential falls and wandering, which is also sometimes judged to be a risk for harm from falls. Restricting the mobility of seniors involves both empirical and ethical questions, since restricting their mobility is both undignified and restricts autonomy and may result in a side variety of medical harm. Further, the assumed benefit of increased safety from lack of falls has been challenged. Often it appears that mobility in seniors is restricted for staff convenience and because of inadequate staffing. Mobility restrictions may also reflect the lack of effective physical therapy, ambulation, and nursing programs and lack of organizational commitment to rehabilitation as the goals of services. As with ID, there is evidence that generally restraint harms seniors through loss of muscle tone and balance, pressure sores, and incontinence and does not result in reduction in injuries, although there may be some exceptions to this generalization.

Nyman and Oliver (2010) briefly reviewed the literature on restraints and safety in seniors, primarily related to prevention of falls, which are a relatively common, significant health risk in some seniors, such as hip fractures and risk of death, and which result in loss of quality of life when seniors are fearful of walking and restricting their daily activity. Oliver et al. (2007) conducted a meta-analysis of five low-quality study of the effects of restraint reduction on injuries and found no effect on injuries. In contrast, one randomized controlled trial that reduced psychotropic medication, which is often associated with negative side effects such as dizziness and sedation in seniors, and increased exercise resulted in a 66 % *reduction* in falls (Campbell et al. 1999). In contrast to the previous forms of restrictive behavior management practices, Nyman and Oliver found evidence, most of which were of poor quality, that elimination of bed rails resulted in increases in falls, but because of the poor quality and limited quantity of the evidence, the authors could not make any firm conclusion that either using or eliminating bed rails resulted in increased or decreased injuries. These authors also discussed the evidence on restrictive behavior management practices on injuries other than falls. They found evidence that bed rails may result in bruising and grazing, and, more seriously, entrapment in the rails resulting in death. This latter risk was more likely when bedrails were not assembled correctly or badly maintained.

Perhaps the most persuasive argument in favor of avoiding using restraints to prevent falls comes from evidence that alternates to restraint may be quite effective. Alternates include lowering bed height, placing mats on the floor, training seniors in safe transfer and exercise training to maintain and improve muscle tone, coordination and balance, alarms, staff education, medication review, environmental adaption, availability of walking devices, etc. The authors concluded that restraint use with seniors should be severely restricted and that generally alternate approaches to ensure individual safety should be implemented in their place.

1.3.2.4 Restraint in Medical Settings

Evans et al. (2003) conducted a systematic review of client safety in from restraint devices in acute care settings, including both direct harms such as lacerations and strangulations from the restraint devise, and indirect harm, such as increased risk of hospitalization or mortality. Based on 12 studies reported in 11 papers, they concluded that, contrary to the rationale for using restraint to promote client safety, restraint devices increase the risk of death, falls, and serious injuries and lengthen hospitalization.

1.3.2.5 Restraint Position and Safety

There have been several calls to ban certain types of restraint based on safety. Most commonly there have been calls to ban face down (prone) restraints. The rationale for this is often unclear and may be based on lurid accounts of deaths during prone restraints. Some evidence to support the view that prone restraints may be more dangerous that other forms of personal restraints comes from Parkes (2000) who found that the physiological recovery time in healthy volunteers following prone restraint was longer than recovery time in other positions. Barnett et al. (2012) replicated this finding and also found that the position of the arms during prone restraint affected physiological recovery time. These effects may be modified by other factors such as struggling during restraint (Barnett et al. 2012). Some have speculated that when people struggle during restraints, the person restraining may increase the applied pressure thereby restricting venous return to the heart. As the person experiences anoxia, they may struggle even more until they are near death and stop struggling, but in some cases it may be too late and the person may die from anoxia. Other risk factors may include recent ingestion of food and the effects of psychotropic medication and PRN medication, which when combined with other risk factors may result in death.

1.3.2.6 Caregiver Risks

Staff, families, and some professional organizations have justified the use of restraints by stating that restraints prevent injuries to caregivers. Several studies that have eliminated restraint have, however, found the opposite. Sanders (2009), for example, reported data on an organization-wide restraint reduction program over a 5-year period which included data on worker injuries and workman's compensation. Over the 5-year period, restraints were reduced from 10.33 to 0.06 restraints per 50,000 adjusted client days. During this time, worker injuries fell from 1.12 to 0.70 injuries per 50,000 adjusted client days for a 37 % reduction. As a measure of the practical significance to the organization and perhaps reflecting the severity of injuries, workman's compensation fell from US$ 171,754.80 in 2004 to US$ 13,154.56 in 2008 for a reduction of 93 %. Thus, this program that achieved a large reduction in client restraint also reported a large reduction in worker injuries and related costs.

Data indicating that also indicate that restraint reduction does not result in increase in staff injuries also comes from Smith et al. (2005)'s report of large-scale reduction in restraint in Pennsylvania's psychiatric hospital system. Over a 10-year period, restraints and seclusion was reduced by 80–90 % (depending on the measure considered) without any increase in the rate of staff injuries.

There are reports of significant staff restraint-related injuries in other contexts. For example, the BBC reported that approximately half of the injuries to police officers occurred during officer safety training (*Police injured due to 'horseplay'* 2009). To date, there are no data on whether training in restraint and/or restraint reduction reduces staff injuries in other contexts, such as police, bouncers, prison officers, deportation staff, etc.

1.3.2.7 Costs

One rationale for using restrictive behavior management practices is that they may reduce costs, for example, by eliminating injuries. Services in fact spend large amounts of money related to restrictive behavior management practices, mostly related to additional staffing and staff injuries from restrictive behavior management practices, leading Lebel and Goldstein (2005) to make the business case for reduction of restraint and seclusion. They argued that the overall costs of implementing restraints were high, and that the initial additional costs of reducing restraint and seclusion, such as those related to additional staff training and supervision, were easily offset by the subsequent savings. The costs of restraint are numerous and include systemic, organizational, and personal costs (Chan et al. 2012).

Other restrictive behavior management practices are also expensive. For example, placing clients on one-to-one or even higher staffing ratios costs a great deal on a daily basis and those costs are incurred indefinitely. This is especially problematic if the enhanced staffing does not reduce restrictive behavior management practices and the challenging behavior that precipitates their use, as may often be the case. Some staff injuries related to restraint may also be expensive, for example, those related to back injuries, as organizations may have to pay for repeated medical procedures and incur higher rates of insurance. Organizations also incur costs related to additional clinical and administrative work; these costs could be avoided if restrictive behavior management practices were reduced. Chan et al. (2012) cited three large-scale studies of a community agency and two state-level agencies that reduced costs by several millions of dollars every year. For example, the Grafton agency claims to have reduced restraints by 98 % agencywide and saved US$ 7M through avoidance of costs associated with staff injuries, workman's compensation, and other reduced staffing costs. (See Sanders 2009).

1.3.2.8 Summary and Critical Issues

Although there are limited data of poor quality on restraints and safety, generally, those data, both from research studies both for people with ID and seniors, tend toward the conclusions that restraint reduction tends to be associated with reduction in client and staff injuries. Interpreting these safety data presents problems for answering research questions and for practitioners. No research studies reported the reliability, accuracy, and validity of the data. Although some studies (Spreat et al. 1986) reported data on reliability of transcription and coding of client records, none reported data on the accuracy of staff records. This is no quibble. For safety data to be meaningful, the caregivers must report data accurately and completely, must accurately and reliably distinguish serious from nonserious injuries, must distinguish injuries due to the target behavior and from restraint, and must also accurately record sentinel events that did not actually result in death.

Injury data must also use a meaning metric. The mere number of injuries tells us little. The number of restraints reflects the number of target behaviors, the number

Table 1.1 An illustration of the interaction of data on number of target behaviors, restraints, and rates of injuries from target behaviors and restraints

Time	Number of target behaviors	Number of injuries from target behaviors	Number of restraints	Number of injuries from restraints	Percentage of restraints with injuries (%)
1	1000	10	5	2	40
2	500	10	4	3	75

of applications or restraints and how safely the restraints were applied. Thus, the meaningful metrics are those related to rate of target behavior and application of restraint rather than frequency. Practitioners also face problems interpreting safety data. For example, if an organization finds that total restraint-related injuries have decreased after staff training and restraint use, should they conclude that the training was effective? Not necessarily. Table 1.1 illustrates this problem. Between times 1 and 2, the number of injuries from both target behaviors and restraints were 10 on each occasion. An organization or therapist might conclude that no change had occurred. The rate of application of restraints to target behavior, however, doubled from 1 to 2% restraints per target behavior. Further, the rate of restraint-related injuries increased from 40 to 75%. Thus, using a more complete dataset, at time 2 one might investigate if (a) caregivers had become lax in implementing prevention strategies, resulting in higher rates of injuries, and (b) there was an issue with unsafe implementation of restraints.

Consideration of restraint and safety data as rate data also has useful implications for practice. Namely, restraint-related injuries can be reduced in three ways: (a) reduction in the number of target behaviors, (b) reduction in the implementation of restraints, and (c) improvements in the safe implementation of restraints. Interventions to reduce restraint-related injuries could do so effectively by some or all of these variables.

A final measurement issue comes from combining data across injuries. Most if not all studies have reported the total number restraint-related or rate of restraint-related injuries per *N* client days. These measures have some intuitive appeal but may belie some complexity because they assume all injuries are of equal concern. For example, suppose prior to restraint an elderly person has 2 serious and 3 nonserious injuries per month for 3 months. Following restraint she has, 0 serious and 0.5 nonserious injuries per month for 2 months, then following a restraint reduction program she has 0 serious and 4 nonserious injuries per month for 3 months. Is this good or a bad outcome? The average rate of all injuries was 5.0, 0.5, and 4 per month before, during and after restraint was eliminated. This might be taken as evidence of ineffectiveness, but the elimination of serious injuries after restraint reduction although accompanied by some nonserious injuries might be considered a good outcome, for example, if the person is mobile, has better quality of life and has reduced risks of long-term harms of restraint. Thus, evaluation of restraint reduction program cannot rely on frequency of restraints alone, but must also consider the overall impact of restraint reduction on person's overall functioning.

1.3.3 Restraint and Stress in Animal Models

When people are restrained they often appear and report being distressed. There is also a literature on restraint and immobilization on stress in animals and the parameters of restraint and immobilization that affect the degree of stress. For example, Kearns and Spencer (2013) exposed rats that had been exposed to a predictable pattern of restraint to an unpredictable change in restraint duration. They found that rats that experienced an unpredictable change in restraint duration showed behavioral signs of stress, such as struggling against restraint, and physiological changes, such as increased plasma cortisol, indicating physiological stress. Unfortunately, there is little data directly evaluating the effects of restrictive behavior management on client stress at this time.

1.3.4 Restrictive Procedures as Treatment

One reason for using RRBPs is that they are legitimate, effective treatments. There are both behavioral and psychoanalytic treatments involving restraint and seclusion.

1.3.4.1 Restrictive Behavioral Treatments

An apparently simple rationale for the use of restrictive behavior management practices is that they are effective and appropriate treatments. If restrictive behavior management practices function as positive punishers, this outcome is expected. (See however Chaps. 6 and 7 which find that restrictive behavior management practices such as restraint may have other functions also.) Thus, there is considerable evidence that restrictive behavior management practices may be effective for many problems and in many populations including children and adults with ID (Harris 1996; Heyveart et al. 2014). For example, O'Brien et al. (1972) taught infants with profound ID in a daycare nursery to walk using personal restraint. In one condition, they restrained the infants holding them at their waist for 5 s when they attempted to crawl, and in another condition, they combining this with response priming by placing them in the standing condition. They found that for two children restraint and priming was effective in teaching the children to walk independently, and they did not need any subsequent restraint. For two children with more severe motor impairments, they regressed after training and only began to walk independently when occasional restraint was used to prevent crawling. Thus, restraint can be part of a package of behavioral interventions to promote desirable skills when sometimes failure to use restraint may be ineffective.

In the most recent meta-analysis of the effectiveness of restraint in people with disabilities, Hayveart et al. (2014a) identified 59 small *N* experiments published between 1990 and 2011 with 94 participants most of whom were identified with severe and profound ID who were treated mostly for self-injury, and also for aggression. Most studies were of reasonably high quality. Their average age was 24 years (range 3–58 years). A total of 52 participants were treated with personal restraint, 32 with mechanical restraint, and 6 experienced some form of environmental restraint. The overall effect size was 3.16 (range 1.27–5.78, with one outlier which did not affect results), that is the average person's target behavior was 3.16 standard deviations lower during restraint than baseline ($p < 0.00001$). The meta-analysis revealed only one moderator—females had larger effect sizes than males. The authors concluded that restraint were on average highly effective. They also noted several mismatches between the literature and practice, namely that in practice restraints are commonly used for aggression, whereas most of the literature is on self-injury and in practice restraints are usually used for safety rather than as a treatment. Others have found mixed evidence in other populations such as people with psychiatric disorders (Nelstrop et al. 2006).

The effectiveness of restrictive behavior management practices does not, however, answer the question of whether or not they are appropriate and there has been much debate over when and if they are appropriate or ethical treatments. This issue is discussed in greater detail in Chap. 3 on ethics.

One strange observation is that sometimes practitioners continue to use restrictive behavior management practices as treatment when those treatments are ineffective or harmful, for example, when they increase or maintain the target behavior, and/or cause distress, physical or other injuries to the individual concerned. It may be that practitioners do so because they do not know any alternative strategies, find alternatives too effortful, and/or do not have sufficient resources to use alternatives. It may be the case that sometimes practitioners experience temporary reduction in aversive client behavior and few negative consequences for such practices and/or support each other in the use of such practices. In other cases, the use of such restrictive behavior management practices is a prelude to removing a difficult client from a program. Perhaps these consequences may be sufficient to maintain practitioners using ineffective/harmful restrictive behavior management practices.

1.3.4.2 Restrictive Psychoanalytic Treatment

Several psychoanalytic therapies also use restraint. For example, "Le Packing" is a psychoanalytic treatment for autism in which the child, nearly naked or naked, is wrapped tightly in damp cloths that have been placed in a refrigerator for up to an hour several times a week (Spinney 2007). The treatment continues for months or years. This controversial therapy is widely used in France where psychoanalysis dominates autism treatment. At this time, there is no evidence that this treatment is effective, no data on child safety and no data on how widely packing is used in France (Mercer 2014). Several scientific papers strongly advice against packing (Amaral et al. 2011), but the French psychoanalytic establishment continues to use it with tacit government support while the French government continues to exclude most children with autism from education.

A second group of psychoanalytic treatments involving personal physical restraint include holding therapy (Welch 1989). Used for children with both autism and emotional disabilities, holding therapy required the therapist and/or parent to hold their child very close to them for extensive periods of time, and for adolescents this may include the parents sitting astride the child's chest. Welch claimed that holding therapy may cure autism, but only provided anecdotal data. Holding therapy appears distressful for both children and adults. Concerns have arisen over the appropriateness and safety of holding therapy, but little data exist on either questions and, thus, many recommend against its use (Mercer 2001; Mercer 2002).

Mercer (2002) noted that holding therapy is but one of several psychotherapies involving child restraint. Other examples include "Z-therapy" that includes restraining the child by the head and across the chest from a few minutes to up to 8 h. Restraints are used for resistant behaviors such as not responding to questions, raising eye brows, looking away, coughing and blinking, and if resistance was present, restraints should be painful. After physical restraints, the child has to identify the therapist as the boss, which, if not done quickly, is also followed by more physical restraint.

Rebirthing is a third form of psychoanalytic therapy for attachment disorder in which the child apparently reexperiences their birth by safety concerns over rebirthing arose when at least one child died due to suffocation during rebirthing. The *Quackwatch* website contains details of the abusive practices used during rebirthing, including multiple physical restraints that resulted in the eventual death of a Candace Newmaker during rebirthing. Mercer (2002) described how Candace Newmaker was restraints for almost 70 min during which she screamed struggled, cried for help and said she was dying. The therapists were sentenced to 16 years imprisonment (http://www.quackwatch.com/04ConsumerEducation/News/rebirthing.html.) There are no systematic data on the efficacy or safety of rebirthing.

Mercer (2002) also describes "strong sitting" and "power sitting" as techniques used in foster care requiring children to maintain correct sitting on the floor. If they do not or the child does not count correctly, then the child is required to sit for up to 2 h before the procedure begins again. Finally, Mercer noted that Federici also advocated two forms of physical restraint as forms of psychotherapy for adopted children to deal with their emotional and behavioral problems.

1.3.4.3 Seclusion as Treatment

Most definitions of seclusion emphasize that it is used for the safety of others, and some laws have indeed outlawed its use as treatment. Others, however, believe that it is a form of treatment that can result in patient improvement (Orr and Morgan 1995) or has other benefits for some psychiatric patients. Advocates of seclusion as treatment have argued that: (1) placement in seclusion reduces stimulation, which for some patients is so aversive or difficult to tolerate, that it allows patients to regain control of their behavior; and (2) seclusion provides feelings of comfort and safety and reassurance. Dix and Betteridge (2001), however, note that although staffs view seclusion somewhat positively, patients are generally very negative about seclusion, which is inconsistent with both of these possible benefits of seclusion. Similary, Dix and Bettenridge's (2001) noted the following arguments in favor of seclusion as treatment: (a) it is effective in reducing psychotic behavior in some people, (b) seclusion reduces stimulation in over-stimulated patients and seclusion enables the patient to experience relief from that excessive stimulation providing feelings of safety and reassurance and a time to reflect.

As noted above, seclusion and time-out can be distinguished on several conceptual, procedural, and practical grounds. Nevertheless, the use of seclusion, if implemented consistently, might set up contingencies between violent and aggressive behavior which might change that behavior. Thus, seclusion might reduce violent and aggressive behavior through a number of learning mechanism. First, seclusion might functionally be a form of time-out from positive reinforcement for some people. Second, it might function as a positive punisher. As noted above, it could also be iatrogenic in that it might negatively reinforce violence and aggression. Thus, the argument for seclusion as treatment is empirically weak except when it functions as a time-out from positive reinforcement or positive punisher.

Comment These arguments are empirically and conceptually weak. For example, there is little non-anecdotal evidence that seclusion reduces psychotic symptoms. Second, the argument that seclusion is a helpful treatment because it provides reduced stimulation to those who are over stimulated, begs the question of why it is necessary to use seclusion to achieve those ends when there are many other ways of doing so, such as teaching effective communication and self-management skills to reduce stimulation. Dix and Brettenridge (2001) noted that although staff tend to see seclusion as calming and therapeutic, patients tend to report it as traumatizing and negative. Interviewed of recently seclude patients confirm that view (Mehan et al. 2000). Further, there is a logical inconsistency in that if seclusion does indeed provide reduced stimulation in people who are overstimulated, then the possibility exists that this procedure is iatrogenic by negatively reinforcing psychotic behavior (cf., Travis and Sturmey 2010).

This rationale raises special ethical and clinical questions. For example, if alternative, effective treatments are available there is little reason to subject someone to restrictive behavior management practices. Further, if restrictive behavior management practices are justified as effective treatments, then there has to be clear evidence that they are indeed effective and not continued indefinitely when ineffective. Chapter 3 on ethics, legal, and professional aspects of RRBPs, and Chaps. 7 and 8 on applied behavior analysis will discuss these issues in more detail.

In short, there is little to justify seclusion as treatment.

1.3.4.4 Rational for PRN Medication

Some services attempt to manage acute agitation or episodes of aggressive and/or self-injurious behavior by using psychotropic medications as needed—mostly antipsychotics or benzodiazepines—to calm the person down, primarily through sedating them and perhaps through reduction of psychotic behavior. Srivastava (2009) conducted a systematic review of studies of PRN medication in psychiatry and found little high-quality evidence that they were effective. Based on ten retrospective studies, she found that approximately 75 % of psychiatric inpatients benefitted from PRN antipsychotics and benzodiazepines for agitation, but only approximately 30 % of non-adults who tended not to have psychotic disorders appeared to benefit. She also found that PRN medication carried risks of negative side effects and that there was little evidence of broader benefits, such as reduced hospital stay. A similar study comes from Stanislaw and Childs (2000) who compared the effectiveness of different forms of PRN medication in terms of time to achieve calmness in acutely agitated patients with brain injury. For example, they found that the average time to achieve calmness varied from 27 min (IM doperidol) to about 43 min (diphenhydramine and haloperidol).

One rationale for the use of PRN psychotropic medication is to increase the safety of the patient who receives them and others. Contradictory evidence comes from studies such as Smith et al. (2008), who reported on the effects of eliminating PRN and standing orders for psychotropic medication in psychiatric hospitals in Pennsylvania in 2004 over a 15-month period. The rate of PRN medication fell from 87.7 to 17 administration of medication per 1000 patient days which was accompanied by *reduced* injuries. Kazunari et al. (2013) conducted a systematic review of 34 similar studies, 17 of which reported positive outcomes; however, Kazunari et al. noted that these studies were largely of poor quality. Hence, the rationale for use of PRN medication either to promote safety or for any other broader patients benefits is weak.

This literature is often weak because the ratings of patient benefit include subjective ratings of calming, often from the people who were involved in the administration of the PRN medication who, thus, were not blind to the treatment condition. The existence of alternate behavior management strategies which also could be used in these circumstances and which do not involve the risks of harm that some psychotropic medications carry strongly suggests that future research should conduct systematic prospective studies comparing more than one approach to managing acute agitation.

1.4 Summary

This chapter argued that restrictive behavior management practices are a group of procedures that forcibly restrict movement in ways that are culturally unacceptable. Rather than being categorically different from other informal and formal behavior management, they differ by degree from other methods to restrict movement, and their acceptability is highly context sensitive. This chapter found that rather than being restricted to institutional settings for people with severe disabilities, restrictive behavior management practices are commonly used in many everyday circumstances and sometimes are desirable and even legally and ethically mandated. What distinguishes problematic from non-problematic restrictive behavior management practices is that they (a) are used when alternate, less restrictive, and effective alternatives exist, but are not implemented or implemented incorrectly; (b) are stigmatizing; and (c) pose unnecessary health risks to clients.

Problematic restrictive behavior management practices are used most often with vulnerable populations, such as seniors in nursing homes, psychiatric in patients, incarcerated youth, and adults with IDs and other developmental disabilities. Their use is incompatible with current service values that emphasize autonomy, respect, and quality of life. They are usually justified in terms of safety of the person or others around them or sometimes as treatment, although the data supporting this are weak.

Chapter 2
Epidemiology

It is easy to assume that restrictive behavior management practices are now used rarely and confined to restrictive settings, such as institutions and youth detention centers, and that such practices are things of the past as we become more enlightened and liberal and more sensitive to the rights of all people. Surely, we have reduced such practices! When journalists and advocates expose these practices at the present time, we want to believe that they represent aberrations—individual services that are badly run, staff members who are bad apples, and family members who are personally bad or dysfunctional. But maybe this is not so. Many service agencies and governments are reluctant to shine the disinfectant light of public data on the use of restraint and seclusion and often only do so when scandals, laws, lawsuits, or freedom of information requests force them to make the data public. Thus, we cannot be certain that restrictive behavior management practices have been reduced. The evidence in this and subsequent chapters show that they in fact continue to be widely used.

Justification for such cause for concern comes from the US Department of Education's (2012) restraint dataset which was publicized not through the action of the US government but rather through an advocacy group of journalists, ProPublica, a not-for-profit investigative journalist organization interested in stories with a "moral force," in collaboration with National Public Radio and exposed the widespread use of restraint in American schools in 2014 (Vogel 2014) (see ProPublica's (2014) restraint website for details).

ProPublica found that in the year 2012, there were over 267,000 reported instances of restraint and seclusion, approximately 163,000 instances of personal restraint, approximately 7600 instances of mechanical restraint, and, surprisingly, approximately 104,000 instances of seclusion. Most schools reported not using restraint or seclusion and those that did use restraint or seclusion an average of 12 times per year. A minority of schools, however, were outliers and used restraint and seclusion sometimes hundreds of times per year. They reported that, although children with disabilities are a minority, they accounted for approximately three quarters of restraint. This dataset is quite limited because the data ProPublica used

P. Sturmey, *Reducing Restraint and Restrictive Behavior Management Practices*,
Autism and Child Psychopathology Series, DOI 10.1007/978-3-319-17569-0_2

to compile it were administrative returns to the US Department of Education by schools, which, as ProPublica acknowledged, are likely to be a gross underreport. For example, several very large school districts reported that no restraint or seclusion occurred at all throughout the year for tens of thousands of children, which is unlikely to be true. Despite these limitations, it seems reasonable to conclude that restraint and seclusion are widely used in American schools today.

This chapter reviews the evidence concerning how commonly restrictive behavior management practices are used and the risk factors for their use. Their prevalence and the pattern of their use obviously change dramatically over time, from state to state, from country to country, and context to context as the society changes its views of their use, as alternative treatments are developed and as regulations and the implementation of regulations that control their use change. Thus, there will be no set answer as to what the exact prevalence of the use of restrictive behavior management practices will be. Because of this, and because of the large number of papers in this area, this chapter focuses on research over the period of 2000–2014. We review the prevalence and risk factors by population including people with intellectual and other developmental disabilities, seniors, children and adolescents, people with mental health problems, incarcerated youth, prisoners, and other populations.

2.1 Specific Populations

2.1.1 Mainstream School Settings

2.1.1.1 Prevalence

There is evidence from statewide and national US databases that restrictive behavior management practices are widely used in educational settings. The US General Accounting Office (2009) cited data from California's and Texas' education systems showing that there were over 30,000 "interventions" in these two states in 1 year. Similar national data were discussed above (ProPublica 2014). Gagne et al. (2014) compared the US national school database on restraints for 2009–2010 and 2011–2012 and found little evidence of change in the use of restraints. Further, in an analysis of restraints rate per 100 students with a disability, they found that rates of restraints varied widely. Many schools did not report restraint use, whereas others reported over 80 restraints per 100 students. If the data are accurate, this may indicate widely varying practices in the use of restraint and associated preventative strategies. The only national information that was available was based on state returns to the US Department of Education, whose accuracy and completeness are unknown. Thus, there are no well-conducted studies that estimated the prevalence of restrictive behavior management practices found from either American or British sources.

2.1.1.2 Risk Factors

Several American reports have focused on disparities in the use of restraint related to ethnicity and disability. These studies have all shown that children with disabilities and nonwhite children are much more likely to be restrained than children without disabilities and White children (General Accounting Office 2009; Office for Civil Rights 2012; Texas Education Agency 2009). Some put this issue of restraint in education as part of a broader literature on unequal use of disciplinary procedures in schools against boys, nonwhite children, and children with disability (Peterson et al. 2013)

2.1.1.3 Conclusion

There is a surprising lack of quality evidence relating to the use of restrictive behavior management practices in mainstream educational setting. The reasons for this are unclear. It may reflect the reluctance of government agencies and private schools to open up a can of worms and subject themselves to liability issues and organizational reforms that would likely result from the publication of such data.

2.1.2 Incarcerated Youth

De Hert et al. (2011) conducted a systematic review of 10 years of research on the use of restraint and its correlates in youth in psychiatric settings. They identified seven studies. The prevalence was high and variable both for seclusion (26% of patients; 67/1000 patient-days) and restraints (29% of patients; 42.7/1000 patient-days). Risk factors included past or current aggression and/or violence, suicidal behavior, more severe psychopathology, nonwhite ethnicity, emergency admissions, out-of-home placement, and poorer family functioning.

A similar illustrative study comes from Pogge et al. (2011) who analyzed 2 years of restraint and seclusion data from a private psychiatric hospital serving 2411 children and adolescents during this time period. Seclusion included seclusion in the child's room and seclusion in an off-unit seclusion annex. Restraints were coded as short term (< 15 min) and long term (> 14 min). They also analyzed data on intramuscular pro re nata (PRN) medication. The most common behavioral precipitants were externalizing behavior problems, such as physical or verbal threats and attempts at self-harm. As in other populations, restraints were distributed very unevenly with only 29% of children experiencing any restraint with a mode of 1 restraint per child, but ranging up to 163 restraints in one case. Risk factors included age: Younger children had more restraints (53%) than older children (19%). Other demographic and diagnostic variables did not predict restraint use.

Thus, among patients, children and youth with psychiatric disorders are at high risk for restraint and other restrictive behavior management practices, primarily related to externalizing behavior problems and self-injury/self-harm. Thus, as with other populations, the opportunities for reducing restrictive behavior management practices lie primarily with the management of these behavior problems and associated professional practice and administrative oversight.

2.1.3 Adults with Mental Health Problems

2.1.3.1 Prevalence

Steinert et al. (2010) conducted a systematic review of restraint databases in psychiatric facilities. They found 12 such databases which included single or multiple hospitals and national data from Norway and Finland. They found that rates of restraint and seclusion varied widely. At one extreme, Iceland, a country of some 300,000 population and only one psychiatric hospital, reported using no restraint or seclusion for decades, but replaced it with one-on-one nursing staff. In contrast, Austria reported that 36 % of patients were exposed to restraint and seclusion, and The Netherlands used seclusion with 12 % of patients for a mean duration of 294 h! Steiner et al. suggested that the high rates of seclusion in the Netherlands might reflect strong legal prohibitions against the use of involuntary psychotropic medications, except in cases of emergency. Thus, restraint and seclusion are commonly used in psychiatric hospitals, and practices vary very widely from country to country.

The rate of restraint varies dramatically over time in some states reflecting the presence programs to reduce restraint and continued commitment to do so. For example, Smith et al. (2005) reported very large reductions in restraint in the Pennsylvania state hospital system between 1990 and 2000. The rate of restraints fell from 4.2 to 0.3 episodes per 1000 patient-days. The mean duration of seclusion decreased from 10.8 to 1.3 h. The rate of restraint fell from 3.5 to 1.2 episodes per 1000 patient-days. The average restraint duration fell from 11.9 to 1.9 h. Thus, the rates of restraint and seclusion vary considerably over time depending upon the quality of the programs used to reduce restraint.

The prevalence among patients in forensic psychiatric facilities may be especially high. Haw and Wolstencroft (2014) reported that in an English secure forensic institution with 242 patients fully 73 % had prescriptions for PRN medications. Within the previous 2 weeks alone, some 542 doses were administered to 37 % of the patients. This resulted in 11 % receiving high doses of antipsychotics and 20 % receiving polypharmacy due to PRNs. Further problems included absent or vague documentation of the reasons for PRN medication.

2.1.3.2 Risk Factors

Some studies have also found that factors related to the facility, rather than the patient, also predict restraint use. For example, Lay et al. (2007) found wide variations between different Swiss psychiatric hospitals in their use of restrictive procedures, but simple structural variables, such as hospital size and staff workload, did not predict the use of restrictive procedures, although van Der Schaaf et al. (2013) found that some physical and architectural features, such as special safety features and access to private space, predicted restraint use. More specific programmatic variables related to restraint use were identified by Smith et al. (2005) who found that in Pennsylvania's psychiatric hospital system that longer restraints occurred at night and restraints were used more frequently during the week.

2.1.3.3 Conclusions

Restrictive behavior management practices, especially restraint and seclusion, are commonly used in psychiatric hospitals and may be used especially liberally in forensic settings. Wide variation in their use occurs between hospitals, over time and across different countries. These variations reflect differences in policy from country to country and programmatic variables correlated with time of day, day of week, and efforts to reduce restraint and seclusion over time.

2.1.4 Persons with Intellectual Disabilities

2.1.4.1 Prevalence

Table 2.1 summarizes several studies of the prevalence of restrictive behavior management practices in children, adolescents, and adults with Intellectual Disabilities. The reported prevalence is quite high. For example, Emerson (2002) reported in his study 3 that just over 10% of a large sample of children with Intellectual Disabilities experienced physical restraint and just over 10% experienced seclusion. Most of the data in this table related to certain at-risk subsamples, such as individuals with challenging behavior and/or those in residential settings. Among these groups, the rates of restrictive behavior management practices are quite high ranging as high as approximately two thirds, although figures of one third to a half were commonly reported. A notable observation comes from Allen et al. (2006) who reported high rates of physical restraint use in some families. Most of these families also reported receiving no or minimal professional assistance, despite the severity of their children's behavioral issues. Thus, within this population, certain subgroups, including some families, have very high rates of restrictive behavior management practices in contemporary services.

Other restrictive procedures, such as PRN medications, are also commonly used in adults with Intellectual Disabilities. For example, Delafon et al. (2010) reported on the prevalence of psychotropic medication in assessment units in Leicestershire, UK, in a sample of 119 individuals over a 1-month period. They found that approximately three quarters of people with Intellectual Disabilities were prescribed psychotropic medication, approximately one quarter also experienced PRN psychotropic medication, and approximately 40% experienced polypharmacy, mostly due to the use of PRN medication.

Table 2.1 A summary of selected papers on the prevalence of restraint and other restrictive behavior management practices in children and adults with Intellectual Disabilities

Reference	Methods	Results
Murphy et al. (1993)	Total population survey of people with intellectual disability and self-injury (N=616)	13 % of sample who were self-injured wore protective devices or mechanical devices. Nearly half used psychotropic medication, but only 2 % had any formal psychological intervention
Emerson et al. (2000)	N=500 adults with Intellectual Disabilities in residential settings	Of 53 % of the sample who had moderate or severe challenging behavior, 44 % experienced physical restraint, 35 % sedation, 20 % seclusion, and 3 % mechanical restraint
Emerson (2002): Study 1	N=107 children and adolescents with Intellectual Disabilities and challenging behavior	67 % "usually" or "sometimes" managed with physical or mechanical restraint, seclusion or sedation
Emerson (2002): Study 2	N=68 children and adolescents with Intellectual Disabilities and challenging behavior	46 % had physical restraint, 67 % had seclusion 2 % had sedation, and 4 % had medication
Emerson (2002): Study 3	Of 909 children, data on challenging behavior were collected on 656. Of these 42 % had at least one form of severe challenging behavior	28 % had physical restraint, 32 % had seclusion, 1 % had sedation, and 3 % had mechanical restraint. The corresponding figures for all children were 12, 13, < 1, and 1 %, respectively
Feldman et al. (2004)	Surveyed 625 clients with challenging behavior in Ontario. Included 96 agencies institutional and noninstitutional settings. Used open-ended questions about how providers managed challenging behavior	12 % had physical restraint, 12 % had confinement time out, and 6 % had mechanical restraint. Many behavior management practices, including restrictive behavior management practices were informal and undocumented
Allen et al. (2006)	N=72 families with children with severe challenging behavior. Data were gathered via postal questionnaire	88 % used physical restraint and 21 % used it frequently
Sturmey (2009)	Analyzed English restraint data from Healthcare Commission and Commission for Social Care 2007 data. N=509 community residential units run by the National Health Service with 3902 residents	Approximately, 80 % of units used some form of restraint, 45 % used physical restraint, 9.5 % reported using seclusion, 8 % reported using mechanical restraint, 6 % reported using other restraint, and 81 % reported using PRN medication. A minority of units used restraint at much higher rates than average, and a minority of individuals experienced high rates of restraint

Table 2.1 (continued)

Reference	Methods	Results
Devreau and McGill (2009)	N=542 managers of residential National Health Service and social service run residential units with 25 % response rates	29 % reported use of breakaways for grabs and bites, 26 % blocks for punches and kicks, 12 % restraint while resident was sitting, and 5 % while resident was lying on floor
McGill et al. (2009)	Used an 8-item survey of N=268 individuals from 100 staff respondents participating in conferences. Settings included residential services (37 %), 30 % in schools 8 % from day services, and the remainder from other services. Respondents included nurses (39 %), teachers (39 %), and social work (6 %)	22 % of clients used protective devices, 50 % used PRN medication, 27 % used seclusion, and 84 % used physical restraint during the previous year. 10 % of clients experienced physical restraint daily
Allen et al. (2009)	N=901 children and adults with challenging behavior and Intellectual Disabilities who were part of a larger sample. Data collected by a screening questionnaire	36 % experienced restraint, 22 % seclusion, and 27 % PRN medication
Chaplin et al. (2009)	Residents (N=68) of a 6-bedded secure assessment and treatment unit over a 6-year period	49 % experienced de-escalation, 35 % restraint and medication, 23 % sanctions or surveillance (e.g., removal of dangerous objects), 20 % "external assistance," and 20 % were transferred to other units
Finn and Sturmey (2009)	N=81 service users of a day program for adults with Intellectual Disabilities and mental health disorders and/or challenging behavior	13 consumers accounted for 100 % of uses of restraint. Incidents included 31 removals, 1 wrap, 7 take downs, and 92 time outs
Merineau-Cote and Merin (2012)	N=81 adults living in community settings. Data were collected using a mail survey	All restrictive measures—63.0 %; seclusion—44.4 %; physical restraint—42.0 % physical restraint; and mechanical restraint—27.2 %

PRN pro re nata

2.1.4.2 Risk Factors

Several studies have robustly found that restraints are concentrated in a small number of individuals with Intellectual Disabilities (Finn and Sturmey 2009; Luiselli et al. 2005; Sturmey 1999; Sturmey 2009; Sturmey and McGlynn 2002). For example, Sturmey (1999) found that in a sample of 300 residents with intellectual disabilities, only 33 clients accounted for all short-term restraints, such as those related to aggression, and 11 clients accounted for all long-term restraints, such as those related to chronic severe self-injury and pica. Thus, approximately 15% of clients accounted for 100% of restraints. Finn and Sturmey (2009) made similar observations when they presented histograms showing that, in a sample of clients attending a day program, only 22% of consumers accounted for 92% of restraints with a handful of consumers having much higher rates of restraints that all other consumers. Thus, there is good evidence that individual differences are large, raising the question as to what might account for these individual differences. Similar data can be presented for differences between settings. For example, restraints are reported much more frequently in residential care than in family setting.

Table 2.2 summarizes a number of studies that have examined predictors of restrictive behavior management practices in people with Intellectual Disabilities. Studies have reported predictors that included demographic and diagnostic variables, behavior problems, and environmental variables. This table shows that restrictive behavior management practices are often predicated by externalizing behavior disorders, such as aggression and injury to others, but not internalizing behavior disorder, such as anxiety and withdrawal. Several studies reported that those diagnosed with autism spectrum disorders were more at risk, although the degree of intellectual disability produced different outcomes in different studies, perhaps because externalizing behavior disorders are more dangerous in physically able individuals who are more likely to have mild intellectual disability, but self-injury is more likely to occur in individuals with profound intellectual disability. One study also found that limited communication skills were also a significant predictor. Some studies reported that high rate behaviors such as stereotypy also predicated restrictive behavior management practices. Behavior severity and indirect measures of behavior severity, such as out of geographical district placement and presence of a behavior support plan, and detention under the British Mental Health Act, are also significant predictors of restraint use. There is some evidence that the failure to implement positive procedures, such as redirection (Chaplin et al. 2009), predicts use of more intrusive management strategies, such as physical restraint. When reviewing these data, it is important to keep in mind that some studies did not distinguish different types of restrictive practices. This might be important as, for example, Sturmey (1999) found that short-term restraints were predicted by hurting others, but long-term restraint was predicted by hurting self.

In contrast with diagnostic and demographic variables that practitioners cannot change, environmental variables, which are manipulable, strongly predict the use of restrictive practices. For example, Luiselli et al. (2005) analyzed the type of activities that predicted the use of physical restraint in a community-based residential school. They found that seat work accounted for nearly 20% of all physical restraints with leisure activities alone, leisure activities with others, transition, chores, and preferred activities, each accounting for approximately 8–11% of incidents of physical restraint. Finn and Sturmey (2009) replicated the effects of environmental variables in predicting restraint use in adults with Intellectual Disabilities in a day treatment program. Although such data show that environmental events pre-

Table 2.2 Risk factors associated with restraint and other restrictive behavior management practices

Reference	Risk factor
Oliver et al. (1993)	More severe changing behavior, multiple forms of challenging behavior, younger, greater impairments than those without self-injury
Sturmey (2009)	Short-term restraint frequency and duration predicted by hurting others, but not demographic or other behavioral variables Long-term restraint was predicted by hurting self
Sturmey et al. (2005)	Impulse control disorder Aberrant Behavior Checklist Irritability DASH-II Elimination disorder Effect sizes were small
Sourander et al. (2006)	Autism
Robertson et al. (2005)	Restrictive management practices were more likely in community settings, where there were many people with challenging behavior rather than few people with challenging behavior
Tasakanikos et al. (2007)	Externalizing behavior problems, such as aggression and pestering staff independently predicted the use of antipsychotic medication and psychiatric services
McGill et al. (2009)	The following demographic variables predicted physical interventions (including mechanical restraint, PRN medication, and seclusion): young, male, not legally restricted, and autism. The following behavioral variables predicted physical interventions: aggression (87 %), intense displays of emotion (79 %), and least predictors were inappropriate sexual behavior (30 %), antisocial behavior such as lying and cheating (32 %), and inappropriate personal habits (36 %). Predictors varied by type of restrictive behavior management practices
Allen et al. (2009)	Detention under the Mental Health Act (restraint and sedation), more severe challenging behavior (seclusion), destructive behavior (restraint and seclusion), placed out of geographical area (seclusion), and had behavior plans (restraint and seclusion)
Emerson (2002) Study 1	More severe challenging behavior, less severe intellectual disability and more restricted expressive communication (physical restraint), and greater self-care ability and more stereotyped behavior (seclusion)
Emerson (2002) Study 2	Injury to other children (restraint)
Emerson (2002) Study 3	Irritability, less anxiety, more conduct disorder and attending special education (physical restraint) and isolated/ritualistic behavior, attending special education, more conduct disorder, more self-injury, more irritability older and Black British (seclusion)
Webber et al. (2010)	Participants on compulsory detention were more likely to be seclusions (44 %) versus a match control group (5 %)
Webber et al. (2012)	Better quality behavior support plans predict less restraint
Webber et al. (2014)	Seclusion predicted by individual variables, such as age, autism, and psychiatric disorders and organizational variables, such as using institutional or community residential services and location of services

PRN pro re nata

dict restraint use, they are relatively crude, in that they do not identify the precise functions of stimuli involved in a high-risk situation. They may be quite useful, however, in that they may direct clinicians where to look when conducting a more detailed functional behavior assessment and may be helpful in designing effective behavior support plans. For example, Luiselli et al. (2000) constructed behavior support plans using antecedent interventions to greatly reduce the use of restraint in two adolescents with pervasive developmental disorder compared to their existing behavior support plan.

People with Intellectual Disabilities may be especially vulnerable to the use of restraints during medical, dental, nursing procedures, and physical and occupational therapy. Newton (2009) reviewed the use of restraints during dental procedures and found a wide range of restrictive practices used during dentistry with people with Intellectual Disabilities. A subsequent survey revealed that although dental practitioners reported being confident in behavior management issues, many general practitioners' knowledge of nonrestrictive management practices was limited, although specialists reported somewhat more non-pharmacological methods of behavior management (Humza Bin Saeed et al. 2012).

Genetic Syndromes

Individuals with certain genetic syndromes, such as Prader-Willi, Cornelia de Lange, and Smith-Magenis syndromes, which are associated with severe self-injury, are at especially high risk for restrictive behavior management practices. For example, Anderson and Ernst (1980) surveyed behavior management practices for 40 individuals with Lesch–Nyhan syndrome, a rare genetic syndrome associated with multiple forms of severe self-injury, such as lip and finger biting. They found that nearly half were restrained throughout the day, and about 80 % were restrained at least half of the day. Sixty percent had teeth extracted to prevent self-biting. People with Prader–Willi syndrome are often subjective to environmental restrictions, such as locked refrigerators and kitchens, because they often eat very large amounts of food and are severely obese placing them at risk for serious cardiac and other health problems and reduced mortality.

2.1.4.3 Conclusion

In sum, although we do not have good demographic data because of the problem of adequately defining and sampling from a population of individuals with Intellectual Disabilities, there is strong evidence that certain groups, service, and perhaps certain families are at high risk of frequently using restrictive behavior management practices. Similarly, a small number of clients and a few settings account for the majority of restraints and seclusions. The strongest and most consistent predictors of restrictive behavior management practices are externalizing behavior problems, such as aggression, tantrums, and self-injury. There is good evidence, which is consistent with the literature on functional behavior assessment, that environmental variables predict use of restrictive behavior management practices on a case-by-case basis and that information can be a useful part of assessment that leads to an effective behavioral support plan.

There is evidence that deficiencies in services, such as the absence of technically adequate behavior support plan and its effective implementation, also predicts the use of restrictive behavior management practices (see Chaps. 10 and 11) which is consistent with many studies that have shown that implementation of an effective behavior plan may reduce their use. Thus, if services wish to reduce restrictive behavior management practices, they should identify and focus on a specific number of individuals and settings, provide effective, evidence-based interventions for externalizing behavior and self-injury, and provide adequate support and oversight for all staff, including professional staff, to do so.

2.1.5 Seniors

2.1.5.1 Prevalence

Services for seniors have varied dramatically from place to place and time to time in their use of restraints. Hence, restraints might be used routinely in one state and rarely in the neighboring state. Likewise, in response to Federal or other legal initiatives (Hawes et al. 1997) or even under their own initiative, services for seniors may change from routine, widespread use of restraints to nearly eliminating them. Thus, individual figures quoted in should be considered in the context in which the data were collected, but should not be generalized to other contemporary contexts.

There are a large number of empirical studies of the prevalence of physical restraints in nursing homes. Here, we consider two reviews. Dube and Mitchell (1986) reported that restraint was used in nearly 100 % of nursing homes. The proportion of residents restrained varied widely from 19 to 85 %. More recently, Schussler et al. (2014) also reported widely varying figures. These authors conducted a systematic review of characteristics of nursing home residents with dementia. The review discussed seven studies published between 2003 and 2013. The prevalence of restraints ranged from 10 to 59 %. Six studies found that the most common form of restraint was bed rails. Figures varied in part due to the definition of restraint and the time period over which restraint was reported (e.g., last 24 h vs. last month).

Psychotropic medications are also used widely in nursing homes, predominantly for behavior management. Simoni-Watsila et al. (2014) using a 5 % sample of Medicare data from 2007 found that two thirds of the sample used at least one psychotropic medication with nearly 60 % taking antidepressants, approximately one third taking antipsychotics, and nearly two thirds taking psychotropic medication from at least two different classes of psychotropic medication.

2.1.5.2 Risk Factors

Hofman and Hahn (2014) conducted a systematic review of the literature to identify risk factors for restraint in the elderly. They identified nine studies that met inclusion criteria published between 2005 and 2011. They identified the following risk factors: lower independence, greater cognitive impairment, greater mobility impairment, and history of fractures and falls, externalizing behavior problems such as verbal and physical agitation. Thus, these predictors reflect the use of restraints, in particular, bed rails to manage wandering and disruptive behavior in seniors.

Differences between nursing homes in their use of restraint are very large. For example, Meyer et al. (2009) found that rates of restraint varied from 5 to 59 %, raising the possibility that nursing homes may differ not only in terms of resident characteristics but also in their practices that may discourage or facilitate the use of restrictive behavior management practices. Hoffman and Hahn (2014) focused on resident individual differences that predicted restraint, but other factors unrelated to the individual are also important. For example, staff turnover, (Hawes et al. 1997) including turnover of nursing home administrators (Castle 2011) predicted higher use of restraints, although not all studies found facility characteristics to predict restraint (Meyer et al. 2008; Tinetti et al. 1992). A gap in the literature is data that specify exactly what care practices determine for the use of restrictive behavior management practices. For example, the group of studies that have shown that staff training and support and state regulation and oversight may reduce restraint in nursing homes suggests that there are many educational and supervisory practices that influence the use of restrictive behavior management practices; hence, the absence of appropriate staff training and support may be one crucial variable that predicts the use of restrictive behavior management practices.

2.1.5.3 Conclusion

The rate of restraints varies considerably from one nursing home to another depending upon professional practices, oversight, and individual differences in residents. Resident behavior that places them at risk, such as wandering and falls, and challenging behavior are the most common individual predictors of restraint use. These data indicate that oversight and staff training, especially related to behavior management and general acceptability of restraints may have a large impact on nursing home use of restraints.

2.1.6 Brain Injury

Some individuals with acquired brain injury may be at risk for agitation and aggression both immediately after injury (McNett et al. 2012) and for some individuals on a longer-term basis (Stubbs and Alderman 2008). This may place them at risk for restrictive behavior management practices.

McNett et al. (2012) reported on the rate of several restrictive behavior management practices in patients with traumatic brain injury in an acute care ward. They found that nearly half had at least one episode of agitation including problems such as pulling on medical devices. Although many such problems were dealt with by reorientation, 32 % were managed by constant supervision, 30 % by benzodiazepines, 21 % by antipsychotic medication, and 24 % by restraints. Agitation strongly predicted all forms of restrictive behavior management practices. Thus, behavior management practices were commonly used to manage agitation in an acute care setting.

Stubbs and Alderman (2008) reported on the rates of restraint in a 85-beded tertiary neurobehavioral unit for adults with traumatic brain injury. Over a 12-month period, there were 1427 applications of restraints at a rate of approximately 118 per month (range 75–168 per month). About 90 % of incidents of restraint were under 10 min in duration. Injuries occurred to patients in 0.98 % of applications and in 6.5 % of application to staff. During the year, the rates of restraints increased somewhat. Similarly, Alderman et al. (2002) found that approximately 10 % of all incidents of aggression in a residential program for traumatic brain injury resulted in restraint. Again, restraints appear to be used quite commonly in some residential units for traumatic brain injury, although large-scale data are not yet available.

2.1.7 Dentistry

Within dentistry, a wide range of behavior management methods are used, some of which are quite restrictive and potentially dangerous. They include voice control, tell–show–do, positive reinforcement, distraction, nitrous oxide, nonverbal communication, hand over mouth, hand over mouth with air restriction, physical restraint, conscious sedation, nitrous oxide, and general anesthesia, although the American Academy of Pediatrics eliminated the use of hand-over-mouth restraint from its clinical guidelines (Oueis et al. 2010). Sometimes dentists practice polypharmacy, for example, combining nitrous oxide with other medications which is sometimes dangerous (Levering and Wellie 2007). In the free market of professional practice in which many wealthy patients pay handsomely for aesthetic and preventative treatments and in which in many parts of the world demand grossly outstrips supply, dentists have considerable latitude over what kind of work they accept and how to practice. Additionally, there is a lack of attention to behavior management during professional training. Further, dentists can also bill for some restrictive behavior management practices, such as general sedation, but not for preventative behavior management practices, such as patient education. Hence, many forces conspire toward unnecessary use of behavior management practices in dental treatment (Newton 2009), although professional guidelines exhort them not to do so and such practices may result in charges of nonprofessional conduct.

2.1.7.1 Prevalence

Little is known about the prevalence of different behavior management strategies during dentistry. Most of the literature has focused on questions only tangentially related to the prevalence such as the acceptability of and practitioner confidence in the use of different behavior management techniques and parental accompaniment (Crossley and Goshi 2002), differences across different practitioners, time periods and countries, and professional training issues (Newton 2009).

2.1.7.2 Risk Factors

Certain groups of dental patients are at increased risk for restraint and other behavior management practices during dentistry including children with dental fears and phobias and other non-fear-related behavior management issues perhaps related to broader noncompliance. For example, dental fears and phobias are commonly related to noncompliance and other behavior problems during dental treatment. Thus, children with fears or other behavioral issues are at high risk for behavior management practices.

2.1.7.3 Conclusion

Although behavior management issues are commonly acknowledged in dentistry, especially related to fears and compliance issues in children and specific populations at risk for behavior management practices, surprisingly little is known about the use of behavior management practices in dentistry.

2.1.8 Detained Immigrants

No systematic study on the use of restraint with detained immigrants was identified for this section of the chapter; however, Kalhan (2010) noted that detained immigrants are often subjected to prison-like conditions prior to trial or removal, including physical restraints. Amnesty International (2009) reported extensive and excessive use of mechanical restraint in the USA. Examples included restraint of pregnant women, widespread and unnecessary use of mechanical restraint during transportation, and illegal use of mechanical restraints when defendants appeared in court, who were sometimes only unshackled in order to take the oath. Chapter 5 of this volume documents similar problems with the unsafe and lethal use of personal and mechanical restraint during deportation in the UK.

2.2 Conclusions

Restraint, seclusion, and other forms of behavior management practices are widely used in contemporary services for many at-risk populations. High rates of behavior management practices are well documented among children and adolescents with disabilities in educational settings, youth in psychiatric in patient services, adults with Intellectual Disabilities in contemporary community settings (as well as in institutions), adults with psychiatric disorders in in-patient units and in nursing homes. Information on the prevalence of restraint and seclusion is lacking, especially related to mainstream education, detained immigrants, and the prevalence of solitary confinement in prisons. In many of the populations reviewed here, rates of behavior management practices varied widely, not only related to individual differences but also between services and over time. This latter observation is important as it implies that the services delivered, professional competence, and service oversight and regulation have a key role in reducing behavior management practices in a wide range of contexts. It is notable that the status of the literature differs from population to another. In some areas, such as Intellectual Disabilities and seniors, this is an extensive literature documenting the prevalence and risk factors for behavior management practices, where as in other populations the literature is very underdeveloped or absent. Thus, in some cases, social science has lagged behind contemporary social issues.

It is apparent from studies of different populations that certain risk factors reoccur across populations. Namely, the effective management of externalizing behavior disorders and self-injury/self-harm is a common risk factor across populations and service often remain sorely deficient in delivering effective evidence-based practices for these problems. In several examples, there are clear hints of the importance of environmental variables related to functional behavior assessment with strong implications for treatment and prevention, such as the management of overall level of positive reinforcement, management of demands, skilled performance from direct carestaff, and the need for adequate training and support for professional and nonprofessional staff in such settings.

Chapter 3
Ethics and Legal Aspects

This chapter reviews the ethics and legal and professional standards of conduct, including family members, regarding the use of restrictive behavior management practices, especially those related to restraint and seclusion. Using interventions that place clients, peers, caregivers, and family members at risk for harm raises special concerns that have been addressed extensively in legal and professional statements regarding everyone's obligations and liabilities regarding the use of restraint and seclusion, including actions that should be taken to prevent the use of restraint and seclusion. At first glance, it might seem that eliminating restrictive behavior management practices should be done without further thought; however, Chap. 1 showed that at times society requires us to restrain ourselves and others, and, even without legal requirements to do so, caregivers, medical and dental staff, and therapists often restrain others, sometimes to prevent possible harm to vulnerable people or sometimes to achieve some desirable outcome that is seen to justify the use of restrictive behavior management practices to some. Indeed, there are circumstances where failure to restrain someone might be unethical and illegal. Because of the risks of injury and death, the demeaning nature of restrictive behavior management practices, the possibility of other alternate, desirable behavior management practices, and the excessive and abusive use of restrictive behavior management practices in services and families, the law and professional bodies have stepped in to control the behavior of professionals and nonprofessionals to reduce and eliminate restrictive behavior management practices. Thus, the aim of this chapter is to review the ethics and legal constraints on the use of restrictive behavior management practices. The first part of the chapter reviews what is meant by ethics. The following sections review a variety of professional guidelines, laws and advocacy organizations, and web sites, mostly on the use of restraint.

Ethical and legal concerns over restraint and seclusion periodically receive considerable public attention. This usually occurs when there is a death, serious injury, or ongoing injuries of a vulnerable person in restraint or seclusion, or when a specific service uses restraints and seclusion excessively, often in the context of more broadly occurring mismanagement, failure of oversight and regulation, and/

P. Sturmey, *Reducing Restraint and Restrictive Behavior Management Practices*,
Autism and Child Psychopathology Series, DOI 10.1007/978-3-319-17569-0_3

or abuse and neglect. For example, in 1999, the *Hartford Current* reported 142 restraint-related deaths in the USA. Over the past 10 years, there have been a number of restraint-related deaths of children in youth facilities in the UK and of adults in immigration. Further details can be found in Chaps. 4 and 5.

3.1 What Are Ethics?

It is useful to distinguish ethics as a branch of philosophy and professional ethics (Sturmey 2005). Ethics, as a branch of philosophy studies, analyzes and codifies right and wrong behavior. It attempts to answer questions such as "What are morals or values?," "How should we behave?," and "How should we behave to be consistent with our moral standards and values?" Ethical questions often involve questions about the right way to behave toward other people. It involves both prohibitions and exhortations to behave well, that is, virtuous behavior that leads to values. In contrast, professional ethics are sets of rules, usually promulgated through professional societies or the law, to control professional behavior that primarily focus on preventing harm to the public through the control of professional training and the punishment of professional misconduct through fines and required activities, such as professional retraining and suspension of professional licenses. Professional ethics often also contain rules to promote positive professional conduct, such as professional competency. Professional ethics are drawn by different professional groups and over a wide span of time. Thus, what one professional group may view as professional, ethical conduct, another group might condemn as unethical. As time changes, that same professional group might change its position. For example, a professional group might permit a certain form of restraint for some time and later prohibit it as unethical. Indeed, several professional groups have split over professional ethical issues related to restrictive behavior management practices, such as the use of restraint and aversive behavioral treatments (see below). Philosophical and professional ethics overlap with laws but do not have a one-to-one correspondence with them. Thus, many laws may be philosophically unethical and sometimes laws may conflict and contradict professional standards of conduct. For example, mental health legislation sometimes permits or even indirectly encourages the use of restraint, whereas some professional ethics may severely limit or even completely prohibit its use.

Philosophical ethics can be divided into three kinds of theories. First, consequentialism judges actions by the overall benefit that results to everyone from an action. For example, examples of consequentialist justification for restraint include that there are medical benefits to the person, such as healing of injuries or recovery from medical conditions, such as stroke, and the reduction of harm and distress to others, such as reducing injuries to the person themselves and to other people, and that these benefits are greater than the harm to the person restrained and others. Deontological ethics holds the view that certain behavior is inherently moral, for example, because God commands it or because there are absolute rules of conduct.

Today, this is reflected in statements of human rights and service values, namely that we must treat each other in certain ways, not because of the benefits to each other, but because we are all human and all humans have a certain inherent value. Finally, virtue ethics focuses on the inherent good qualities of a person, rather than specific actions, and emphasizes the internal consequences for our actions over external sanctions. Accordingly, by practicing these common sense virtues such as courage, temperance, justice, and wisdom, people will achieve happiness and their full potential.

Philosophical ethics raises many questions regarding restrictive behavior management practices, such as "When is it right to restrain another person? When is it right to injure another person? What are my responsibilities to another person who is aggressive or in danger of hurting themselves or others and to potential victims? If I take money for a job to treat behavior that may result in restrictive behavior management practices, what are my responsibilities? If the organization I work for fails to prevent harm or causes problem behavior or engages in harmful practice, for example, fails to train or fails to train staff effectively, or supports staff who provoke problem behavior, and these problems result in restrictive behavior management practices, what should I do? If I am not competent to treat a problem and my continued incompetent behavior continues to place a client at risk, for example, when a new staff is assigned a highly challenging client, with restrictive behavior management practices and/or injury, what should I do? When restrictive behavior management practices are used inequitably, for example, people with disabilities, boys or non-Whites are at greater risk for restrictive behavior management practices, what is my right course of action?"

3.2 The Law

There are many laws regarding restrictive behavior management practices including restraint and seclusion in many countries and states. They may derive from international law, such as the Declaration on Human Rights and agreements on torture and national, state, and city laws. They vary substantially over time and in different countries. Generally, they have become more numerous, more detailed, and more complex, or sometimes laws that operate within the same geographical location, are confusing because they use different language and may directly contradict each other.

3.2.1 International Law

Human rights legislation and most contemporary services have statements regarding the rights of people at risk for restrictive behavior management practices. For example, the *United Nations Convention on Persons with Disabilities* (2006), including legal protection against discrimination on the basis of disability status and racial origin, freedom from exploitation, violence and abuse, liberty of movement, living independently in the community, personal mobility, access to education, health, habilitation, and rehabilitation, among others. These rights have direct implications to severely restrict the use of restrictive behavior management practices since their use is incompatible with certain rights such as personal mobility. Further, effective treatment may include the use of restrictive behavior management practices for some people who severely restrict access to education and typical community settings at least temporarily. Often the use of restrictive behavior management practices is associated with failure to provide adequate habilitation and rehabilitation to prevent the use of restrictive behavior management practices effectively. Thus, from a human rights perspective, the use of restrictive behavior management practices, especially those that result in injury and that restrict mobility and access to typical educational and community settings, is problematic and often incompatible with several of the rights enshrined in this convention.

Such declarations are only binding on countries that sign and ratify the treaties. Often countries are reluctant to do so due to concerns for their own sovereignty or that the treaties impose additional responsibilities And/or costs on the country. For example, the United Nations *Convention on the Rights of Persons with Disabilities* (2006), negotiated under President George Bush, calls for relatively noncontroversial actions, such as nondiscrimination, equality for women and children with disabilities, accessibility to education, transport and housing, etc.; yet, the USA has declined to sign due to opposition from a minority of legislators concerned over interference with US sovereignty, opposition to the United Nations, concerns for potential implications for access to abortion and the possibility of states interfering with parents' rights. Thus, at this time, the convention is not a law in the USA, although many other countries have already signed and ratified the treaty.

3.2.2 American Law

American law comes from several sources including the Constitution, its interpretation in relationship to specific situations from the Supreme Court, state and city laws, regulations that attach to federally funded service, etc. The American Constitution guarantees right to all Americans, including people with disabilities and children, the most significant of which here is the due process clauses of the Fourth and Fifteenth Amendments to the Constitution which state that "[N]or shall any person… be deprived of life, liberty, or property, without due process of law." Clearly, restraint and seclusion specifically, but many other restrictive behavior management practices generally, also restrict people's liberty and access to their property. The legal requirement in the USA is that such restrictions are done with due process of law, for example, with informed consent from the person themselves, their parent or legal guardian, or action of a court. Chapter 5 provides some examples of the evolving interpretation of constitutional rights as related to people in institutional settings. Johnson (undated) provides a concise summary of legal aspects of restraint and seclusion, and Peterson et al. (2013) review legal aspects of restraint and seclusion in American school settings.

3.2.2.1 Special Education

Up to the 1960s, many American children with disabilities were excluded from education being deemed "trainable" or "ineducable," but not "educable". This resulted in many children with disabilities being segregated and not benefitting from education. The *Individuals with Disabilities Education Act* is the principal Federal law controlling education for children with disabilities generally, and special education in particular is *Individuals with Disabilities Education Act*. It includes several provisions that directly related to restrictive behavior management practices. Some of these include an Individualized Education Plan that describes the services, the student's current level of performance, the accommodations and modifications to the student's education, which must be provided in the least restrictive environment, meaning in the most integrated setting possible. The student must have a "free, appropriate, public education." A child cannot be disciplined due to their disability and cannot be coerced by the school to take psychotropic medication.

If a child's challenging behavior interferes with his/her education or another child's education, or places themselves or others in harm, then the school must conduct a functional behavioral assessment. A functional behavioral assessment must be a comprehensive assessment that includes identifying the target behavior, its function, reinforcers, its antecedents, and alternate appropriate behaviors, such as communication skills that serve the same function as the target behavior.[1] The school may then implement a behavior support plan. *Individuals with Disabilities Education Act* and the US Department of Education have expressed very strong support for positive behavioral supports based on the child's functional behavioral assessment, such as environmental and curricular modifications, teaching skills, and positive reinforcement.

When it comes to restraints, *Individuals with Disabilities Education Act* has both strengths and weaknesses. Since the constitutional protection of due process applied to restricting someone's movement, the use of restraint requires due process, such as that involved in developing the child's individual education plan. Further, the Supreme Court in *Youngberg v. Romeo* specifically rules that citizens have a liberty interest to be free from restraints. (See below for further discussion of *Youngberg*.) Further, a school that used restraint repeatedly over a prolonged period of time would have difficulty as it used restraint only as an emergency. Further, failure to develop a functional behavioral assessment, design and effectively implement a positive behavior support plan in a timely fashion to protect the students from further harm and ensure their freedom from restraints might be seen as a breach

[1] For example, if tantrums have been positively reinforced in the past by access to music, then we might teach the child to request music in some acceptable way such as pointing and use of sign language or words.

of both *Youngberg* and *Individuals with Disabilities Education Act*. In reviewing special education law related to restraints, Johnson (undated) concluded that most organizations that have taken a position agree that: (1) restraints should be used in emergency situations to ensure safety from injuries to the student or others; (2) restraints should be used after other methods have been tried as a last resort; (3) staff should trained in de-escalation methods; (4) only by staff trained to use restraints should use them; (5) the least restrictive and harmful methods of restraint should be used; and (6) restrains should be documented.

Despite its strengths, *Individuals with Disabilities Education Act* has some major weaknesses. First, *Individuals with Disabilities Education Act* has been widely criticized for the lack of effective oversight and enforcement resulting in widespread failure to implement preventative strategies, such as the use of functional behavioral assessments and training staff in preventative behavioral strategies. Second, although *Individuals with Disabilities Education Act* discourages restraint and seclusion, it does in fact permit their use.[2] Third, *Individuals with Disabilities Education Act* and *Youngberg* case law on restraints presume that professional judgments about restraint are sound unless they are a *substantial* departure from professional practice standards. Recent national restraint data (ProPublica 2014) indicated that both restraint and seclusion are currently widely used in educational settings, and hence we may question the effectiveness of *Individuals with Disabilities Education Act* in safely minimizing restraints.

Section 504 of the *Rehabilitation Act* and *Americans with Disabilities Act* (ADA) cover students more broadly than *Individuals with Disabilities Education Act*, and both may also have implications for nondiscriminatory use of restrictive behavior management practices. Finally, there are laws and regulations in individual states and common law that may also govern the use of restrictive behavior management practices. In merging the list of common requirements relating to the use of restraint in schools, Johnson (undated) also added the following to the above list: (1) restraints should not be used to force compliance where there is no imminent danger to anyone; (2) staff making decisions about restraint should be qualified to do so; (3) parents should be included in such decisions and should be promptly notified of the use of restraint; (4) schools should meet with parents after restraints are used and evaluate if the current plans need to be modified; and (6) restraint use should be reviewed as part of the individual education plan process which is part of the review for the development of a behavior support plan.

3.2.2.2 Institutional and Community Services

Civil Rights of Institutionalized Persons Act Following prolonged and repeated institutional scandals from the 1940s to the 1970s in the USA (Blatt and Kaplan 1966) and the failure of American states to address the problem effectively on their own,

[2] Arnie Duncan, US Secretary of State, while expressing general disapproval of restraints and seclusion of children in American students, also noted in response to specific questions that restraints and seclusion are not prohibited by *Individuals with Disabilities Education Act*.

despite repeated exposes of gross underfunding and decades of neglect and isolation of services, the Federal government passed legislation to protect the civil rights of people in institutional settings including state and locally operated jails and prisons, juvenile correctional facilities, public nursing homes, mental health facilities, and institutions for individuals with Intellectual Disabilities. Civil Rights of Institutionalized Persons Act states that "Whenever the Attorney General has reasonable cause to believe that any State… is subjecting persons residing in… an institution… to egregious or flagrant conditions which deprive such persons of any rights… protected by the Constitution or laws of the United States causing such persons to suffer grievous harm,… pursuant to a pattern or practice of resistance to the full enjoyment of such rights… the Attorney General… may institute a civil action… against such party for such equitable relief… to insure the minimum corrective measures necessary to insure the full enjoyment of such rights." The Civil Rights of Institutionalized Persons Act requires annual reports to be sent to Congress on these actions. The Department of Justice investigated numerous institutional scandals which included excessive and abusive use of restrictive behavior practices, and this effort continues to this day and has been instrumental in improving the worst conditions in institutions and has resulted in the closure of many institutions as part of settlement agreements between the Department of Justice and states. A series of federal lawsuits established the right to freedom from unnecessary restraints and restrictions on movements, such as locked wards, and the right to safety, such as safety from the harm that may come from restrictive behavior management practices. The Civil Rights of Institutionalized Persons Act also requires annual reports to be sent to Congress on these actions.

A Civil Rights of Institutionalized Persons Act investigation has three parts: investigative findings, complaints filed in Federal court, and settlement and court decisions. Members of the public can report possible problems to the Department of Justice. Their 2008 annual report indicated that they had received over 7000 letters and hundreds of phone calls reporting possible violations that year. If the Department of Justice suspects a possible violation, it conducts an on-site investigation into the allegation. The attorney general then writes a report to the governor of the state concerned stating its legal authority to make the investigation, describing how it conducted the investigation, summarizing its findings, and what actions must be taken to remedy the problems. The investigation letter then offers copies of their experts' observation, hopes that these matters can be addressed promptly, and then lets the state governor know that, if the matter is not addressed, the US Department of Justice may sue the state in Federal court. Often the state and the US Department of Justice enter into a written settlement agreement which involves an extended period of monitoring by court-appointed experts until the state has remedied all the problems to the satisfaction of the court monitor and the court. If the state does so, the case may be resolved. If the state continues to fail to address the issue in either the letter of investigation or the settlement agreement, then the US Department of Justice may file suit in federal court and sue the state. This can result in substantial expenses to the state in terms of the cost of protracted litigation and court fines. In fact, states rarely litigate these cases. The US Department of Justice has sued many US states in Federal court from the 1960s onwards and continues to do so to this day. (See the Civil Rights of Institutionalized Persons Act web site[3] for reports from historical and ongoing investigations.)

After complaints, media exposes, or on its own initiative, the Department of Justice hires qualified professional experts to investigate evaluate whether or not services conform to minimal professional standards. (Note that this is not the same as typical professional performance, which may often be below minimal professional standards.) This initial investigation might conclude that there is no finding, might lead to a negotiated settlement to cure the legal harm, or might result in a Federal lawsuit in which the Department of Justice sues a state in court. Such lawsuits have resulted in substantial changes in services, Federal takeover of state services and substantial financial costs, such as large-scale hiring of staff, institutional closure, and the development of community services; thus, often states prefer to settle.

With regard to restraints and other restrictive behavior management practices, common issues include whether or not a competent functional behavioral assessment was conducted, whether the behavior support plan was based on that functional behavioral assessment, whether the facility adequately trained their staff to implement the plan, including teaching replacement behavior that serves the same function as the target behavior, and whether the facility had adequate oversight and took effective action to reduce client injury and restraint. Often these investigations include both observations of services and interviews with clients and staff. It also includes extensive analysis and cross-referencing of documentation, especially relating to clients with self-injury, aggression, pica, clients on one-on-one staffing, client with gait problems and clients injured by other clients, especially those who have been injured frequently by others. For example, in the case of a client with self-injury that involved personal and mechanical restraints, an expert might record all incidents of restraints and all injuries of cross-referencing, direct care, nursing, medical, psychology, other professional notes, and minutes from administrative functions, such as the Human Rights Committee, safety and quality assurance, and other administrative committees. These would be used to evaluate the effectiveness and safety of the use of restraint and the adequacy of service performance in conducting a functional behavioral assessment and developing a behavior support plan and for service responses to increases in client target behavior and increase in client injury. Civil Rights of Institutionalized Persons Act investigations often require institutions to substantially improve their behavior management services and to implement safe restraint reduction programs.

Youngberg v. Romeo (1982)

Several specific Civil Rights of Institutionalized Persons Act cases are often cited for establishing certain specific rights or standards that flow from broader constitutional rights. In *Youngberg v. Romeo* (1982), Nicholas Romeo was a man with profound Intellectual Disabilities who lived in Pennsylvania state hospital. Staff restrained him many hours a day, and he was injured frequently due to restraint and ineffective behavior management resulting in continuation of dangerous behavior.

[3] http://www.justice.gov/crt/about/spl/findsettle.php

The court interpreted the Fourteenth Amendment of the Constitution Due Process Clause as establishing a constitutional right to safety, "reasonably adequate training," and "safety and freedom from unreasonable restraints" for people living in institutions. Since this was passed in federal court, this decision applied to all persons in institutional settings and became the precedent for all subsequent Civil Rights of Institutionalized Persons Act lawsuits related to the right to safety, adequate habilitation, and freedom from restraints.

Wyatt v. Stickney (1973)

In 1970, Bryce Hospital, Alabama moved to lay off staff. In response, a staff who was the aunt of Ricky Wyatt, a resident labeled a "juvenile delinquent," complained to the Department of Justice that the state was infringing upon the minimum constitutional rights of Bryce residents. The case expanded to a large class action suit involved three state facilities. The state commissioner argued that the court-mandated staffing levels were impossible to meet and were too restrictive and not in the best interested of the patients (Stickney 1974).

The case established the right to four general rights including: (a) humane psychological and physical environment, (b) qualified and sufficient staff for the administration of treatment, (c) individualized treatment plans, and (d) minimum restriction of patient freedom. As with *Youngberg,* these standards directly relate to behavior management strategies, such as skills training generally as well as training specifically related to behavior programming. This lawsuit also commented upon safety issues related to restraint. It required a physician or other health profession to write orders for restraint or seclusion which are only valid for 24 h. Thus, safety and restraints are central to Civil Rights of Institutionalized Persons Act investigations and are one of their most common elements. After 30 years, the case was dismissed in 2003 and cost Alabama millions of dollars to litigate the case and remedy the problems.

Americans with Disabilities Act (1990)

A significant change in legislation occurred with the passage of the *Americans with Disabilities Act* (1999), which made it illegal to discriminate against someone on the basis of disability, including denying them access to community settings on the basis of their disability, and required public services to "administer services, programs, and activities in the most integrated setting appropriate to the needs of qualified individuals with disabilities." Thus, a well-run, clean, safe, restraint-free institution is probably illegal because it violates the *ADA*'s mandate for community integration. In *Olmstead v. LC,* the Supreme Court confirmed that two women with Intellectual Disabilities and schizophrenia had a disability within the meaning of *ADA* and that their placement in an institutional setting was a violation of *ADA*. Subsequently, states developed Olmsted plans to limit institutionalization and develop integrated, community services.

The US Department of Justice has aggressively pursued ADA's integration mandate, which has resulted in the development of community services and pushed deinstitutionalization in the USA still further. ADA has had a broad impact on deinstitutionalization and community mental health and disability services in the USA. States now have few defenses for institutionalization and failure to develop and maintain adequate community services. The *ADA* did not address restrictive behavior management practices directly. If states, however, fail to provide accessible and effective community behavioral services resulting in institutional placement and thereby unnecessarily discriminate against people with disabilities by institutionalizing them, then this might be part of an *Olmstead* case. Likewise, to the extent that remaining institutions continue to use ineffective behavioral interventions resulting in a failure to place people with disabilities in community settings, thereby discriminating against people with disabilities at risk for institutionalization, then, ADA supports effective behavior management, including safe elimination of restrictive behavior management practices, albeit indirectly.

3.2.3 British Law

The most specific review of physical interventions and British law comes from Lyon and Pimor (2004) who provided a comprehensive review of the topic. In Britain, the law is complicated due to different laws operating in the differing parts of the UK. Thus, laws and legal proceedings are different in England, Wales, Scotland, and Northern Ireland. Further, the development of new laws from the European Community and other international bodies and treaty obligations also influence British law (most of the specific examples below related to English law) and may not apply to other parts of the UK.

Lyon and Pimor (2004) noted that there are three types of laws. First, common law refers to long-established legal principles set out in case law, such as one's "duty of care." Case law refers to long established legal principles that are derived and developed from individual cases. Second, there is legislation, which is the law passed by Parliament or legislative action by the secretary of state or other government entities. Finally, government departments issue guidance, regulations, and "circulars" that offer advice. The term "advice" is perhaps misleading as the term may seem to imply a mere suggestion; this is not so. If people or agencies do not follow the advice, their behavior may be illegal and they have to have substantive reasons to deviate from this advice.

Lyon and Pimor noted that a basic concept in British law is that individual liberty may not be infringed upon *without lawful excuses;* however, individual liberty may be restricted if a person commits a criminal offence or a civil wrong (or "tort"). A tort is a "wrongful act or failure to act for which damages can be obtained in a civil court" (p. 265) which occurs between two private individuals where one person has a "duty of care" to another. We have a "duty of care" to our "neighbors," broadly defined. We should behave in the way a "reasonable person" would do, so as to prevent harm to our neighbors, both from our acts of commission and acts of omission.

For example, if a client refuses to eat and might starve to death, but a staff failed to act, then the staff might be guilty of a tort because her negligence caused harm to the client when the staff had a duty of care to the client. If the staff intervenes against the client's will and physically restraints her in order to force her to eat, then the staff may be guilty of assault and battery. If the staff goes to court to get an order for the treatment, then the treatment may legally proceed (pp. 243–244).

Parents also have legal challenges with regard to restraint and seclusion of their children. In the past, emphasis was placed on parental rights over their children as their chattel, but today the law emphasizes parental duties toward their children. These include duties to protect their child, provide for their child's care and upbringing, ensure they attend school, consent to medication, and administer the child's property, all of which may impinge on the use of restraint and seclusion. For example, because of their duty to ensure their child's care and upbringing, parents of a child with challenging behavior may have a duty to seek out and obtain effective treatment and education, and if they use restraint or seclusion in their home, they must do so for the paramount benefit of the child, but not for personal convenience or as punishment. If parents hire other people, such as baby sitters and the baby sitter harms their child, the parent may be liable and have committed a tort. For example, if they hired a child minder for their child who was aggressive, but failed to inform and/or adequately prepare the baby sitter, then the parents may be held accountable for the injuries that the child minder caused when restraining their child because the parents had a duty to their own child and were negligent because they failed to act. If accused of assaulting their child, parents might raise the defense that parents have a right to "reasonable chastisement," but only so long as the punishment is "reasonable" and does not violate the European Convention on Human Rights which gives children protection from "cruel, inhuman, or degrading treatment or punishment" (p. 29). The questions that all parents face are complicated by issues such as evolving definitions of who is a parent, what is a reasonable standard of behavior for parents with regard to discipline, and at what age children can make legal decisions, such as consent for treatment.

Staff, including professional staff, also have obligations to safeguard and promote child welfare. Professional staff who violate their contract of employment, professional code of conduct or who violate generally accepted standards of professional conduct regarding restrictive behavior management practices might also face legal consequences. Specific English educational legislation specifies that school staff have to provide "full-time and efficient" education and that they are not exposed to harm. An example of a staff legal issue related to restraint is that of documentation (incident recording) of restraint and restraint-related injuries. For example, if a parent complained about their child receiving injuries from restraint, but there was no documentation, this might be taken as evidence of abuse (pp. 246–247). Further, the lack of documentation means that the child's behavior and their treatment cannot be adequately assessed and a functional assessment cannot be adequately performed, thereby potentially depriving the child from the protection of an effective, less restrictive, and less harmful intervention. (The issue of documentation of restraint and injury was an important issue during the investigation into the Gatehouse school in England. See Chap. 5.)

Recently, there has also been more legislation relating to the work environment and the responsibilities of employers regarding liability in providing services and their responsibilities to provide a safe work environment to employees. An employer is vicariously liable for the actions of his employee if the employee commits a tort; the person doing so is an employee rather than an independent contractor, and does so during the course of his work. The last two elements require further clarification. A person may be an employee, even though he signed a contract stating he is a contractor. If the person produces an independent product not under the supervision or direction of the employer and is not integrated into the running of the business, then they are not an employee and the employer is not vicariously liable for the person's actions. When is a person working in residential care? If they commit sexual offences against children after regular work hours, even though the employer has trained them not to do so, their employer may be vicariously liable because the person's actions are so closely tied to their employment of caring for children. If someone is injured by an employee, they usually sue the employer, rather than the employee, for damages because the employee probably has more assets and insurance to cure the harm done.

An employer also has a common law duty to their employees' safety. This includes competent staff, a safe place of work, proper plant and equipment, and a safe system of work. All of these four elements impinge directly on the use of restraint and seclusion and behavior management generally. For example, failure to provide competent staff in a school—including all staff members from classroom assistant, teacher, professionals to principal—may place employees in danger of injury from students and/or other staff. Consider the case of when a teacher has their retina detached during a restraint and the child is bruised from an improper restraint. The injured *employee* might sue the employer for failing to provide them with effective and sufficient staff training. Even though the employer might point to the employees signature on a piece of paper stating that they had training on restraint before hiring, the employee might claim that the training was inadequate because it was merely classroom-based training and did not involve scenario-based skills practice to competency and, in any case, if that training was a long time ago, then the employer should have retrained the staff, especially after other staff had been trained in similar situations with the same client. The injured *employee* might also sue the employer for failing to provide competent behavioral services, because the child's behavior plan was written by someone not trained to write a behavior plan and the employer failed to train that person to competency or failed to hire someone to do so. So, the injured *employee* might claim that the employer failed to protect them from harm by not having competent behavioral staff. The employer might claim that the fault lies with the employees who did not act safely in line with policy, and her training did not implement prevention strategies as they had been trained to do and that their training was indeed sufficient. If an employee is injured due to an unsafe work place, such as slippery surfaces, that result in employee injuries while restraining someone in a bathroom, or if the employer fails to provide safe restraint devices that result in staff injuries, then the employer may be liable for the injuries to their employees.

The idea of a "safe system of work" is somewhat nebulous. British law has decided that it must be defined on a case-by-case basis, but might include elements such as the physical layout of the job, the sequence in which work is done, warning notices, and instructions. Consider, for example, a staff in a day program, who is injured at work by an aggressive client because a fellow staff failed to restrain a dangerous client while taking clients off the bus. Suppose the place was crowded so that staff had difficulty using emergency restraint safely. Suppose also that the arrival of several buses at one entrance resulted in crowding and noise that irritated some clients, and that staff responsibilities were unclear because there were new staff, untrained float staff, and untrained interns present who did not know about prevention strategies or specific behavior management procedures for each client, and that the regular supervisor was absent. This combination of physical layout of the job, the sequence of having to take everyone off the buses at the same time, and the lack of instructions for new staff on how to manage the situation might all constitute an *unsafe system of work*. The employer might be found negligent due to their failure to identify and fix these problems. The fact that the employer set up a committee to deal with this issue 6 months ago, who did an incompetent job, does not absolve him of responsibility. There are now legal cases in England that have applied these principles to specific cases where employees have successfully claimed damages from their employer due to absence, insufficient, or ineffective training.

There are other British laws related to safety at work. British law also requires employers to conduct risk assessments and act prudently to ensure their employees' safety. This includes identifying and minimizing employee risks from violence and aggression from clients. In sum, in order to discharge their duty of care to their employee, an employer must have a clear policy, a risk assessment system, clear procedures to specify what actions to take in risk situations, provide appropriate training, provide a safe work environment, provide staff support relating to violence, ensure that the procedures are workable and review them, and provide debriefing after an incident.

3.2.3.1 Influence of European Convention on Human Legislation

Since the publication of Lyon and Pimor's book, the *European Convention on Human Rights* has begun to influence British legislation related to restraint, seclusion, and other restrictive behavior management practice (Karim 2014). The *European Convention on Human Rights* guarantees a number of rights and fundamental freedoms including prohibition of torture, the right to liberty and security, and the prohibition of discrimination. European and British courts are now interpreting the use of such practices with reference to European laws, which are now evolving rapidly (Karim 2014).

3.3 Professional Ethics

3.3.1 General Principles

There are now numerous position statements from professional bodies regarding restrictive behavior management practices. For example, Scheuermann, Ryan, Peterson and Billingsley (2013) analyzed 15 position statements on restraint and seclusion related to schools and found substantial differences in the content of many statements and also disagreement over required conduct. They coded the statements into two broad areas. The first area was their content such as reliance on research-based practices, maintaining child dignity, and professional competence. The second area was positions on restraint and seclusion such as opposition to nonemergency restraint and seclusion, opposition to seclusion, leaving decisions to use restraint and seclusion to professionals, providing guidelines on the use of restraint and seclusion, supporting or opposes legislation to limit or ban their use, and required monitoring and oversight.

Scheuermann et al. found that of 15 statements ten opposed all nonemergency use of restraint and seclusion, nine had an ethics code for members, and seven supported legislative control of restraint and seclusion. There was least agreement on the following issues: Legislation banning all use (1 policy), policy supporting leaving decisions to use to professionals (2 policies), providing guidelines for use (2 policies), reliance on research-based methods (3 policies), legislation to require monitoring and oversight (3 policies) and opposing legislation to restrict use (3 policies). Thus, position statement varied widely in both what they addressed and whether or not they agreed on certain key issues, such as the role of legislation. Such a variety of positions from different professional organizations reflects the professional differences on the professional ethics of restraint and seclusion.

Scheuermann et al. went on to discuss five ethical problems specific to restraint and seclusion in education. The first was risk of death and/or injury. Death from some forms of restraint is now well documented (see Chap. 5) as is the risk of injury. Thus, most restraint policies and training courses require some form of monitoring during restraint and seclusion. Failure to provide sufficient and competent monitoring raises issues of professional ethics, namely, the competent performance of professionals and whether they acted with beneficence to their client. It also raises legal issues, such as liability for the persons concerned and their organization. In many organizations using restraint and seclusion, the procedures are often carried out by nonprofessional staff, such as classroom assistants, nursing assistants, or nonprofessional residential staff, although professional staff many have trained them and may be involved in their supervision and be present during restraint and seclusion. Organizations have a responsibility to their clients and staff to ensure that their staff is trained to competency to carry out these procedures safely. All courses of action, or equally decisions not to act, such as delaying or failing to implement a behavior support plan, involve risks and benefits including risks of injuries from restraint. Thus, the professional ethical question becomes whether the benefit of restraint and seclusion outweighs the benefits and risks of not acting and alternative courses of action, such as nonrestraint interventions, or other forms of less dangerous restraint or seclusion. When working with a new client with no history of restraint or seclusion, it may be difficult to predict the risks of restraint and seclusion, but if the client had relevant risk factors, such as asthma, medication resulting in increased risk of bruising, then professionals could make some assessment of the risks and benefits or restraint and seclusion. In other situations, such as when the client comes with a history of restraint and seclusion or restraint and seclusion has recently been used repeatedly, then professionals and the team have information on at least the common risks of restraint and seclusion. A significant challenge to everyone is evaluating the risks of low-frequency, serious injuries to self or others.

A second ethical issue is the disproportionate use of restraint and seclusion among certain disadvantaged groups including non-White students, students with disabilities, and boys. Peterson et al. (2013) presented national data that each of these groups experience greater rates of restraints in American education settings than would be expected. (Other research has also found similar results with other populations and in other contexts.) An important aspect of this issue is that repeated use of restraint and seclusion removes the child from education and may result in violations of the *Individuals with Disabilities Education Act*, since the child did not receive a free, appropriate public education. There are two especially problematic examples here. The first is that some children with high rates of restraint and seclusion do not receive any meaningful education at other times of the day when not in restraint, and this contributes to the inappropriate use of restrictive behavior management practices. For example, it is not uncommon to observe a challenging child placed on one-on-one staffing, but the one-on-one staff is an inexperienced, underpaid, and untrained classroom assistant who physically contains the student by limiting their movement, but the student receives little or no effective teaching because the assigned one-on-one staff does not know how to teach and is untrained to do so. The second example, which is similar to the first, is a small number of children in chronic mechanical restraints for self-injury. The mechanical restraints prevent self-injury, but the child is unable to interact with the environment and learn due to the restraints. (See Chap. 8 for examples of how to empirically evaluate safety and restrictiveness in this situation.) A third related issue is the repeated use of ineffective restraint and seclusion when alternate intervention methods may have worked. This is especially important in the context of two of *Individuals with Disabilities Education Act* requirements—the mandate for schools to conduct adequate functional behavioral assessments in such circumstances, and it strongly recommends the use of positive behavior support and the right to a free and appropriate public education.

Peterson et al.'s final ethical issue is the problem of implementation problems, referring broadly to not only effective and safe implementation of restraint and seclusion but also the child's education more generally. Thus, when caregivers implement restraint and seclusion and injuries occur, they may have to demonstrate that they implemented these methods accurately; likewise an organization may have to answer for its actions, if an untrained staff is not well trained and clients are injured during restraint or seclusion. While discussing this issue, Peterson et al. raised an important point regarding caregivers' ability to recognize emergencies. Well-trained staff may perceive a mild behavioral escalation as confirmation of their functional behavioral assessment and an opportunity to teach a replacement behavior; untrained or poorly trained staff may perceive the same event as a sure sign of imminent danger and respond with restraint or seclusion. Thus, untrained staff might restrain or seclude following a minor behavioral escalation, honestly believing their actions to be ethical. Organizations should guard against this possibility as it may lead to excessive use of restraint and seclusion and should train their professional and nonprofessional staff to use effective behavior management strategies, including preventative strategies to avoid the need for restraint, and to apply them only when there is a true emergency.

3.3.2 Some Examples of Restraint Position Statements

There are now numerous position statements on the use of restraint and seclusion and a comprehensive review of them is beyond the scope of this chapter; however, it is useful to consider a few in detail to illustrate the issues, the range of public opinion, and points of professional disagreement. Table 3.1 provides a partial list and summary of some of these statements from organizations such as Applied Behavior Analysis International, American Association of Intellectual and Developmental Disabilities, The Association for the Severely Handicapped (TASH), and British Institute for Intellectual Disabilities.

Applied Behavior Analysis International has issued three related policies on the right to effective treatment, right to effective education, and restraint and seclusion. American Association on Intellectual and Developmental Disabilities has issued two statements, one on aversive procedures and one issued jointly with the ARC for People with Intellectual and Developmental Disabilities[4] on behavior supports. TASH has issued many position statements including those on positive behavior supports and aversives.

The statements agree on several key issues. All agree on the key goal of ensuring client safety and in treatment that enhances the person's access to less restrictive settings. Interestingly, one point of agreement is the key role of functional assessment in behavioral treatment that should be used to develop behavioral supports. The statements agree on the important of other key strategies such as preventative strategies and staff training and professional competency in reducing restraint and seclusion safely. Thus, although disagreements between the statements have generated considerable professional tension and, at times, animosity (Foxx 2005), there is substantive agreement on several key issues.

These statements differ and disagree in several important points, but perhaps more importantly they disagree in terms of how to frame the question of restraint and seclusion. Applied Behavior Analysis International acknowledging some of the reasons for managing and reducing restraint and seclusion are safety and treatment efficacy, the questions mainly framed are one of science, research evidence, and technology to transfer that research knowledge to practice. Hence, Applied Behavior Analysis International's statements include appendices of research articles that are the basis for their statement. Further, their statements are especially detailed and describe what specific actions professionals and services should take to limit the use of restraint and seclusion and promote appropriate behavior, including detailed statements on the right to effective treatment and education. In contrast, the other statements frame the question primarily as one of human rights. For example, TASH's statement describes the reduction of restraint and chemical restraints as one of dignity, rights to safety, different treatment of people with disabilities, and right to access to community living. Unlike, Applied Behavior Analysis International, these other statements do not provide a research base for their decisions and do not provide details of how to manage restraint; indeed, American Association on Intel-

[4] A US national advocacy group for people with disabilities.

Table 3.1 A summary of some position statements on restraint and seclusion

Organization (year)	Summary
Association for Behavior Analysis International (1989a). *Right to effective treatment*	The statement calls for access to effective behavioral treatment to protect clients from harm due to the lack of effective or use of ineffective behavioral treatment. The statement declares that individuals who receive behavioral treatment have six rights including: (1) therapeutic social and physical environment; (2) services whose overriding goals are personal welfare, (3) treatment by a competent behavior analysts, (4) programs that teach functional skills, (5) behavior assessment and ongoing evaluation, and (6) the most effective procedures available
Association for Behavior Analysis International. (1989b). *Right to effective education*	Calls for all children's education to encourage academic achievement, use empirically validated curricula and objectives, use criterion references assessment to guide placement, use individually paced instruction from competent teachers, use measurement-based decisions, and that administrators also have responsibility for student progress. This statement does not address RBMPs directly, but does describe the characteristics of an appropriate education that would greatly reduce or eliminate the need for such procedures
Association for Behavior Analysis International (2010). *Restraint and seclusion*	Opposes inappropriate and/or unnecessary use of restraint, other restrictive procedures, and seclusion. They should only be used under limited circumstances with meticulous oversight, controls and high standards of practice. These practices should be based on three principles: (1) the welfare of the individual served is the highest priority; (2) individuals (and parents/guardians) have a right to choose; and (3) the principle of least restrictiveness. Applied Behavior Analysis International described how restraint, time out and rarely seclusion might be incorporated into a behavior support plan, including addressing a specific target behavior, be based on functional assessment, incorporate reinforcement for positive behavior, be used for only brief duration, be evaluated by objective data, be based on current scientific practice and supervised by a Board Certified Behavior Analyst of other professional with equivalent training and experience with informed consent. States that emergency restraint may be required for dangerous behavior that is unpredictable, but must be carried out by well-trained staff using clear procedures considering the risks and benefits of use and nonuse of emergency restraints. Repeated use of crisis management is not a substitute for the treatment and indicates that a functional assessment and behavior plan should be developed. Finally, there should be rigorous oversight and evaluation including oversight by a qualified Board Certified Behavior Analyst or similar professional, conducted by fully trained staff, and monitored with reliable and valid data. Restraint and seclusion should only be used if effective and safe and should be eliminated or reduced if possible

Table 3.1 (continued)

Organization (year)	Summary
American Association on Intellectual and Developmental Disabilities (2012) *Aversive procedures*	Addresses aversive procedures generally which are defined as procedures that cause obvious signs of physical pain, physical side effects such as tissue damage, and are dehumanizing, for example through social isolation. The statement does not address restraint or seclusion directly. The statement calls for the immediate elimination for the use of such procedures and calls for "reducing the actions by professionals and others that compromise the lives of persons with intellectual and other developmental disability and their families." The statements calls for further research into effective and humane forms of positive behavior support
Joint Statement by American Association on Intellectual and Developmental Disabilities and The Arc (2010) *Behavioral supports*	This statement addresses behavioral supports generally, and calls for the treatment of challenging behavior through positive behavior supports that improve the person's quality of life and reduce challenging behavior. It stated that "children and adults with intellectual and/or developmental disabilities are frequently subjected to physical restraint, including the use of life-threatening prone restraint and seclusion" and that these procedures "do not reduce challenging behavior… [and] inhibit the development of appropriate skills and behavior" and are dangerous, undignified, and unacceptable. The statement supports the use of positive behavioral interventions in naturalistic settings such as choice making in family settings and opposes all aversive procedures such as seclusion and stated that "physical restraints should only be used as a last resort to eliminate the danger of physical injury to self or others." Rather, positive behavior supports should use evidence-based practices such as basing interventions on functional behavioral assessments and positive reinforcement, be humane, caring, and dignified; carried out by well-trained individuals, and monitored for effectiveness and modified as needed
TASH (2000) *Positive behavior supports*	States that "services must employ instructional and support strategies which are consistent with the right of each individual with severe disabilities to effective support without compromising their equally important right to freedom from harm. Access to strategies that humanely assure physical safety is an important part of this right." First calls for the cessation of procedures that are dehumanizing, would not be used with persons without disabilities, causes obvious signs of physical pain, injuries, illness, tissue damage, severe stress, ambivalence, or discomfort on the part of family members or caregivers, peer repulsion or stress upon seeing the procedures, use for purposes other than emergencies and imminent harm, and the use of sedative drugs for behavior management. It then calls for interventions which are developed in collaboration with the individual, are culturally sensitive and foster self-determination, are based on a functional assessment, and develop interventions that are constructive and comprehensive involving medical, education, communicative, and environmental interventions and are provided in a manner that maximizes participation in community settings and personal well-being

lectual and Developmental Disabilities specifically admonishes professionals for their use of such practices.

Another key difference between these statements is that Applied Behavior Analysis International's statement explicitly leaves the door open to the use of such procedures, albeit under very limited circumstances. For example, the *Right to Effective Treatment* statement acknowledges that "decisions on the use of potentially restrictive treatment are based on consideration of its absolute and relative level of restrictiveness, the amount of time required to produce a clinically significant outcome, and the consequences that would result from delayed intervention." Subsequently, Van Houten et al. (1988), in an expansion of this statement, commented that exposure to nonrestrictive but ineffective treatments is unacceptable and that slow acting, nonrestrictive treatments are also questionable as they continue to expose the person to risk of harm and denies them the benefits of more effective faster acting treatments including access to more better environments. Van Houten *et al.* conclude that sometimes a temporarily restrictive procedure that is quick acting is the least restrictive alternative. Similarly, Applied Behavior Analysis International's position statement on restraint and seclusion acknowledges circumstances in which nonemergency restraint and seclusion might be required when they permit the inclusion of restraint and indeed seclusion in behavior support plans under limited circumstances.

The statements differ on the interpretation of the evidence on treatment effectiveness. Both American Association on Intellectual and Developmental Disabilities and TASH asserted that these procedures are ineffective. For example, AAIDD (2010) stated that "[restraints] do not reduce challenging behavior… [and] inhibit the development of appropriate skills and behavior," and TASH asserted that "current research and practice have demonstrated the practical efficacy and benefits of functional behavioral assessment and positive interventions for helping to resolve the challenges of problem behavior affecting people with severe disabilities," although neither position statements supported these assertions with research citations.

Finally, the statements differ on the role of legislation restricting or banning restraint and seclusion. Applied Behavior Analysis International stated that "decisions related to treatment selection are based on information obtained during assessment about the behavior, the risk it poses, and its controlling variables; on a careful consideration of the available treatment options, including their relative effectiveness, risks, restrictiveness, and potential side effects; and on examination of the overall context in which treatment will be applied" (p. 114). In contrast, TASH calls for the banning of all such procedures, except under emergency circumstances.

3.4 Conclusions

The use of restrictive behavior management practices raises numerous ethical and legal issues. The two most common approaches underlying ethics and restrictive behavior management practices are consequentialist ethics—do the least harm and the most good for the most people you can—and deontological ethics—restrictive behavior management practices are wrong because all people should be treated with respect and dignity and should be autonomous and restrictive behavior management practices are incompatible with these principles. Although there is professional agreement on several aspects of ethical practice related to restraint, such as the use of preventative strategies, functional assessment and adequate staff training, there is disagreement over whether restraints should be completely banned under every circumstance, used only in emergencies or sometimes incorporated into behavior plans but carefully regulated and supervised by competent professionals.

Professionals, including administrators, have special obligations, since they contract with employers, the state or family members to provide effective services and have an obligation of beneficence to their clients. This almost always translates into safe reduction in restrictive behavior management practices and improving client's quality of life more broadly. Unfortunately, many professionals and administrators are not competent to discharge this duty and are thus obliged to seek consultancy or training to ensure they can behave competently. Many professional and administrators may even believe themselves to be competent when they are not and thus fail to seek additional help. Others fail to seek help because they seek to avoid the public embarrassment involved in revealing the use of restrictive behavior management practices or the own incompetence and/or avoid the strenuous extra work required to reduce restrictive behavior management practices safely.

Over time, the amount of legislation in many countries has increased and become more prescriptive, addressing both institutional and community settings; however, the effectiveness of such legislation is often limited. This reflects ambiguities within legislation, such as failure to define emergencies clearly, and failure to include essential elements of good practice, such as uniform public reporting of the use of restraint, as well as failure of government to follow up and enforce legislation.

Chapter 4
Nineteenth- and Early Twentieth-Century History

The aphorism that "there is nothing new under the sun" is nowhere more true than when it comes to restraint reduction. Perhaps surprisingly, the themes of contemporary efforts to reduce restraints and other restrictive procedures are clear and present in accounts of restraint reduction in the eighteenth and nineteenth centuries. At that time, restraint for many people meant being chained to a wall or floor in an asylum. Other forms of mechanical restraint and treatments involved being tied down into various devices. From Vincenzo Chairugi in Italy to Pinel in France, the notion of reducing restraints developed in response to both ethical concerns based primarily on religious beliefs and responses to restraint-related deaths, mostly in patients in asylums. As a result, moral treatment, perhaps better thought of as a form of psychosocial as opposed to medical treatment, originating with Pinel spread quickly to the UK and across the rest of Europe and to the USA in the early nineteenth century.

Eliminating restraints was controversial from the get go. Reports of eliminating or reducing restraints were met with doubt and even accusations of exaggeration and data forgery. This chapter describes various historical efforts to reduce and eliminate restraint and draws parallels between those efforts and our own today. Many of these eighteenth- and nineteenth-century examples were individual physicians who were superintendents of the new asylums. Others were religiously inspired people, such as Quakers, who were committed to social justice, pacifism, and nonviolence while interacting with the world rather than retreating from it.

4.1 Chiarugi

Attempts to reduce restrictive procedures, especially mechanical restraints, can be dated back at least to the middle of the eighteenth century. Vincenzo Chiarugi (1759–1826) was a *primo infermiere* in a large psychiatric facility in Florence. Prior to his appointment there, he had removed all chains at the Santa Dorotea where he worked from 1785 to 1788; he was ahead of Pinel in removing restraints by several

P. Sturmey, *Reducing Restraint and Restrictive Behavior Management Practices*, Autism and Child Psychopathology Series, DOI 10.1007/978-3-319-17569-0_4

years, but was not as well-known as Pinel. Gerard (1997) characterizes Chiarugi's writings as less psychological and more biologically oriented than Pinel's. Nevertheless, he quotes Chiarugi as saying "The patient is to be treated with respect... no physical pain to be inflicted under any circumstances...the application of restraints...must be applied in accord with humanitarian and hygienic practices..." (Gerard 1997, p. 391), although Chiarugi also suggested that beatings might be necessary in some cases of mania. Chiarugi also replaced metal chains with cloth restraints to reduce injuries (Denunzio and Hogan 2012). Chiarugi also emphasized walks, hygiene, and good food, although he apparently made no link between humane treatment and management of restraints, at least as indicated in this quotation. He also advocated seclusion and methods other than chains as restraints where necessary. Chiarugi mentioned both medical care and an early version of moral treatment, but the accounts are not as systematized as later ones.

4.2 Pinel

Pinel became an icon of liberal care for people with mental illness. The two images of releasing people from chains at the Salpêtrière, recorded in painting, and the development of moral treatment made him a symbolic figure in psychiatry. Jarvis and Clark (1969/2013, pp. 10–14) described how Pinel began to remove chains from people with mental illness in 1792 during the French Revolution. After a member of the Commune visited the Bicetre and washed his hands of the endeavor, Pinel began by removing the chains from 12 people (with groups of staff and vest restraints on hand if needed). Before doing so, Pinel talked to the persons, promised them liberty from their chains, and also threatened them with personal and mechanical restraints if they became violent. He also asked for their agreement not to be violent. In the first few days, he released 53 people from chains and reported that "the whole discipline was marked with a regularity and kindness which had the most favorable effect on the insane themselves" (p. 12); thus, concerns over client and staff safety were allayed.

Through case descriptions, Pinel described the possibility that psychological approaches might change mental illness. These included both treating the patient in a kind and benevolent manner and threatening the patient with extreme punishment to scare them into changing their behavior. His work subsequently inspired others to reduce mechanical restraints.

4.3 Tuke and Moral Treatment

In response to the death of a Quaker woman in the county asylum in York in 1790, the Society of Friends (Quakers) founded the Retreat in York in the early and mid-1790s. Since it was founded by the Society of Friends, it reflected the nonviolent values of that society and aimed to provide care for friends in the company of other friends. The Retreat accommodated 30 persons, although over time the number increased. The program was originally run by William Tuke. Subsequently, Samuel Tuke (1813/2009), William's grandson, published his account of the founding of the Retreat.

In 1815/1816, the British government conducted investigations into conditions in asylums including the abuse of restraint in Bethlem Asylum, London, and elsewhere. This inquiry found that patients chained for months or longer in part due to the lack of staff and the practice of leaving asylums unstaffed at night. These reports were probably instrumental in promulgating institutional reform, the development of new asylums, and moral treatment.

Samuel Tuke (1813/2009) described both moral treatment and ways of reducing restrictive procedures. Even from its proposal, the Retreat emphasized "mild treatment" in contrast to the treatment in the county asylums which often used extensive chaining and physical punishment. He noted that pharmacological treatments were largely ineffective and thus unwarranted. Moral treatment assumes that people with mental illness were not entirely without mental capacity and ability to control one's own behavior, and this residual mental capacity could be harnessed in various ways. Thus, moral treatment consisted of treating the person kindly and respectfully which included removing irritations, such as restraints. Tuke (1813/2009) stated that moral treatment has three components: (a) strengthening and assisting the patient to control their disorder, (b) using restraint and coercion appropriately, and (c) providing general comfort to the patient. The Retreat arranged patients "in classes…according to the degree in they approach rational and orderly conduct" (p. 141). Tuke (1813/2009) described this under the rubric of "exciting fear"; perhaps he means that patients could work their way up a progressively less system or might be dropped to more restrictive groups, as in a token economy; but Tuke was not specific here. He did write that "they are informed on the first occasion, that their treatment depends, on great measure, upon their conduct" (p. 141), but again he did not spell out any particular system for doing this. Tuke emphasized that attendants must approach the patients "with soft and mild persuasion" (p. 150), but should not dispute with them concerning delusions and hallucinations. Staff who worked with patients who were depressed should not focus on their depression, but rather "seduce the mind from its favorite but unhappy musings, by bodily exercise, walks, conversation, reading and other innocent recreations" (pp. 151–152). Tuke also noted the effectiveness of engaging patients in topics of which they know a great deal and could display their competence. Tuke also recommended religious activities as part of strengthening and assisting the patient to control their disorder. Concerning "coercion," Tuke did not recommend that all restraints could be eliminated, but did recommend "only as a protecting and salutary restraint" (p. 168) and never restraints that irritated the patient; hence, they never used chains at the Retreat, as the county asylums did at that time. Despite its commitment to "mild treatment," the Retreat did include a seclusion room "for the entire seclusion of a violent patient…furnished with a bed, securely fastened to the ground. Light is…not entirely excluded; and care is taken to have the room properly ventilated" (p. 98). Tuke also noted some use of mechanical restraints to force-feed patients who refused to eat and could not be induced to eat by other methods. Tuke did, however, note that manic patients might be kept in dark rooms wearing a "strait waistcoat," and suicidal patients may be restrained to their beds (p. 164). Tuke also described the use of mechanical restraint to feed patients who refused to eat on rare occasions. Tuke's commitment to monitoring and reducing seclusion and restraint is reflected in his noting that "during the last year, in which the number of patients has generally been sixty-four, there has not been occasion to seclude, on average, two patients at one time" (p. 166). He went on to note that at any one time, no more than four patients were mechanically restrained; thus, a simple data collection was part of his treatment package. Thus, in the early nineteenth century, moral treatment attempted to reduce restraint, but did in fact use it, although they did not use some of the restraint methods used in the county asylums, such as chains.

The third aspect of moral treatment was to provide for the patient's comfort. Moral treatment saw this as part of the cure. It included tea parties for the women, visits to the city, visits from members of the Retreat's committee, employments, and amusements, other than those that worsen the patient's mental illness, and carefully selected books to read, especially on topics that the patient formerly enjoyed.

Moral treatment was influential elsewhere. In the early 1800s, Ireland began establishing a statewide system of asylums (McClelland 1988) in response to the poor conditions of people with mental illness in community settings, for example, some people were kept in holes in the ground in their family homes. Since Ireland had only one asylum at that time, the program was set up anew. It adopted moral treatment with its near prohibition on restraint use in part because several key figures were exposed to Quaker ideas of pacifism and social responsibility during the education and contemporary exposes of abuse of restraint in Bethlem Asylum, London, as well as Tuke's work. This led to local politicians to brag that "there is not in the Richmond Lunatic Asylum to the best of my knowledge, a chain, a fetter or a handcuff" (quoted in McClelland 1988, p. 106).

Moral treatment included a system of treatment of people with mental illness, although its authors did not specify it as clearly as they might have. It did not commit to eliminating restraints and other restrictive procedures but did attempt to minimize their use through its three-part treatment program and some, at least, informal use of data. Tuke's account did not provide any systematic data on restraint use, but did indeed use some simple forms of data to monitor restraint and seclusion.

4.4 Gardiner Hill

Gardiner Hill became the house surgeon for the Lincoln Asylum in 1829. In 1829, a patient at Lincoln Asylum had died when strapped to a bed at night unattended. Consequently, the asylum rules were changed that no one should be restrained at night unless a staff was also present in the room. The rule resulted in a reduction in restraint according to Connolly (1956/1973, p. 177). (This incident parallels similar recent events in the USA, such as *The Hartford Current's* publication of deadly restraints which also resulted in changes in regulations. Unfortunately, it is unclear if these revised rules resulted in reductions in restraints. Efforts to reduce and eliminate restraint included: (a) requiring a written record of every instance of restraint; (b) destruction of all iron hobbles, handcuffs, and straitjackets; and (c) provision of clothing and bedsheets made of material that was not easily torn, so that some forms of property destruction that previously had been the reason for restraints were reduced. By August 1834, the facility had eliminated mechanical restraints in all residents for days at a time. By 1835, the facility, now with Gardiner Hill in place, had eliminated mechanical restraints and confinement to rooms for all residents for 24 consecutive days. By 1836, the facility had been restraint free for 3 months and this was apparently still the case in 1837 (Connolly 1856/1973, pp. 177–178). Gardiner Hill (1838/1971) subsequently published his account of this as *Total abolition of personal restraint in the treatment of the insane.*

4.5 Thomas Prichard

Gardiner Hill gave credit to Thomas Prichard at the Northampton Asylum (now St. Andrews Hospital) for the initiation of the restraint-free movement. In 1840, the asylum's record stated that restraint had only been used one time and then in Prichard's absence. These records may have been inaccurate (Haw and Yorston 2004) as they excluded at least one case of restraint used for "some months."

To evaluate the veracity of these claims, Haw and Yorston (2004) reported a detailed analysis of the use of restraint before and immediately after admission in the first 50 cases. They found many examples of complete elimination of restraint. Of these 50 admissions, 18 % had a history of restraint and 16 % were admitted in restraint. Of these, 7 of 8 (88 %) had restraints removed upon admission and 4 (8 % of the sample) had some temporary application of restraint. Haw and Yorston concluded that Thomas Prichard was unaware of Gardiner Hill's contemporary efforts at restraint in reduction. They also concluded that restraint reduction was ongoing broadly at several asylums at this time.

4.6 John Connolly

John Connolly was a physician who in 1839 became the resident physic at Middlesex Lunatic Asylum in Hanwell, a facility for 800–1000 people, primarily, but not exclusively, with mental illness. Many facilities used mechanical restraints, which in this context meant shackling someone to a wall or bed, shackling people's ankles together, restraint chairs in which the person was kept for days at a time, and restraint jackets. Additionally, facilities often used restraints due to staff shortages such as on Sundays and engaged in inhuman practices, such as bathing people with mops while in restraint. Connolly described how "In some of the old asylums I have seen rows of chairs filled with these poor creatures, in rooms having a sloping floor and gutter…. They sat in these chairs all day, and they were fastened down on straw all night. They were rudely washed in the morning—perhaps with a mop; they were carelessly fed; they were clothed in the refuse clothing of the house" (p. 61).

As we have seen, Connolly was not the first person to eliminate restraint but he was aware of previous models to do so such as Pinel's work, Tuke's work at the Retreat in York described in a publication by Samuel Tuke in 1813, and Gardiner Hill's work at Lincoln Asylum. Thus, Connolly's contribution comes from his extensive writings and his attempt to systematize interventions into his "new or no restraint system" (Connolly 1856/1973). He did not describe his new or no restraint system in a very ordered way, but rather gave a discursive account of that system. He was clear, however, that the system did not merely include abolition of mechanical restraint, but rather was "a complete system of management" that began the moment the patient was admitted (p. 35). Connolly first emphasized that the asylum must already be well run. This meant that staff was effective, there was a good diet, clothing was clean, and the place was cheerful. Second, the aim of the facility, irrespective of the severity of the patient's problems, was to be to cure, or if cure was not possible, to protect, take care of, keep out of mischief, and tranquilize the patient (here "tranquilize" meant to keep calm and free of distress, rather than sedate the patient). Third, upon admission, the facility must immediately release the patient from all restraints. The facility's medical officer must immediately visit the new patient and assure the patient that they need not fear ill-treatment. The staff then gave the patient a comfortable warm bath, dried the patient, gave them comfortable dry clothes, and gave them a good meal in the day room. Connolly noted that this treatment would often greatly contrast with patient's treatment in other facilities where people were often restrained, kept dirty, ill-clothed, and harshly treated. He noted that these initial steps were often, but not always, sufficient to begin a change in the new patient. Fourth, after admission, if the patient was very active, but not dangerous, then staff should not interfere with them. Connolly noted that when staff frequently prevented patient movement and blocked their impulses, patients were likely to become angry.

One controversy related to the new or no-restraint system was that others alleged that it merely substituted seclusion and personal restraint for mechanical restraint. Connolly was very much aware of this criticism from those opposing the new or nonrestraint system. Connolly described the use of personal and mechanical restraints in this way. Recall that staff should not interfere or restrain patients who were merely active, but not dangerous to themselves or others. Connolly noted that if "repression by holding the patient's hands and arms is never resorted to except when some sudden impulse requires such immediate interposition for a few minutes, after which the impulse usually passes away; or the patient is removed, and his attention occupied with something that makes him forget it…. Continued holding, or struggling, or violent overmastering of an irritable patient belongs to the older system of treatment, and is quite inconsistent with the new" (p. 41). Connolly also noted that seclusion was part of the new or nonrestraint system. Connolly designed a specific seclusion room which he had padded with thick coconut fiber from floor to ceiling, a thick mattress covered the entire floor, and there was no furniture in the room. There was a guarded window to let in air and light and an observation window for staff to observe the patient. Staff was to ensure that the patient had food and water and to document each use of seclusion, including its duration, and the physician was to review each record at the end of each day.

He described the use of the seclusion room as follows. A group of three to four staff is quietly assembled. If possible, staff should attempt to distract the patient and persuade him to go to his room or padded apartment. If this is ineffective, the staff should swiftly hold and escort him to the seclusion room and place him there without injury. During seclusion, staff should make food and drink available. Once calm, one staff member should explain that people at the asylum have good intentions and that the incident will not be held against the patient. For the management of agitation in patients who cannot sleep and might become violent, Connolly recommends fresh air, cold water, sitting up, diversion, drinks, or tobacco to ensure they do not become agitated.

Connolly emphasized the importance of recruiting good staff and careful staff supervision, the importance of order, cleanliness, and respectful treatment of patients at every point in the daily routine. Connolly also emphasized active treatment which included attending the chapel, walks in the garden, and pleasant meals. A work program included men gardening and attending workshops and women working in the laundry, bakery, or "the busy and cheerful, and scrupulously clean kitchen" (p. 58).

Connolly also noted organizational variables that helped or hindered in the management of restraint. These include having sufficient staff, clear supervision of the program from a chief physician, good supervision of attendants by officers, and a board that does not interfere too much with the medical officer's work.

There are two other aspects of Connolly's work that, although he did not acknowledge them as parts of his system, may have been crucial. First, he required a written record of each mechanical restraint. Staff had to turn this record in to him each day, and he copied it into a book. Hence, he was made aware of each instance of restraint. Second, he wrote annual reports to the facility board in which he committed himself to care free of mechanical restraint publicly for the next year directly and indirectly. He also reported the numbers of mechanical restraints to the board and other statistics, such as the number of days or years since the last mechanical restraint. Unfortunately, he did not also report data on the numbers of seclusions or other forms of restraints and injuries to patients and staff, but provided a narrative, nonquantitative account of these measures. Hence, Connolly engaged in a form of self-control (cf. Skinner 1953) in which he engaged in several behaviors (controlling behaviors) to make other behaviors (his management and intervention strategies resulting in the reduction of mechanical restraints) more likely. Specifically, he publically stated his goal which was explicit and quantifiable, recorded the outcome of his own management efforts in the form of daily and annual records of mechanical restraints, and reported his behavior and its outcomes to others in the annual reports to his board.

Connolly's intervention is like many efforts to reduce and eliminate restraints, including both later and contemporary attempts to do so. His intervention included many components. He measured his performance and his organization's performance by measuring the daily and annual frequency of restraint. He engaged in self-management and publicly stated a goal; in so doing he designed an environment where failure to reduce mechanical restraint would have been aversive through professional embarrassment and humiliation from many colleagues. His intervention also focused on staff performance through both selection and training. From the moment a patient entered his asylum, staff was expected to behave in a certain manner, not unlike some of the practice we today call relationship building. From admission, staff paired themselves with the removal of potentially aversive stimuli—removal of restraints—paired themselves with appetitive stimuli in the form of pleasant baths, clothes, and food, and minimized presenting unnecessary aversive stimuli by refraining from interfering unnecessarily with ongoing activity and from presenting unneeded demands. Further, Connolly's program included gradually promoting alternate behavior. He initially promoted easy behavior, such as sitting in the chapel and walking in the gardens, but later encouraged more effortful behavior in the form of work program. Finally, he taught new skills, such as work and academic skills, to compete with the aggressive behavior likely to result in mechanical restraints.

4.6.1 Reaction to Connolly's Work

Connolly's work inspired some and was vilified by others. It provoked vigorous debates in *The Lancet* and other journals of the time between 1840 and 1870 and was referenced from time to time thereafter. On the one hand, many other asylums adopted his system of nonrestraint, including John Langdon Down at the first institution for people with Intellectual Disabilities (ID) (Connor-Ward 1999), such that 20 years later, some 24 mental institutions housing 24,000 patients may have eliminated the use of mechanical restraint. On the other hand, his critics suggested that he merely substituted other restrictive procedures such as physical restraint, seclusion, and sedation (Deutsch 1946; Walk 1970); Connolly was acutely aware of this criticism. He was completely honest in describing that limited physical restraint and seclusion were part of his system. His narrative accounts of his program indicate that he carefully, if informally, monitored the use of seclusion and attempted to reduce its unnecessary use. Unfortunately, he did not take data on personal restraints and seclusion, so we do not have the data to back him up on this point.

Jarvis and Clark (1869/2013) reported that Connolly's work was highly influential in the development of new asylums in Britain, other parts of Europe, and the USA. Adoption of the system of nonrestraint was highly variable with several British and other European asylums reporting complete adoption and subsequent eliminations of restraint. Asylums in the USA prevaricated, not as to the efficacy of eliminating restraint, but as to the desirability of adopting the system. In other parts of Europe, the adoption of nonrestraint appeared to reflect the opinions of the superintendent with some adopting it wholeheartedly and others dismissing it as nonsense or at least impractical.

Others argued that mechanical restraints were necessary in some cases. Deutsch (1946) noted that some American psychiatrists obstinately and irrationally opposed restraint-free care, sometimes because of the criticism of American psychiatry from British visitors. Sometimes they only removed mechanical restraints but did not implement the rest of Connolly's program, and thus the heart-hearted attempt at restraint-free care failed because the program was not implemented completely (Colaizzi 2005).

Connolly's program was designed intuitively, rather than scientifically, but it contained many of the elements of subsequent effective restraint reduction programs and used many of the elements of contemporary efforts to reduce restraints. It is remarkable that 170 years later services still struggle to implement effective practices such as those Connolly developed in situations that were perhaps much worse than many contemporary services in terms of staffing resources and the size of the service he worked with.

4.6.2 Community Services

Restraint is often portrayed as a problem of large Victorian, overcrowded asylums, but even historically that is untrue. As we have already seen in the example of development of Ireland's system of asylums in the early 1800s, poor care including prolonged restraint by families was an important motivation in developing this new program. Thus, one of the motivations for the increase in the number of asylums, both for people with mental health problems and persons with ID, was the protection from restraints for people living with their families, people cared for by others under a contract, poor people living in workhouses, and people living in private madhouses (Deutsch 1946; Parry-Jones 1972).

Dorothea Lynde Dix, well aware of the work of Pinel, Tuke, Gardiner Hill, and Connolly (Tiffany 1890), conducted a statewide survey of community care for people with mental illness during 1840–1841 in Massachusetts. At that time, towns contracted with local families to provide care for people who were poor and mentally ill and could not care for themselves. Community care contracts were auctioned off to the lowest bidder in a manner not unlike slave auctions (Deutsch 1946). She also visited the jails where some people with mental illness were also locked up.

She found widespread use of shackles and chains including people chained to logs. In her laconic notes, she wrote "Lincoln. A woman cadged. Medford. One idiotic subject chained, and one in a close stall for 17 years etc." (cited in Deutsch 1946, p. 166). She published her report to the Massachusetts legislature in which she raged "I proceed, Gentlemen, briefly to call your attention to the present state of Insane Persons confined within this Commonwealth, in cages, stalls, pens! Chained, naked, beaten with rods, and lashed into obedience." Ironically, it was this failure of community care and use of restrictive procedures in community services which impelled Massachusetts to expand institutional care for people with mental illness as a more humane alternative to unregulated and unsupervised community services. She then repeated the exercise in Rhode Island, New Jersey, and in many states and was responsible for setting up state hospitals, poorhouses, and reformed jails in many states. She then took a 2-year rest in Europe during which she inspected the asylums of Scotland, set up an asylum in the Island of Jersey, and then persuaded the Pope to build an asylum in Rome (Deutsch 1946.)

4.6.3 Other Examples

By the mid-nineteenth century, it appears that practice in many institutions had regressed. Many now actively voiced their opposition to restraint-free care and others pointed out that institutions, which formerly were relatively small, had expanded from a few tens or hundreds of people to several thousands (Jarvis and Clark 1869). After the American Civil War, when Dorothea Dix returned to the institutions that she had previously helped found, she was deeply disappointed to see that they had deteriorated and become nests of interprofessional debate and rivalry, rather than humane places of care (Deutsch 1946).

The data we have suggest that restraints were used extensively. For example, Esther (1997) analyzed the historical records of the St. Louis Insane Asylum from January through June 1885. She found that 53 patients accounted for 2537 incidents of restraint, almost exclusively for violent behavior, property destruction, and self-injury. Nearly, 10 % of all patients were restrained each month. Esther commented that this rate of restraint is similar to the contemporary data in mental health institutions, perhaps indicating more than a century of lack of progress in this regard. This situation continued in some places until the 1970s when early behavior modifiers went into backwards armed with token economies to teach skills and manage behavior where restraints had been used grossly excessively (Thompson and Grabowski 1972).

One way in which restraints may have increased was the development of mechanical restraints as treatments. For example, Colaizzi (2005) listed the following forms of mechanical and other restraints: (a) metal, leather, and cloth manacles and wristlets; (b) the "composing chair," designed to reduce stimulation in agitated patients, which later became known as the "coercion chair"; (c) various forms of straitjackets, invented by the Quakers, as a more humane alternative to chaining people; (d) the "protection bed" or "Utica crib" with a lid to confine the person to a wooden bed; (e) various forms of hydrotherapy, including ducking chairs and packing people in wet, cold sheets; and (f) "chemical restraints" (a term used at that time and by Deutsch 1946), such as opiates, bromides, alcohol, and chloral hydrate, to put people to sleep or sedate them.

4.6.4 From 1860 to 1940

After the death of John Connolly and the expansion of asylums, little new appears to have occurred on the issue of restraint reduction. A perusal of the contemporary medical, psychological, and disability-related journals, such as *The Lancet, British Medical Journal, British Journal of Psychiatry, American Journal on Intellectual and Developmental Disabilities,* and *The New England Journal of Medicine,* reveals fewer publications and little new material on the topic. Thus, although there were occasional publications on successful restraint reduction, obituaries for mentors, and discussion of the issue of whether or not restraint reduction was possible or desirable, such publications became much sparser. This issue was only taken up again in the 1940s beginning with the work of Deutsch (1946) in the USA and subsequent institutional scandals from 1960 onwards.

4.7 Learning from John Connolly

The nineteenth-century literature on restraint reduction demonstrated a pattern that will become depressingly familiar in the next chapter that we continue to repeat to-day. Exposes of abuse of restraints and restraint-related deaths in the context of other widespread abuse provoked public attention to the issue. The exposes came not from within the system, but from outsiders who in the nineteenth century were religious agitators committed to social justice and action to correct those injustices. Subsequently, individual practitioners in senior supervisory positions often with opposition from some of their board members, fellow professionals, and politicians forced through programmatic changes to eliminate mechanical restraint. Moral treatment and Conolly's own version of restraint-free care were broad packages of staff selection and supervision, active treatment, and the use of data to guide and evaluate intervention. Although there were consistent reports of large and rapid elimination of mechanical restraints, data on other restrictive behavior management practices, such as seclusion and personal restraint, are largely lacking, although anecdotal reports do not describe large-scale substitution of seclusion and personal restraints for mechanical restraint.

Such an approach was replicated across many asylums in the UK, Ireland, parts of Europe, and some American asylums. Implementation was uneven. This reflects the individual opposition of some superintendents in the UK and cultural and economic differences between the UK and its colonies and the other parts of the world.

In the mid-eighteenth century, the zealotry of the new asylum movement with its commitment to moral treatment dissipated and its heroes and their dedicated trainees died. Subsequently, institutions grew too large and optimism gave way to pessimism. Funding probably no longer facilitated previous high-quality care. Indeed, given the very large increase in the number of people in asylums and the associated increase in costs, some saw the job of asylums as self-support through cost reduction rather than treatment. Thus, restraint became a necessary evil or a justified clinical practice.

Chapter 5
Recent History

The story of enlightened nineteenth century psychiatry releasing the insane from chains has been told many times, yet its lessons have gone unheeded throughout the twentieth and twenty-first centuries. Our contemporary concern with reduction in restrictive procedures is not so different from that of William Tuke's and the concerned of The Society of Friends. This chapter continues the history of the use of restrictive procedures in the twentieth century to current times.

5.1 Mid- and Late-Twentieth Century Institutions

Relatively little is written about institutional exposes before the 1960s, but Taylor (2009) presented an interesting account of American World War II pacifists, many of whom were Mennonites and Quakers, who worked in psychiatric institutions. While engaging in that work, their commitment to pacifism and social justice led many of them to document their experiences, which sometimes resulted in public scandals. During the World War II, the nineteenth century institutions not only faced unmaintained and dilapidated buildings, but also grossly inadequate staff due to inadequate findings and the effects of World War II drawing workers to do war work sometimes leaving institutions with 30% of staff positions vacant. In the context of broader neglect, such as gross overcrowding, inadequate staff, and basic concerns of lack of safety and medical treatment, restrictive behavior management practices were unsurprisingly widely used, including locked doors and mechanical restraint. (Taylor provided several photographs of this.).

One of the earliest exposes of excessive restraint use in mental health facilities comes from the work of Albert Deutsch who was a journalist and popular writer on mental health and a variety of topics. His interest in restraint included writing a piece in 1943 reporting that the US armed forces were returning mentally ill veterans in wire cages. Rather than publish it, he handed the piece to the US War Department and decided not to publish it after the practice ceased.

P. Sturmey, *Reducing Restraint and Restrictive Behavior Management Practices*,
Autism and Child Psychopathology Series, DOI 10.1007/978-3-319-17569-0_5

It is perhaps surprising that in the midst of institutional abuse neglect, inadequate finding, and oversight failure some people reduced restraint effectively. Jacoby et al. (1958) implemented a program of restraint reduction in a psychiatric hospital. In 6 weeks, they abolished all restraint in an inpatient psychiatric unit for "disturbed service." Perhaps this example shows that even in grossly underfunded and neglected systems, heroic clinicians can sometimes be effective in eliminating restraint.

5.1.1 Christmas in Purgatory

Concerns over restraint were commonly expressed in numerous scandals in institutions for people with Intellectual Disabilities from the 1960s to current times. Taylor (2009) argued that, although the exposes of the 1940s and 1950s resulted in increased financing and improved institutions, they remained very bad: A few extra chairs and benches and a few extra staff were still grossly inadequate and people were still locked in the buildings and tied to the new benches. Echoing Deutsch's work in mental health, Blatt and Kaplan's (1965) photographic essay *Christmas in Purgatory,* contained many photographs of naked children and adults with Intellectual Disabilities in overcrowded wards with many illustrations of extended mechanical restraints. These problems continued when Hidalgo Rivera went into the wards of Willowbrook, Staten Island in New York to expose the disgusting treatment which were broadcast on camera to the American public, including medical staff deliberately infecting children and adults with Intellectual Disabilities with hepatitis. The institution was subsequently closed as a part of the Department of Justice's class action lawsuit against the state.

5.1.2 US Department of Justice

As discussed in Chap. 3, *Civil Rights of Institutionalized Persons Act* authorized the Department of Justice to investigate violations of the constitutional rights of classes of persons living in institutional settings. Over the last 30 years, these investigations have often exposed abusive and excessive use of restrictive behavior management practices, especially related to injuries and deaths from restraint. Two cases will illustrate that work, although there have been many similar lawsuits throughout the US states and territories.

5.1.2.1 Texas 1974–Present

The ongoing Department of Justice's investigations into facilities in Texas which has taken place, with a short break, for 40 years, illustrate the central role of restraints in *Civil Rights of Institutionalized Persons Act* investigations. In 1974,

Johnny Lelsz was a boy with Intellectual Disabilities and self-injury who had been living in a locked ward in a Texas institution. Parents complained asking for habilitation in the least restrictive environment (i.e., community settings). Following investigations, the Department of Justice investigated and several Texas institutions were involved in the subsequent *Lelzs v. Kavanagh* lawsuit which alleged broad problems including excessive use of restraint and ineffective behavior management resulting in injuries to residents and restrictions on their movement. After closure of two institutions, significant increase in funding for other institutions and some downsizing of the remaining institutions, the state exited that lawsuit in 1999.

Only 6 years later, during the week of June 13, 2005, the Department of Justice investigated Lubbock State School and on December 11, 2006 issued its letter of finding. This letter cited broad deficiencies threatening the safety of Lubbock State School residents including: (a) inadequate nursing, infirmary, physical and nutrition management, physical and occupational therapy, clinical care, neurology, pharmacy, dental, psychiatry services; (b) failure to protect from harm, including injuries, inadequate management of incidents; (c) inadequate psychology and psychiatry services related to behavioral assessments, behavioral interventions, implementation of behavior plans, and restraint use, inadequate quality assurance, and inappropriate chemical restraints; (d) inadequate speech therapy services; and (e) failure to serve residents in the most integrated settings. Examples of citations for restraints included the excessive number of clients in restraints and the failure of the facility to adequately monitor restraints.

On August 20, 2008, the Department of Justice announced that it had expanded its investigation to include all 13 facilities in Texas and thus on June 26, 2009, giving Texas the unique distinction of having all of its facilities investigated simultaneously. The State entered into a settlement agreement with Department of Justice which included extensive provisions related to the use of restraint such as: (a) immediate elimination of prone restraint; (b) release from restraint when the person is no longer a danger to themselves; (c) detailed documentation of each incident of restraint; (d) prohibition of the use of restraint for the convenience of staff or due to lack of alternate treatment; (e) prohibition of restraints other than for emergencies; (f) a requirement that if medical or dental restraints are used then the facilities must also implement strategies to minimize the use of restraints; (g) observation by a professional staff of the client no later than 15 min of the beginning of a restraint; (h) reviews of treatment plans for anyone who is restrained three or more times within any 30 day period; and (i) review of each incident of restraint by the facility within three days of the restraint occurring. The court appointed monitors and monitoring teams to ensure compliance with the agreement.

In the midst of attention from state newspapers and advocacy groups, further fuel was thrown onto the fire. Videotapes of some staff at Corpus Christi State School inciting "Fight clubs" between residents emerged taken on staff cell phones during the fights. It was unclear whether staff were also betting on the fights. Video clips of the fight club was posted on Youtube[1] and the incident made national TV news

[1] https://www.youtube.com/watch?v=nzGJAC6XGzk

which resulted in suspension of admissions to Corpus Christi State School. Police investigated and staff were taken to court and at least one was imprisoned.

During the current Department of Justice's investigation, the monitoring teams have continued to investigate the State's compliance with the agreement and the use of restraint at all of the State's facilities. Their detailed reports are posted online at the state agency's website[2] and some progress in reduction of restraint and other restrictive procedures is documented, but with overall very low levels of compliance with the agreement's standards. In 2014, the State recommended closure of 6 of the facilities reflecting increasing costs of such facilities and ongoing problems at the institutions; it is unclear if the recommendations will be acted on.

5.1.2.2 Howe Developmental Center, Illinois 2009.

Consider this second example of the findings from Department of Justice's investigation into the Howe Developmental Center, Illinois conducted in 2009. The Department of Justice's letter to The Governor of Illinois, citing previous Federal cases that establish the constitutional right to safety, the report stated that "… the state of Illinois fails to protect Howe residents from harm and risk of harm, and to provide residents with a reasonably safe environment" (p. 6). The stated standard of professional performance is that restraints should only be used for imminent danger and the person should be released immediately when they are no longer in imminent danger. Regarding Howe's use of restraint, Department of Justice concluded that "restraint practices at Howe deviate substantially from generally accepted professional standards, specifically in the facility's use of four, five and six-point restraints … Many restraints were applied consecutively, resulting in individuals being restrained for hours at a time … Howe's procedures to review the appropriateness of restraint were frequently untimely and cursory …" (p. 15). Noting that professional staff took 14–40 days to review increases in restraint use, the Department of Justice concluded that "Howe's indiscriminate use of restraints, and untimely and cursory reviews of whether they are appropriate, constitute an unlawful deprivation of resident's constitutionally protected liberty interests" (p. 16).

One facet of protection from harm, including protection from the harm from restraints, is minimally adequate training, broadly defined. Thus, the Department of Justice cited Howe for deficiencies in both behavioral programming and training generally. The Department of Justice found that the behavior programming was inadequate because functional behavior assessments were absent, did not involve sufficient client observation and failed to identify the function of the target behavior clearly. Behavior support plans were also inadequate because they did not identify a replacement behavior, identified incorrect and/or replacement behaviors, such as "waiting" or "compliance," taught skills out of context and continued training sometimes for over 18 months when the training was ineffective. Behavioral treatment of pica was especially weak and restrictive, as it mostly involved removing pica items and blocking to prevent consuming the item, but did not teach replacement

[2] http://www.dads.state.tx.us/monitors/reports/

skills. Oversight by the Human Rights Committee was ineffective as it appeared to approve restrictive behavior plans and restriction on client mobility routinely without analyzing the problems or requiring remedial actions when restrictions were approved. Data collection and analysis were also largely absent, rendering evaluation of behavior plans impossible. Finally, habilitation was generally ineffective or absent, including select of nonfunctional goals, failure to match programs to resident needs, failure to collect outcome data, using the same treatment plan for large number of clients without individualization of the teaching plan, and ineffective and largely absent speech/communication training.

This dire catalog of poor and absent training that places clients at risk for restrictive behavior management practices is found in almost all Department of Justice investigations into developmental centers. It is interesting to note that the quantity, quality, and degree of analysis in Department of Justice reports and the extensive follow-up on initial investigations, sometimes going on for decades, contrasts greatly with similar investigations from other countries, such as the report of the British Ely Hospital scandal in 1968. (See below). Similar institutional scandals involving restraints have been reported in other countries such as the UK and recently in Canada and The Netherlands. It might be tempting to assume that such problems are restricted to institutions in the past; this is false. Excessive use of restrictive behavior management practices have been exposed by the media in community services for people with Intellectual Disabilities over the last 30 years, including contemporary community services in the USA, UK, The Netherlands, and Canada amongst others and continues at the time of writing this chapter.

5.1.3 British Institutions

The UK does not have a Federal system of government and so there is no Federal oversight and investigation of services. Rather, its institutional problems tend to be exposed by the media. Only over the last 15 years, mostly in response to scandals in community services, are a patchwork, ad hoc oversight mechanisms gradually developing (see below and next chapter).

5.1.3.1 Ely Hospital Scandal, Cardiff, UK (1968)

One of the earliest British scandals was the Ely Hospital inquiry (Ely Hospital Report 1969) which found widespread neglect, violence and threats of violence between nursing staff, violence from nursing staff to residents, understaffing, dirty conditions and lack of programming and education, lack of professional training for medical and other staff, and lack of curiosity or motivation to seek such training. Within this context, the report also noted abuse of seclusion and PRN (pro re nata, "as needed") medication by nursing staff, including seclusion for extended periods of time, failure to seek medical approval for these procedures, and lack of oversight from medical and administrative staff. This inquiry prompted the subsequent publication of *Better Services for the Mentally Handicapped* in 1971.

The inquiry was limited in that the method used was interviewing witnesses. Many of the witnesses refused to show up or testify. When the report was written there was considerable pressure on the British government to suppress it, but finally it was published. Unlike US Department of Justice investigations, the extent of restraint, seclusion, and PRN medication was never systematically investigated in the document; in any case it may have been impossible to do so since nursing and medical records were very incomplete.

5.1.3.2 More Institutional Scandals

Between 1969 and 1979 there were further ten investigations, often conducted following the investigations by newspapers and television (Brend 2008) and in one case involved the only strike by staff in a National Health Services hospital. The airing of the TV program *Silent Minority*[3] in 1981 revealed dreadful conditions in mental handicap hospitals, such as dirty conditions, lack of activities, lack of family contact, many children, and residents working unpaid due to lack of staff. One individual was photosensitive due to psychotropic medication probably used to manage behavior problems leading to sunburn.

Misuse of restraint featured in many such investigations. For example, *Silent Minority* included people with Intellectual Disabilities restrained for 4–5 h a day, unregulated seclusion, including one individual secluded more or less continuously for most of 6 months and resident movement was restricted by placing wire cages around recreational areas. Investigations into Darenth Park, a large mental handicap hospital, revealed an individual whose guidelines required him to be restrained by six staff.

These and other exposes were instrumental in development of community services for people with disabilities beginning in the 1970s in the UK.

5.2 Deadly Restraint

Hartford Current's 1998 expose of restraint-related deaths echos the death of a Quaker woman in a county asylum nearly 200 years earlier. It was not state oversight or mental health professionals that exposed restraint-related deaths. Rather, it was investigative journalists at the *Hartford Current,* Eric M. Weiss, Dave Altimari, Dwight F. Blint, and Kathleen Megan who exposed them. These journalists compiled a database of 142 restraint- and seclusion-related deaths that occurred between 1988 and 1999. Most deaths occurred in developmental centers, for people with Intellectual Disabilities, and in psychiatric hospitals. They believed that the true number of deaths was approximately three times higher or about 50–150 deaths per due to underreporting and misclassification of cause of death. Approximately 60% of restraint-related deaths occurred in hospitals, including psychiatric hospitals and

[3] *Available on Youtube* https://www.youtube.com/watch?v =az2fTYud0us

psychiatric wards of general hospitals, and approximately 40% occurred in community group homes and large residential facilities for people with developmental disabilities and troubled youth. The deaths they reported occurred throughout the USA. About a third died from asphyxia and about a quarter died from cardiac related events. Of the 114 cases in which ages were confirmed, 26% were children.

This series uncovered several disturbing practices. First, there was no national requirement to report restraint-related deaths and only three states required services to report them. Weiss noted that "The federal government—which closely monitors the size of eggs—does not collect data on how many patients are killed by a procedure that is used every day in psychiatric and mental retardation facilities across the country" (p. A1). Often the information on death certificates and related investigations was poor or absent. For example, often the cause of death was recorded as "positional asphyxia" or "natural causes," without referencing restraint. Many cases involved minimally or untrained staff. Often incidents were covered up by staff, administrators, or law enforcement. Rarely did cases result in any kind of prosecution of staff or facilities, police were often not called and families often had to resort to civil prosecutions that were often unsuccessful or resulted in minimal damages. Oversight from states was generally poor or absent and few states published any statistics on restraint-related death rendering it difficult to hold state agencies accountable or for the agencies themselves to take any effective action as they often were unaware of the extent of the problem.

The second article highlighted staffing and staff training issues. They noted that almost all staff who administered restraints are direct care staff and only three states at that times required any licensing of direct care staff. Staff were often poorly paid, sometimes earning less than employees at local grocery stores, often got injured on the job, and echoing some of the findings of British inquiries into restraints, may have to work under difficult conditions when short of staff. Imprecise and incomplete state regulations and poor staff training left the door open for staff to misapply restraints and, if legal charges are filed against them, they may claim to be doing their job as they were trained to do so. For example, one state worker successfully defended themselves against a charge of negligent homicide because the state regulations did not specify that they should have observed the child's face for signs of distress during restraint. In the remaining articles in the series and in follow-up article, the authors called for better use of preventative strategies, less use of frightening clients, and better oversight and regulation of restraints.

5.3 Response to Deadly Restraint

5.3.1 Databases

Deadly Restraints precipitated a number of similar articles including a database from the National Alliance on Mental Health, a review of restraint-related deaths in the UK (Patterson et al. 2003), reports of restraint-related deaths in seniors (Miles and Irvine 1992) and a more recent report of restraint-related deaths in people in the USA (Coalition Against Institutionalized Child Abuse 2011; Quip for Equality 2011). For example, Patterson et al. (2003) reported a series of restraint-related deaths in the UK. Searching the academic literature and contacting Mental Health Commissioners in England and Scotland yielded only two cases; however, a search through a large database of newspaper articles resulted in a total of 12 deaths being identified. Again, government sources on this matter appeared incomplete and obscure. In a similar vein some 10 years later, the BBC reported that, at least 10 deaths had occurred following restraints at bars and clubs in the UK. In response, the British government required bouncers to receive training in restraint methods (Reed 2010).

These reports confirmed the findings of *Deadly Restraints;* namely, restraint-related deaths which occurred surprisingly frequently, were underreported and underinvestigated by government agencies. Oversight by agencies and governments was lax, depriving vulnerable populations of alternate effective interventions that might keep them safe and continuing to place them risk of injury and death.

5.3.2 *The US Response*

5.3.2.1 General Accounting Office Investigations

There were several responses from the US Federal government, including those related to mental health and Intellectual Disabilities (General Accounting Office 1999a, b), and to public and private schools and treatment centers for children and adolescents (General Accounting Office 2009). The General Accounting Office's investigation into restraint and seclusion uncovered at least 24 restraint or seclusion-related deaths in 1998, but believed that this was a large undercount. Disturbingly, they found that only 15 states had any systematic reporting system, but these systems were inadequate and that Federal reporting requirements differed across different Federal agencies, such as developmental disabilities, mental health, drug and alcohol abuse, and residential settings for children and adolescents. Only recently had there been any Federal regulation of restraints and seclusion in psychiatric facilities, residential centers for children and group homes. Even when deaths were reported to relevant state agencies, the agencies concerned only investigated a minority of these deaths. They also noted that even in states that had strong regulation of restraint and seclusion in the public sector, they did not make the same requirements of private sector providers, again resulting in different lives of protection depending where a client receive services. Thus, the General Accounting Office recommended uniformity across Federal agencies in the protections offered to service users, uniform reporting protocol, reporting and oversight of deaths, maintenance of adequate records, and adequate staff training on alternatives to restraints.

In response to General Accounting Office, the Health Care Facility Administration published a new restraint rule for Medicare and Medicaid programs. This rule specified that a licensed physician or other health care profession conduct a face-to-face patient assessment within 1 h of a restraint being initiated, codified staff training, and required more stringent documentation of each restraint. This series of articles had many repercussions both in the USA and elsewhere.

On a positive note, the General Accounting Office found that some states had effective procedures in place to reduce restraint- and seclusion-related deaths in some of their agencies. For example, the General Accounting Office cited a 90 % reduction in restraint in Pennsylvania in their state mental health facilities and Delaware's Medicaid Federally funded Intermittent Care Facilities/Mental Retardation residential program for Intellectual Disabilities had reduced restraint by 81 % between 1994 and 1997. Similarly, effective programs exited in some of Massachusetts' and New York's agencies. They noted that "successful strategies to reduce the use of restraint and seclusion have similar components: defined principles and policies that clearly outline when and how restraint or seclusion may be used; strong management commitment and leadership; a requirement to report the use of restraint or seclusion; staff training in safe use of, and alternatives to, restraint and seclusion; and oversight and monitoring" (pp. 3–4). No states were cited that had reduced restraints comprehensively across multiple state agencies and none had imposed these regulation on the private sector.

In the same year, the General Accounting Office (1999b) also reported that the extent of physical and other harm, such as might occur in a person with a history of physical and/or sexual trauma, from restraint or seclusion to clients and care givers was unknown. This was primarily due to the lack of reporting requirements and lack of Federal and State oversight of this issue resulting in piecemeal monitoring of restraints and seclusion nationwide. For example, five states accounted for more than two thirds of deaths and 28 states reported no deaths, which is extremely unlikely to reflect the truth. Several Federal laws were proposed to Congress. Following opposition from health care professionals and some health care industry lobbies, the legislation was never passed.

5.3.2.2 Nursing Homes and Health Care Finance Administration

The Health Care Finance Administration, currently known as Centers for Medicare and Medicaid Services, is a US agency which administers Medicare (the Federal health insurance program for seniors) and Medicaid (the Federal needs-based program), and has oversight over the Children's Health Insurance Program among other things. In 1999, the Health Care Finance Administration issued new regulations governing restraint, seclusion, and behavior management which were broadly similar to the *Joint Commission on Accreditation of Healthcare Organizations* regulations described in the section above. As with the *Joint Commission on Accreditation of Healthcare Organizations* reforms there was much consternation when the new rules were proposed.

Despite the complaints from the health care industry and some professions, the effects on restraint use were good. Currier and Farley-Toombs (2002) reported that following the introduction of the new rule that the frequency and duration of restraints fell by over 50 % in 4 months on four psychiatric units with 80 beds in a university-based medical facility serving children, people with substance-related disorders, adults, and seniors. Weintraub and Spurlock (2002) reported similar data on restraint reduction and also reported no increase in falls or injuries. There are also data showing large nation-wide reduction in restraint over much more extensive periods of time. For example, Centers for Medicare and Medicaid Services (2008a) reported that the percentage of nursing home residents with restraint fell from 21.1 % in 1991 to 5.0 % in 2007. The one worrying trend is that the proportion of nursing home residents who take atypical antipsychotic medication, which is often used and misused for behavior management, is very high: 25.5 % (Centers for Medicare and Medicaid Services 2008b). Thus, it is unclear if Centers for Medicare and Medicaid Services has reduced restraint but replaced mechanical and personal restraint with pharmacological restraint. (More recent data confirms that may have in fact occurred. See Chap. 11).

5.3.2.3 Joint Commission on Accreditation of Healthcare Organizations

The Joint Commission on Accreditation of Healthcare Organizations is an American, not-for-profit organization that certifies quality of care in over 20,000 health care facilities, such as hospitals, including general and psychiatric hospitals, nursing homes and other health care entities voluntarily join. The organizations are accredited on performance measures, such as appropriate coronary and pneumonia care and their measures now include measures of quality of care related to restraint. The Joint Commission on Accreditation of Healthcare Organizations awards prized to top performing health care organizations every year.

In 1996, prior to the publication of *Deadly Restraints*, the *Joint Commission on Accreditation of Healthcare Organizations* had already revised their accreditation standards to make them much more specific and extensive regarding restraint use (Zusman 1999), but following *Deadly Restraint, Joint Commission on Accreditation of Healthcare Organizations* revised the standards making them even more specific and extensive than before (Zusman 1997). A partial listing of some of these included: "[1] … [a] restraint or seclusion … is limited to those situations with adequate, appropriate clinical justification; … [b] Organization leaders support limited, justified use of restraint or seclusion through appropriate … plans policies and priorities … human resource planning … [c] staff orientation and education creating a culture emphasizing prevention and appropriate use and encouraging alternatives … [d] patient and … family education … [e] assessment processes that identify and … prevent potential behavioral risk factors … [f] design and delivery of patient care … [g] the development and promotion of preventative strategies and use of safe and effective alternatives … identify and … prevent potential risk factors … [h] design and delivery of patient care and … the development and promotion of preventative strategies and use of safe and effective alternatives … [2] Performance-improvement processes identify opportunities … to reduce restraint or seclusion use … [3] [a] when restraint and seclusion or restraint is used, organization policy and procedures guide appropriate and safe use … [b] the least-restrictive safe effective restraint or seclusion method is employed … correctly by competent, trained staff … [c] ordered by a licensed independent practitioner … orders … [d which] define specific time limits … " (Zusman 1997).

These modest requirements, which surely John Connolly would have approved of, caused consternation to some in the health care industry. The new regulations required extra work, such as quality assurance plans to reduce restraint and required physicians or other health care professionals to observe patients face-to-face within an hour of restraint. Some were also concerned that the scoring criteria were subjective and that some of the rules conflicted with other Federal rules. The health care industry was right to be concerned. Zusman (1999) reported that in the first year of the 1996 regulations that "problematic" standards—those that 5 % or more of hospitals did not meet—included: lack of implementation of performance improvement processes to reduce restraint or seclusion; lack of organizational policy and procedures to guide safe use; lack of time limits on restraint orders (38 % of hospitals), and inadequate documentation of restraint orders (15 % of hospitals). Perhaps most telling was the lack of organizational plans and follow-up to reduce restraint since this is often one of the key elements in reducing restraint on an organization-wide basis (See Chap. 11).

Data questioning the effectiveness of *Joint Commission on Accreditation of Healthcare Organizations*' new system comes from the General Accounting Office's (1999) audit of restraint- and seclusion-related deaths. They detected 21 restraint- and seclusion-related deaths in *Joint Commission on Accreditation of Healthcare Organizations*-accredited facilities in 1998 *after* the new regulations had been implemented. Only 15 of these deaths had been reported by facilities as sentinel events, 3 were not, and *Joint Commission on Accreditation of Healthcare Organizations* did not know if 3 other deaths had been reported or not.

5.3.2.4 Substance Abuse and Mental Health Services Administration

The Substance Abuse and Mental Health Services Administration is the US Federal agency responsible for behavioral health including substance abuse and mental health including prevention and treatment at individual, family, and community level and includes all US entities including states, territories, and tribal communities. The Substance Abuse and Mental Health Services Administration's commitment to reducing and eliminating restraint came from the top. In 2003, the agency organized a nationwide conference on eliminating restraint and seclusion. They wrote a national policy to do so, opened a center for promoting alternatives to seclusion and in The Substance Abuse and Mental Health Services Administration's newsletter there have been many articles continuously since 2003 to assist providers with reduction and elimination of restraint and seclusion. The Substance Abuse and Mental Health Services Administration recognizes organizations that are effective by giving them awards and national recognition in their newsletter.

Currie (2005) noted that The Substance Abuse and Mental Health Services Administration had used the methods used in Pennsylvania as a model for restraint reduction throughout The Substance Abuse and Mental Health Services Administration and highlighted the use of data and transparency in the use of restraint as a key component in reducing restraint on a large-scale. The Substance Abuse and Mental Health Services Administration's work on reducing and eliminating restraint has resulted in a plethora of publications describing the uneven distribution of restraint and interventions to reduce and eliminate it. It also published national data on use of restraint and seclusion identifying at risk populations and trends across time (Huang 2011). The Substance Abuse and Mental Health Services Administration developed a six-component program which included: (1) involvement of leadership to promote organizational change; (2) use of rigorous debriefing after incidents of restraint and seclusion; (3) use of restraint and seclusion data to inform practice; (4) workforce development and training; (5) Use of seclusion and restraint prevention tools such as crisis plans, identifying triggers, and use of alternatives to restraint and seclusion such as comfort/sensory rooms; and (6) full inclusion and participation of consumers and family members.

The Substance Abuse and Mental Health Services Administration's ambitious and continuing efforts on restraint reduction are noteworthy because they have taken strategies used at the level of facilities and states and attempted to apply them on a national level. For example, Wieman et al. (2014) found that implementation of The Substance Abuse and Mental Health Services Administration restraint and seclusion guidelines resulted in reduction of proportion of persons secluded by 17% ($p<0.0002$), hours of seclusion by 19% ($p<0.0001$), proportion restrained by 30% ($p=0.03$) and restraint hours by 55% ($p=0.08$). Huang (2011) presented national data at a conference suggesting quite large reductions in restraint and seclusion between July 2000 and July 2007. For example, in 2000, the number of hours of restraint for children aged less than 12 years was approximately 3 h/1000 patient hours and this fell to less than 1 h/1000 patient hours. More recent data indicates little change in restraint use, some evidence of increase and disturbingly nearly 30% of children aged 13 or under being restrained (National Association of State Mental Health Program Directors Research Institute, *undated*). Thus, it seems that most change mostly occurred early in between 2000 and 2001 but since that time there is evidence of gradual increase in restraint in some younger patients.

These data illustrate an important question regarding restraint reduction programs, namely, some restraint and reduction may be insufficient. Even if the initial reduction in restraint occurs and is both impressive and statistically significant, service providers must continue to pursue the reduction and elimination of restraint vigorously over extended periods of time, especially for interventions that take place in large organizations.

5.3.2.5 Veterans Health Administration

The Veterans Administration (VA) provides medical and long-term care for US veterans. Following media reports of poor nursing care and insanitary conditions at some VA facilities, the General Accounting Office conducted several surveys of

Veterans Administration facilities and analyzed how the Veterans Administration Headquarters responded to the identified deficiencies in care.

In 2001, the General Accounting Office found widespread poor medical and nursing care as well as problems in basic sanitation and cleanliness. With regard to restraint, of 116 facilities surveyed, 47 % had deficiencies in administration of psychotropic medication including nurses administering psychotropic medication outside the scope of physicians' orders to calm patients without using alternate methods, and failure to track resident behavior to ascertain if psychotropic medication was appropriate or effective. In 28 % of facilities, staff were untrained as to what constituted restraint, using bed rails, seat belts, and tables to restrict resident mobility without physician's orders. Disturbingly, the General Accounting Office found that the Veterans Administration Headquarters did a poor job of quality assurance. The General Accounting Office had access to multiple sources of information, but did not analyze and integrate information across sources and thus missed opportunities to improve services. Finally, the Veterans Administration Headquarters did not effectively follow-up on plans of correction with facilities when deficiencies were noted.

In addition to the Veteran's Administration, the Veteran's Administration Office of Inspector General also investigates individual VA facilities including their use of restraints. Examples of their reports can be found at www.va.gov/oig. As with other agencies, the Veteran's Administration has undertaken initiatives to reduce the use of restraint (Gillies et al. 2005).

5.3.3 British Response

These reports of restraint-related deaths in people with Intellectual Disabilities in the UK prompted the British Institute of Learning Disabilities, the lead not-for-profit organization for people with Intellectual Disabilities in Britain, to take action which has continued over the last 15 years. This has included several literature reviews (Allen 2002, 2009; Harris et al. 1996), reviews of legal aspects of restraint (Lyon and Pimor 2004), a code of practice that has been revised four times (British Institute of Learning Disabilities 2014) and practical guidelines for nonprofessionals (Barksby and Harper 2011; British Institute of Learning Disabilities 2002). Two interesting developments have also been the certification of certain forms of staff training to reduce restraint use and promote safe use of restraints and the promotion of Positive Behavior Supports as methods to reduce restraint. British Institute of Learning Disabilities now accredits a number of staff training organizations as approved to provide training in behavior management, restrain reduction, and implementing certain forms of restraint.

Both of these initiatives are interesting responses to the issue of restraint-related deaths that may promote client safety, but both beg empirical questions. Have these initiatives in fact reduced restraint and seclusion and reduced restraint-related deaths and injuries to clients and staff? For example, certification of certain staff training packages as approved to reduce restraint and promote safety assumes that these outcomes do indeed achieve these outcomes; however, reviews in the next chapter on randomized controlled trials finds that such approaches *may* reduce restraint, but may also be ineffective or may *increase* restraint use. Likewise, the promotion of Positive Behavioral Supports to reduce restraint begs the questions of what constitutes Positive Behavioral Supports and whether or not there is evidence that the procedures implemented under the rubric of Positive Behavioral Supports are effective in achieving these outcomes (Sturmey and Didden 2014).

5.4 Summary

Between 1970 and 2010, much attention was paid to restraints in the context of institutions for people with disabilities, which played a part in accelerating deinstitutionalization in the USA and Britain, and in nursing homes and youth facilities, predominantly in the USA. *Deadly restraints* played a key role in this both in the USA and Britain. There is some evidence, especially from nursing homes and some psychiatric facilities in the USA, that such publicity may have led to policies that were both implemented and effective in reducing restraints. One might hope that this attention may have resolved or at least reduced restraint today, but the next chapter will show that restraint and restraint-related death remains with us in much of the same way as it has been for the last 200 years.

Chapter 6
Failing to Learn from John Connolly: Current Use of Restraint and Seclusion

Despite a 200-year-old model of how to reduce restraint and restrictive behavioral practices effectively, and despite recent restraint-related deaths documented clearly in British, American press and academic publications, contemporary services and some families continue to tie people up, use physical coercion, and keep people in cages. This chapter provides an overview of contemporary use of restrictive behavioral practices in educational services, services for young people, community residential care for people with Intellectual Disabilities, and nursing homes.

6.1 Contemporary Education

6.1.1 British Education System

The use of restraint and seclusion in the British education system has received attention in the press. In 2006, Jade Chambers, a 6-year-old girl with ID, had been restrained at least 25 times and dragged without the school informing her parents (Asthana 2006). Her parents subsequently sued the school. In a second case of restraint in British schools, a former head teacher was cleared of professional misconduct by the professional conduct panel of the National College for Teaching after she provided a 19-year-old girl with Asperger syndrome, who had been restrained repeatedly, with blades and sterile wipes to allow her to self-harm in a more mis controlled way than she had used in the past. This had been done in consultation with the girl's mother and a psychiatric nurse. The panel found that the head teacher was "naïve" and "inexperienced," failed to seek out professional assistance (*Unsted Park* "self-harm blades" *head teacher cleared*, 2014).

Following allegations of school-wide abuse of restraint and systemic problems in the running of The Gatehouse School, an English special education school, Stone (2009) conducted a review of the use of restraints at the request of the local city

P. Sturmey, *Reducing Restraint and Restrictive Behavior Management Practices*,
Autism and Child Psychopathology Series, DOI 10.1007/978-3-319-17569-0_6

council. Stone found that restraint was used as the first rather than last resource, classrooms were locked during lessons, restraint was not recorded and reviewed accurately, medication use was not recorded consistently, the school did not respond to complaints concerning restraints, staff were hired without background checks, staff and the Board of governors were largely untrained. Ofsted, the British national body charged with reviewing schools, inspected the school in 2006 and failed to detect any such problems. Stone also documented allegations of bullying and intimidation of staff by school management. Staff, including professional staff, failed to report abuse and neglect. Members of the school's management board apparently had made weekly oversight visits, but there was no evidence that they had reviewed restraints in any way; Stone described them as untrained "well-meaning lay people." These changes took place within a local city that was undergoing tumultuous changes and turnover of senior administrative staff. Stone concluded that there was organization-wide dysfunction, both in the school and the city council departments responsible for overseeing the school.

In 2014 an art teacher was suspended for taping 20 students' lips together because they giggled and talked in class (Morris 2014). Some students' lips bled when the tape was removed and some students reported they had difficulty breathing. The principal informed the parents by letter and the teacher was suspended.

6.1.1.1 Government Response

The British government's response to these problems has primarily been to pass laws and guidance outlining the circumstances in which restraint may be used with little attention to oversight and prevention. For example, despite the continued attention to restraint and seclusion and injury to children in British schools from restraint, there are no nationally available statistics on use of restraint, seclusions, and related injuries. The disinfectant function of daylight is sorely missing. The only data close to national statistics on restraint come from the BBC's investigation into complaints about using school staff using the *Freedom of Information Act*. They found that there were approximately 1700 complaints about school staff and about half related to assault and "inappropriate restraint" (*School staff get 1700 complaints* 2010). Such data, however, are inadequate as it is unclear how accurate and complete they are, and restraints that do not result in a complaint would not be included in such data.

The 1996 *Education Act* specifically prohibits no contact policies and instead authorizes school staff to restraint students to prevent aggression between students, property damage, and injury, to ensure a student leaves a classroom when they persistently refuse to follow instructions to do so, to prevent disruption in the classroom, and elsewhere. Subsequent guidance from the Department for Children, Schools and Families (2013) is permissive on several key issues. For example, it leaves it up to each school to decide if staff training is needed, who should be trained and what kind of training should be delivered and how. Although the law requires the school governing body to have a procedure in place to record "significant incidents," it fails to define what constitutes a significant incident, how it should be recorded and what training is needed to make an adequate record. Similarly, it requires the school board to "take reasonable steps … to ensure that parents are kept informed" (p. 5), but fails to define what constitutes a reasonable step, and when and how parents are to be informed. The law also is weak on prevention. Although it references the need to have a "well-run school" and "creating a calm, orderly and supportive school climate" (p. 5), but unlike the US law, does not require the adaption of evidence-based practices such as functional behavior assessments (FBA) or related positive interventions based on functional behavior assessments. Similar advice was circulated to teachers from their union (National Union of Teachers 2012).

6.1.1.2 Summary

The British education system uses restraint to an unknown extent and almost nothing is known about seclusion in British schools. The lack of national data leaves this problem hidden. The British government has made ambiguous response. On the one hand, advice is given that the restraints and seclusion should be the last resort, staff should be trained and alternate intervention methods be used, serious incidents should be recorded and parents should be kept informed, but the details are left up to the schools and their governing bodies. Although individual incidents and reports into misuse of restraint (Stone 2009) illustrate the negative consequences of failing to address these problems effectively, current British legislation fails to provide clear protection to children from the misuse of restraints and seclusion. At this time there is no clear initiative from the UK government to reduce restraint in educational settings.

6.1.2 US Schools and Treatment Centers

We tend to think of restraint and seclusion as a problem for institutions for people with Intellectual Disabilities and mental health needs and in nursing homes as not as something that happens to children in school. Thus, Federal attention to restraint- and seclusion-related deaths in schools occurred relatively late. The now familiar pattern repeated itself once more. The National Disability Rights Network is a federally funded organization that provides support and technical assistance to state protection and advocacy and client protection programs in the USA. In January 2009, they reported dozens of cases of restraint, seclusion, children being pinned down to the floor for hours at a time, handcuffed, locked in closets that resulted in child injuries, trauma, and death. Around the same time, The Council of Parent Attorneys and Advocates (2009) also published a similar report. Individual scandals in schools continue to emerge from time to time. For example, Grove (2012) reported that in one school system restraint was used excessively as a part of widespread use of coercive practices in a special education school. These included denial of food, a time-out/seclusion room described as being "the size of a refrigerator," and physical restraint with up to five staff restraining one child.

In response, the General Accounting Office's (2009) reported hundreds of cases of alleged abuse and death related to restraint and seclusion in American schools. The General Accounting Office's (2009) investigated selected cases in public and private schools and treatment centers excluding child psychiatric facilities and juvenile facilities. Their remit and methods were broadly similar to their investigation 10 years earlier and their conclusions were depressingly similar to those it had already at that earlier time. Namely, as there were no Federal regulations restricting or governing restraint or seclusion in public and private schools, regulations varied substantially from state to state. For example, some states had no laws related to restraint and some state laws only covered some settings, but not others. Differences between the state laws were substantive. For example, eight states banned prone restraints, but others permitted them. Almost no states required reporting of restraints. Because of incomplete reporting, the General Accounting Office's was unable to determine how widespread restraint-related deaths were, however, they did identify hundreds of allegations almost all of which involved children with disabilities. Data from those states that did report restraints centrally indicated that restraints might be used quite commonly. For example, Texas restrained 4202 children 18,741 times and California reported 14,354 instances of student restraint or other emergency procedures in 2007–2008.

When analyzing ten cases in which restraint resulted in death in detail, the General Accounting Office's found several disturbing practices. Often staff involved were untrained in restraint methods. Sometimes schools failed to conduct criminal background checks and hired staff with criminal backgrounds. For example, one teacher's aide, who had a criminal history of burglary and cocaine procession, taped first grade students to a blackboard and taped their mouths shut. Sometimes, teachers who had been found guilty of excessive force continued to teach and keep their teaching licenses.

In response to this, Arne Duncan, the US education Secretary, wrote to all states on July 31, 2009 encouraging (but not requiring) them to develop or review their current policies and offered the Illinois state rule as a model for states to consider. The letter asked for all states to minimize the use of restraint, ensure that staff are informed of policies and ensure that parents are informed when restraints are implemented. The letter also advocated for the use of positive behavior support as a preventative approach to behavioral challenges.

Following another death in prone (face down) restraint of a 17-year-old girl in a youth facility on December 13, 2009, the Governor of Ohio, Ted Strickland, issued an executive order banning prone restraint in all state human service agencies. The order also restricted restraint use to trained staff and established a state oversight committee on restraint and seclusion to establish a single-state rule for the use of restraint and seclusion.

Follow-up National Disability Rights Network reports in 2010 and 2012 were discouraging and understandably frustrated. For example, in 2012 National Disability Rights Network reported that within the American education system between 2010 and 2012 children had been stuffed into duffle bags and placed in a hallway, tied to desks, restrained in duct tape, and restrained in chairs designed to be used as devices for physical disabilities. Several states used dangerous and unmonitored seclusion and locked room time-out on some occasions against parental wishes and without parental consent. On several occasions these practices resulted in child injuries and on at least one occasion a child attempted suicide while unmonitored in a seclusion room. There were also examples of children being restrained and/or secluded without an Individualized Education Plan (IEP) and without a functional behavior assessment or behavior support plan in place, even when restrictive practices continued for extensive periods of time in violation of the *Individuals with Disabilities Education Act*. The report also provided that in some instances children with disabilities were treated differently because of their disability, for example, when some schools had instructions from superintendents that only children with IEPs could be restrained or secluded. An especially egregious example of the abuse of physical restraint and seclusion was exposed in newspapers and national TV in 2012 in Middleton, Connecticut whose school district used seclusion of children excessively; the seclusion rooms were colloquially called "scream rooms" which made the headlines (McGaughey and Bell 2013).

The National Disability Rights Network (2013) was critical of the US Department of Education. Although seemingly promising in 2009, by 2013 little concrete had been done. For example, although the Department of Education collected national data on use of restraint and seclusion in 2009, it failed to publish, analyze, or use the data to keep children safe or provide them with a better education. In addition, the National Disability Rights Network was of the opinion that Department of Education Secretary Duncan had issued ambiguous guidance by stating, in writing, that under certain circumstances restraint and seclusion were not banned by *Individuals with Disabilities Education Act* and had failed to take leadership and develop, implement, and evaluate national plans to eliminate restraint and seclusion in schools as other Federal agencies, such as The Substance Abuse and Mental Health Services Administration had done in 2003. (See below for a discussion of The Substance Abuse and Mental Health Services Administration, and restraint reduction.)

6.1.2.1 Response from Advocacy Organizations

In response to specific incidents and the general issue of restraint and seclusion-related deaths, several advocacy organizations, lawyers, coalitions of lawyers, advocates, and family members have been active in advocating for reduction or abolition of restraint. Examples include the National Alliance on Mental Illness, Coalition for Against Institutionalized Child Abuse, Council of Parent Attorneys and Advocates, Alliance to Prevent and Restraint, Aversive Interventions and Seclusion, state organizations, and websites from individual parents and blogs. Some law firms and their websites, such as Wrightslaw, also offer advice and resources to parents concerned about special education, including restraint- and seclusion-related injuries and deaths. These organizations have been influential in provoking state officials to pass laws to protect individuals from restraint- and seclusion-related injuries and are important resources for concerned parents and advocates.

6.1.2.2 In Favor of Restraint

Although some sit on the fence on the use of restraint, few explicitly support its use. Thus, an unusual position from the American Association of School Administrators (Pudelski 2012) reported the results of a survey of school administrators provided some rather rosy data, but no details or accuracy of the methods used on the use of restraint and seclusion. It also provided some anecdotes of parents and teachers who supported the use of restraint and seclusion.

The position of the American Association of School Administrators was that misuse of restraint and seclusion does occur, but only in rare cases due to a few bad apples, but that most staff are benevolent and competent. They concluded that "We believe the use of seclusion and restraint has enabled many students with serious emotional or behavioral conditions to be educated not only within our public schools, but also in the least restrictive and safest environments possible."

6.1.3 Australia

In 2011, Australian TV ran a program on use of restraint and time-out in Australian schools, both in special and mainstream education, in Victoria and other parts of Australia.[1] The program included parental complaints that their concerns were minimized by the Department of Education. In response, the Australian Primary Principals Association claimed that restraints were not used systematically.

Some 3 years later, however, Dean (2014), in the Australian *Daily Mail,* presented a series of photographs of children with autism in special educational classes in which the children are physically restrained to chairs and strollers during routine activities such as eating and teaching. The article documents numerous examples of restraint and some examples of seclusion/time-out rooms in Australian special education and complaints from parents concerning the use of restraint and schools ignoring their requests to stop using restraints and regarding restraint-related injuries. Schools denied any improper action. At this time there are no data on the extent of restraint use in Australian schools.

6.1.4 Conclusion

Despite the repeated scandals and concerns regarding the use and safety of restraint and seclusion in educational settings, their use appears to be widespread, at least in those countries in which some kind of data are available. Interestingly, in all three examples, the information came from the media, rather than government departments and government education departments have tended to deny any wrong doing, and/or assert the rights of staff to restraint children, but have failed to initiate effective action to reduce restraint and seclusion in schools.

---

[1] Details can be found here http://www.abc.net.au/7.30/content/2011/s3219518.htm.

6.2 Youth Facilities

6.2.1 *British Youth Facilities*

Concern over behavior management in British youth has been precipitated by a number of child injuries, deaths related to behavior management practices including those approved of by the Home Office such as using "distraction techniques" such as blows to the nose. In 2004, Gareth Myatt, a 15-year old at a private youth facility run by G4S, Rainsbrook Secure Training, England, died in restraint. After refusing to clean a sandwich toaster, staff removed almost all his personal processions from his room, but when they took the piece of paper with his mother's phone number on it, Gareth became aggressive which resulted in several staff restraining him. The facility's training materials referred to staff members as "Clubber," "Crusher," and "Mauler." During the subsequent investigation, the facility director stated that he has not read the facility's restraint manual and was unaware of the risks of the approved restraint methods. There were no prosecutions, even though the coroner concluded that "Inadequacy in the monitoring of the use of Physical Control in Care at Rainsbrook by Rebound management caused or contributed to Gareth's death" (Sambrook 2013). One of the staff involved was subsequently promoted. At around the same time, a second teenager, Adam Rickwood, also died in restraint after staff used a "distraction" technique (a blow to the nose) (Wainwright 2011).

Four years after these children died in restraint, in 2008, the UK Minister of Justice commissioned an independent review of restraint which established a board to advice and review the use of restraint in British youth facilities. In a subsequent report, Smallridge and Williamson (2011) reviewed progress and found some evidence of changes in policy and implementation, such as implementation of staff training. They reviewed data on restraint use and, unfortunately, found that overall restraint use had remained widespread. It had fallen only 13 % from 7909 in 2008/2009 to 6904 in 2009/2010 and the proportion of children and youth restraint *increased* from 11 to 12 %. There was some evidence of modest reductions of restraint use in some parts of youth services. They also concluded that restraints using pain were sometimes required but were unsure whether handcuffs were appropriate or not. Sadly, other than discussion of staff training, the report contained little discussion of prevention strategies, functional assessment, or treatment.

6.2.2 *US Facilities for Troubled Youth*

The General Accounting Office's published three reports into restraint in residential facilities for youth (2007, 2008a, b). They first (General Accounting Office's 2007) investigated abuse and deaths in private residential programs such as wilderness therapy programs, boot camps, boarding schools (or "academies"), and ranch programs for youth. In three of eight deaths, the General Accounting Office's found that staff physically restraining youth was prominent. For example, one death related to an individual restrained over 250 times and on at least two occasions for over 12 h. He was also tied up to prevent him leaving the camp. This continued after he was 18 years old and a legal adult. A second death related to a youth with asthma who was restrained, but staff claimed they did not know he suffered from asthma. Problems related to use of restraint included ineffective management and lack of trained staff to deal with challenging youth. The General Accounting Office's also found evidence of deceptive marketeering and corrupt, and probably illegal practices. The General Accounting Office (2008a) reported two further deaths in services for troubled youth in which restraint paid a part.

The next month, the General Accounting Office's (2008b) reported that regulations in private youth residential facilities and residential programs related to restraint were inconsistent across different Federal programs with respect to data reporting and monitoring, staff training, on-site inspection, etc. For example, not all state agencies relating to youth residential treatment required approved restraint and seclusion to be in place or to monitor restraint and seclusion data. Further, they found that regulations often excluded juvenile justice facilities and boarding schools. The General Accounting Office's recommended that Federal agencies should come together and agree to uniform minimum requirements related to restraint and seclusion and then require state programs to follow these new uniform standards as a condition of participation in the program.

6.2.3 Rikers Adolescent Unit 2011–2014

While writing this chapter, the US Department of Justice (2014) issued a 79-page report into pervasive staff violence and abuse against New York's treatment of male adolescents aged 16–18 years, many of whom (51 %) had mental health diagnoses, in the city's jail at Rikers Island, including excessive physical force and excessive use of punitive segregation from 2011 to 2013. It concluded that there was a pervasive culture of violence at Rikers and that the state had failed to keep the adolescents safe. Specifically, Rikers staff used excessive force such as "head shots" (blows to the head), used force as retribution and in response to disrespect, taunts, insults, and verbal altercations with staff, used brutal specialized response teams, and used force as the first response to both minor and major behavioral incidents. Staff also attempted to justify their use of violence by yelling "stop resisting" when adolescents had never resisted or had stopped resisting. Staff also covered up assaulting inmates, by failure to document, false documentation, and assaulting inmates in areas where cameras did not record. Rikers staff also used punitive segregation (locking inmates in their cells) excessively and inappropriately. Staff also deliberately used painful escort techniques, such as applying flex cuffs tightly to needlessly inflict pain when no danger to others existed, sometimes resulting in serious injuries such as broken wrists.

The report found that Rikers uses segregation excessively—on any day approximately 15–25 % of inmates are segregated in 6-by-8 foot cells for 23 h per day or longer. Many of those segregated are mentally ill and appear to be segregated because of behavioral issues related to their mental health problems. Some inmates, including those with mental illness, are sentenced to such segregation for months at a time for behavioral infractions. Rikers implemented a primarily punishment-based levels system whereby inmates earn time-out of segregation, but the facility administration admitted that the program was a failure. Rikers had attempted to use 2-h restrictions to cells as an alternative, but had abandoned this somewhat less restrictive program.

These problems with use of inappropriate and dangerous use of restraint, escorts, seclusions, and other restrictive behavior management practices took place in the context of broad systemic problems. These problems included inadequate programming and education leaving inmates idle for most of the day, staff codes of silence, teachers and doctor failing to report abuse, inadequate incident investigations, failure to provide medical care when inmates were injured, and multiple problems with videotape surveillance. The Department of Justice identified pervasive staff problems including high staff turnover, lack of staff professionalism, inadequate and ineffective staff training, ineffective staff supervision and disciplinary systems, untrained investigators, investigations taking months or over a year, and ineffective managers who lived in a corporate world divorced from the daily running of the facility. These problems had been documented some 10 years previously, in an earlier lawsuit, but date back to the 1980s.

The Department of Justice (2014) called for broad reform to address these issues. This included relocating the program elsewhere to be run by competent staff with adequate supervision, increasing the number of cameras, strengthening and implementing Riker's own policies prohibiting excessive use of restraint and isolation, and requiring adequate incident documentation and investigation, providing adequate inmate supervision to ensure their safety, provide adequate and effective staff training, improve staff and management accountability.

Gilligan and Lee (2013) also conducted an investigation focusing on seclusion at Rikers. They reported that the number of punitive segregation beds had increased from 614 to 998 (+61.5%). On January 1, 2004, 2.7% of inmates were in punitive segregation but by June 30, 2013, this increased to 7.5%. At the same time, force incidents increased from 7.0 in 2004 to 24.7 per 100 inmates per year. They concluded that seclusion was widely misused and contributed and exacerbated existing mental health issues in a population that already had a very high rate of mental health issues. New York City has now proposed to eliminate seclusion for adolescents at Rikers, but the current status of implementation is unclear.

6.2.4 Conclusion

Some youth facilities today continue to use restraint, seclusion, and physical violence from staff to adolescents almost with impunity. Despite exposes from the media, the US Federal and British government investigations, there is little evidence that these restrictive practices are being reduced to any meaningful extent. Indeed, in some circumstances, they are increasing. Rather than promoting acceptable, effective alternatives, government reports fuss over the details of whether or how much pain should be used to control behavior.

6.3 People with Intellectual Disabilities

6.3.1 Institutional Scandals

Scandals related to restraint in institutions continue today. Four examples from The Netherland, Greece, Serbia, and the Czech Republic illustrate this continuing problem. These examples were compiled in an ad hoc manner and, doubtless, this is an under-report of the extent of this problem. A systematic survey might reveal many more such contemporary examples; The Disability Rights International website[2] catalogues many examples of such problem all over the world.

In 2007, an investigation into institutions in Serbia revealed that children with disabilities were routinely tied to cribs not merely for days but apparently for all their lives until they died. Stojanovic (2007) reported that children were kept in cribs from birth, tore off their ears and blinded themselves while staff stood by and did nothing. This situation took place in the context of extensive defunding of health and social care and civil war, when the lives of people with disabilities are most vulnerable. When the situation was made public, the Serbian minister for health, who admitted that he had not in fact read the report, stated that "I'm not saying that everything is ideal, far from it, … But… I don't think that the problems (listed in the report) are illustrating the true situation."

In January 2011, the BBC reported that a teenager, Brandon, had been tethered to a wall in a Dutch institution for over 3 years (Morris 2011). The Dutch minister for health supported this practice when she stated "I take my leave of Brandon and his careers with my mind at ease." The Dutch government reported that there were, in fact, approximately 40 other people restrained continuously in a similar manner. Subsequently, the Dutch government proposed legislation, but as in other countries that have done so, there is little evidence of changes in service practice (Romijn and Frederiks 2012). Currently there is no publically available information on the use of tethering people to walls in Dutch institutions.

In 1984, the European Community identified that the Greek mental health system was totally inadequate and the institution on the Island of Leros, where 1350 people including 300 children were warehoused, neglected, sedated, and tied up (Ekdawi 1987), came to symbolize this problem. Laws were passed, but little seemed to happen in the ensuing 20 years (Hadjimatheou 2009; Holt et al. 2000). So, it is perhaps unsurprising that in 2014 the BBC reported that children with disabilities were be-

[2] http://www.disabilityrightsintl.org/.

ing kept in cages in Greece in order to reduce costs. Following a report in 2010 to the Greek government that inadequate staffing resulted in at least two deaths, the solution was to place children in cages to prevent access to dangerous objects that they might choke on. Some children have spent most of their lives in cages and are fed through the bars by staff. This takes place within the context of the economic crisis in Greece in which there is insufficient fund to pay staff, including the facility director.

Mental Disability Advocacy Center (2014) described the use of cages in The Czech Republic, Hungary, Sovenia, and Slovakia in around 2003. Some of these countries have since banned their use, but not the Czech Republic. For example, Holt (2004) reported on the use of metal restraint cages and netted beds based in mental health facilities, including children in the Czech Republic. Of 9657 mental health beds in the Czech Republic, around 100 were reported to have nets and 20 to be caged. Some physicians reported reducing the number of such restraints over the years. Reading, much like the accounts of restraint in the nineteenth century asylums, some modern superintendents supported the use of metal cages and netted beds on the grounds that they were more humane than the alternative and necessary for safety due to the lack of staff and effective treatments for violent behavior. At the time Vaclav Klaus, the President of the Czech Republic, stated that he "refute[d] the idea that the use of [cage] beds is abusive, or worse, that mentally handicapped children are tyranised in our country." In 2012, the European Court of Human Rights ruled against the Czech republic's excessive use of restraint in 2007 with a man with mental health issues who was restrained, injured, but no prosecution ensued/ The European Court of Human Right ruled that the use of restraints and failure to prosecute were violations of the European Convention on Human Rights (Mental Disability Advocacy Center 2012). Recent reports indicate that, although the Czech Republic has signed a number of treaties regarding rights of people with disabilities, the use of cages in The Czech Republic largely continues unabated, despite a number of deaths of people in cages (Mental Disability Advocacy Center 2014).

In these contemporary examples of institutional abuse and restraints, it is interesting that when these situations were made public that the national governments supported or excused the use of restraint in three cases. In the cases of Greece and Serbia, and some of the examples on The Disability Rights International website, but not The Netherlands, they take place in the context of economic crises, civil unrest, or war.

6.3.2 Current Community Scandals and Restraints

Over the last 10 years, a number of scandals in community services for people with Intellectual Disabilities, reminiscent of past institutional scandals, have included reports of inappropriate use of restraints. Three took place in the USA and all took place in the late 1990s in the context of rapid deinstitutionalization and transition from institutional to community care. Other more recent scandals are related to

British community services that had been operating for many years but in poorly regulated, sometimes isolated community services with poorly trained staff.

6.3.2.1 Washington DC

In 1999, just after the publication of *Deadly restraints,* Katherine Boo, a *Washington Post* investigative journalist, uncovered systematic and widespread abuse in community services for people with Intellectual Disabilities in Washington DC for which she earned a Pulitzer Prize for Public Service.

Boo published a series of articles on scandalous conditions including companies' failure to implement daytime and leisure programs to prevent deaths, dirty and dangerous group homes, widespread client abuse, and profiteering by private group home. Following the closure of its institution, the District of Columbia had rapidly established group homes with private providers. After the group home programs had been set up, however, the District of Columbia government failed to investigate deaths, including suspicious deaths, and at one point ceased auditing services completely.

Despite numerous violations of standards, the district government never levied any fines and continued to pay providers millions of dollars to private companies enriching the company owners. Boo noted that "… there are 11 bathrooms in the million-dollar Upper Marlboro "Manor Farm" where the Washingtons [owners of the group home company] make their home. A city report recently noted that the home they provide for Elroy [a group home resident] had no toilet paper." Other low points in these community services included a psychologist billing services for treating a client who had died and paying go-go dancers as group home consultants. One resident was sexually abused in the group home, but staff failed to report it. Subsequently, police arrested him when he sexually abused a 12-year-old boy with Intellectual Disabilities. He ended up in a county jail in a fortified white cage. (Someone should have called Dorothea Dix.) As one lawyer, ironically also named John Connolly, noted "I haven't seen an advocate in years."

Within this broader context, Boo noted several examples of inappropriate restrictive procedures. One group home company locked a man in a euphemistically termed "private treatment room" for months. A group home owner confiscated a resident's shoes to prevent him from running away in the name of "reality therapy." Tragically, one client was given pro re nata (PRN) Ativan for a medical appointment that the group home cancelled. He was so sedated that later that morning he could not even drink without assistance. The next day he died. Staff failed to call a physician. One client was restrained for making noises and asking for cookies. Another resident received two head injuries and had been physically restrained by staff whom State response inspectors described as "hostile."

Following Boo's articles in 1999, the District of Columbia issued a report on July 7, 2000 on the District's Mental Retardation and Developmental Administration, the state agency responsible for oversight of community services. The report acknowledged that elimination of monitoring services contributed to the problems and that service administrators had the knowledge of the problems, but failed to act. Even when the district was aware of these scandalous conditions, it failed to act and dodged the issue by: (a) treating the incidents as a public relations problem, (b) claiming that the problems were historical, rather than current, and (c) that they had already taken action to fix the problems. The investigation also revealed chaotic documentation of critical incidents, including four client deaths. Even though there was documentation of client deaths in some District agencies, other District agencies were unaware of the death. This poor communication between agencies was illustrated by the death of Patrick Dutch who died after staff left him in a van for 7 h in 99°heat. Group home staff assumed he had been taken to his day program and the day program assumed he had a doctor's appointment. The group home failed to ensure that their resident arrived safely at the day program and the day program failed to call the group home when Mr. Dutch failed to arrive at the day program. Only after continued public exposure concerning the inability of the District to manage its community service, did it begin to address the issues, for example, by setting up a fatality review program coordinated across all District agencies.

The problems with the District of Columbia's community services do not appear to have been resolved. In February 2006 people with mental retardation were remaining in hospital for months because of the lack of community placement (Barker 2006a). In June 2006, the District of Colombia was back in Federal court regarding abuse in its group homes and grossly inadequate medical care also contributed to client deaths (Barker 2006b). Again, the District of Columbia attempted to limit information becoming public by only issuing redacted documents and requiring *Freedom of Information Act* requests to release information to the *Washington Post.* Given the lack of available public information, it is not possible to determine the use of restraints and restrictive procedures at this time.

6.3.2.2 Georgia

In 2001, *The Atlantic Journal-Constitution* published a series of exposes on client deaths and abuse in group homes in Georgia. Physical and mechanical restraints did not feature prominently in these accounts of group homes, although pharmacological restraints did. Journalists Ken Foskett and Ann Hardie reported that state investigators had documented many cases of heavy sedation to control challenging behavior. Day program and residential staff repeatedly mentioned overmedication in the case of the death of Stephen Bennett. There were many other factors that might also have been related to his death, but the state failed to conduct an autopsy, so the cause of his death was unclear. In an earlier article, Hardie also reported sedation in many residents living in the Mi Casa group home.

This excessive sedation took place within the context of systemic problems within Georgia's group homes at the time. As with Washington DC, Georgia had closed Brook Run, a state institution, and rapidly established a network of group home providers. Unfortunately, some providers had little or no experience. For example, former managers of McDonalds and housekeepers ran group homes for working with people with complex needs. There was also a lack of regulations and oversight. For example, some group homes were unlicensed and there was no requirement to report deaths and conduct investigations or autopsies into unexpected deaths. Even when deaths occurred it took the state 15 months to implement a rule requiring reporting of deaths within 3 days of the event, and then approximately service providers reported deaths late on approximately 40 % of occasions. Absent regulation and oversight, there were many cases of abuse and neglect, staff did not attend mandated staff training and sometimes staff who had been found guilty of client abuse were rehired to work with residents with the most challenging behavior.

6.3.2.3 Connecticut

In 2001 *The Hartford Courant* published a second series of articles into deaths in community group homes in Connecticut. There was at least one death that was directly related to/restraint. Michael Sniadecki, a 25-year-old man with Intellectual Disabilities, died in a group home in Naugatuck when his head was trapped between his mattress and his bedrails. A state investigation revealed that the group home had installed the bedrails improperly. The state refused to release incident reports and autopsies, if they conducted any, so it is not possible to determine how widespread restraint-related deaths were in community services in Connecticut at the time.

As in the previously reviewed community scandals, this investigation revealed serious deficiencies in state oversight of community services, in this case specifically related to monitoring of deaths. *The Hartford Courant* revealed that the state did not investigate most deaths: In 2000, the state only referred 53 of 197 deaths for review. Ghoulishly, the state routinely sent some corpses of group home residents to a University of Connecticut pathology class for dissection in class. The physician who conducted the autopsies was unfortunately not a trained forensic pathologist and so made errors resulting in determining the causes of death of group home clients. More seriously, the state of Connecticut routinely denied release of investigations of deaths and autopsies to family members and the press, citing confidentiality of client information. *The Hartford Courant's* investigations of 774 group home deaths suggested suspicious circumstances in about one in ten cases, including deaths due to choking, medication overdoses, preventable pneumonia, falls, burns, drownings, and preventable medical conditions. Many of these circumstances point to deficiencies in staff supervision, medical and nursing services, and oversight and regulation of group homes, but it is difficult to determine the true nature and extent of these problems due to the state refusing to release most information.

6.3.2.4 Canada's Institutional and Community Services

Feldman et al. (2004) surveyed the use of formal and informal management practices in 625 persons with ID in both community and institutional services in Ontario, Canada. They found that 55 % of interventions, including highly restrictive interventions, were informal, undocumented, lacked professional input, and were unevaluated. These informal interventions included both dangerous and non-dangerous highly restrictive interventions such as PRN medication, various forms of restraint, seclusion, and even aversive conditioning. Such informal interventions were especially likely in relatively unsupervised community settings where there was no psychotropic medication or formal behavior management support plans. They concluded that most interventions, including restrictive interventions, were largely unsupervised. Although the study was conducted over 10 years ago, there is little information about the continued use of restraints in Canada's community services.

6.3.2.5 Cornwall

Following complaints from the East Cornwall Mencap Society in October 2004, the British Healthcare Commission and Commission for Social Care Inspection investigated the services for people with Intellectual Disabilities in Cornwall in 2006—some 2 years after the initial complaints. They found widespread abuse and neglect including misuse of restraint both in community group homes and in Budock Hospital. These included residential staff locking internal and external doors to prevent resident movement, removal of taps to prevent a resident flooding the house and removal of all light switches in one home so only staff could turn on the lights. Excessive restraint use included one man, who was blind and deaf, tied up 16 h a day and excessive reliance on PRN medication to control behavior. Other problems included staff physically abusing residents and, reminiscent of eighteenth century practices in asylums, the use of cold showers. The Healthcare Commission could not determine the use of restraint and PRN medication at Budock hospital due to lack of documentation and record keeping.

This excessive use of restrictive procedures took place in the context of wider mismanagement of services and organizational problems. For example, some group homes and one unit on Budock hospital were barren, lacked planned activities, failed to implement any systematic care planning of any kind, and had little or no professional input. In some parts of the service staff were largely untrained and inadequately supervised. For example, unqualified staff carried out invasive procedures, such as rectal PRN medication.

Service mangers failed to identity or respond to these problems. For example, managers sometimes failed to respond to complaints or dealt with them informally. Some managers appeared to use assigning staff to some units as punishment. Managers had not dated some policies so it was impossible to determine when these policies had been approved, implemented, and reviewed. Management had also made poor decisions. For example, it was difficult to provide staff annual compulsory training, such as training in food hygiene. Rather than improving staff training, managers changed their policy so that essential training was only required every 3 years. Record keeping by managers was poor. For example, managers were unable to provide records of critical incidents, including one where a staff member has been dismissed. Some staff worked with children without criminal background checks, even though national and local policy required these checks before they did so. Remarkably, even with oversight from The Healthcare Commission and the attention of national press service, mangers still failed to respond for many months. The Healthcare Commission wrote that "progress has not been achieved as swiftly as the Commissions, or the external team, would have like. The Commission have had to maintain an exceptional level of monitoring and surveillance and press for improvement throughout the investigation… due in part to the trust's denial of the seriousness of the situation" (p. 72).

6.3.2.6 Sutton and Merton, South London

On the heels of the Cornwall inquiry, The Health Care Commission (2007) also investigated allegations of physical and sexual abuse in National Health Service run community services for people with Intellectual Disabilities in Sutton and Merton, South London. The investigation found excessive use of restraint, no policy on the use of restraint, and no monitoring of restraint use. Staff believed they did not use restraint, however, observation of services showed in fact they did, including wheel-chair straps and splints. For example, one woman had been restraint with splint to prevent hand mouthing for many years. Once staff implemented a simple plan to increase time out of restraint its use was reduced to only 3 h per day. (One can infer that there was no treatment plan in place for hand mouthing prior to the investigation). There were also unnecessary environmental barriers in the group homes making movement in and out of the houses and around the houses difficult for residents in wheelchairs, thereby restricting resident mobility.

The Health Care Commission made extensive commentary on services for challenging behavior. They noted a lack of basic preventative strategies, lack of interaction between staff and residents, lack of client choice, even over whether or not to have sugar in one's tea, and rigid routines set for staff convenience. Staff turnover was high and the homes used agency staff a lot. Many staff did not know that the residents and old staff continued to engage in custodial rather than individualized care. There were environmental restrictions, such as high door handles that limited client access to their own bedrooms. Although some staff training had taken place as many staff members had not been trained. Staff who had been trained stated that they had to use restraints because de-escalation techniques were ineffective. Observations during the audit indicated that staff continues the use of restraints, such as pushing a client back into their seat. Staff also used PRN medication to control behavior, but The Commission did not report details of this. A record review found that one client had been restrained in a chair 33 times for 10–15 min, but sometimes up to 30 min without efforts to de-escalate prior to use of the restraint. When staff revised the client's care plan to eliminate this practice the restraint was no longer needed. A third resident was strapped to his wheelchair because he picked things off the floor. There was no indication of the degree of danger of this behavior and not any indication of whether less restrictive interventions could be used. These observations suggest that staff were inadequately trained to manage client behavior using simple preventative strategies and that the care plan was inappropriate because it included an unnecessary and ineffective restrictive procedure that was easily eliminated. For example, only a quarter of staff had received training on "manual handling" (p. 57), but the descriptions of training did not describe any examples of staff training on positive behavior management strategies.

The report contained details of several serious incidents, several of which included client to client injuries due to aggression. These included a client attacking two other residents resulting in bruising to the other client's face. This was a repeat of an earlier incident that had also resulted in a client injury. One man bit another client requiring treatment in the emergency room. Although meetings took place on these incidents, sometimes to attempt to place the clients concerned in other services, there was no indication that services took appropriate action such as retraining staff, conducting a functional assessment or developing a positive behavior support plan to address these problems.

These problems with restraint took place in the context of broader problems, such as lack of client community activities, poor client engagement, lack of person centered planning, insufficiently available professional services, and client physical and sexual abuse. There had been a lack of staff training and supervision, low staffing levels, and low morale. Additionally, there had been significant management problems including high turnover in senior managers and several reorganizations of services one after another leading to fragmentation of services. This resulted in poor management of services and poor service coordination. Interestingly, service managers did have access to information about behavioral incidents and staff and resident injuries, including injuries from restraints; however, there was no indication that they took any effective action based on these data.

6.3.2.7 Norfolk, the UK

There were similar findings in St Luke's Hospital, Norfolk, a privately run service for adolescents with Intellectual Disabilities in 2006 in which staff used restraint excessively and failed to adequately document restraint use (Care Quality Commission 2012). There is only limited information on this incident publically available at this time.

6.3.2.8 New York State

In 2007, Johnathon Carey, a 13-year-old teenager with autism, was killed in restraint by a residential staff in the back of a van while the driver continued driving and failed to intervene to protect Johnathon (Hakim 2011a). The staff who restrained him has worked for 15 consecutive days, had a history of previous allegations of abuse against Johnathon and had a conviction for selling marijuana. The driver had been fired by four previous jobs working with people with developmental disabilities. The state settled two lawsuits with the family for $ 5 million.

Subsequently, Hakim (2011b) published a series of articles in the *New York Times,* which were highly reminiscent of the earlier scandals in Washington DC and Georgia, revealing wide spread abuse and neglect and failure from the New York State Office of Persons with Developmental Disabilities to protect residents of nearly 2000 group homes from harm. Problems included the state failing to investigate in a timely fashion, substantiating few allegations, unions successfully protecting staff from disciplinary actions, the state reassigning staff rather than reporting them to the police for assault or rape, failure to fire staff, probable victimization and retaliation against whistle blowers. Consequently, the two state commissioners resigned, most allegations were turned over to the police and New York State Office of Persons with Developmental Disabilities underwent significant reform. The state governor Cuomo then commissioned a report (Sundram 2011) which reviewed the state's procedures into abuse and neglect across multiple agencies and found numerous inconsistencies in definitions of abuse and neglect, reporting requirement, failure to track allegations in some agencies, and training requirements for staff to investigate abuse and neglect. Special education regulations were extremely weak providing few protections to children.

6.3.2.9 Winterbourne

After a former nurse approached the BBC, the BBC sent an undercover reporter who was hired as a direct care staff into Winterbourne View, a privately operated hospital opened in 2006 by Castlebeck, a private for profit corporation. Subsequently, he covertly videotaped widespread neglect and abuse, including misuse of restraint including staff engaging in verbal abuse, threatening residents, slapping residents in the face, pulling their hair, dragging them out of bed, pulling their hair and physically restraining them, and restraining them using furniture. Following broadcast of the TV program by Panorama in May 2011, 12 staff were found guilty in court, six were sentenced to prison, two nurses lost their licenses, and two city employees responsible for monitoring abuse and neglect were fired. A subsequent newspaper report *(Winterbourne View: Earlier abuse at hospital* 2012) revealed that previously a Winterbourne staff punched out a resident's front teeth and although this had been reported to police, they declined to investigate it or reopen the investigation in the light of the subsequent events. The concerned nurse had been suspended and then reinstated. Further investigations revealed multiple reports to the local city and police of potential abuse and neglect. Castlebeck was broken-up and then sold to other private companies (*Timeline: Winterbourne View abuse scandal* 2012).

In response, the government conducted an investigation, entitled *Transforming Care,* (Department of Health 2012) which concluded that many people with Intellectual Disabilities had been misplaced in hospitals for many years and the report recommended their removal to community settings by June 2014. They found 588 recorded restraints between 2010 and the first quarter of 2011 for a rate of 1.2 restraints per day; one person was restrained 45 times in 3 months. There were also numerous indications of serious problems that went unheeded by Castlebeck management, the police, and the local city, including 78 emergency hospital visits, 29 calls to the police, and 27 allegations to the local city of staff assaults on residents. These problems took place in the context of expensive, yet overall poor quality of services, such as lack of client activities, high staff turnover, and lack of staff training. There was also a failure to meet licensing requirements and failure to enforce licensing requirement, for example, the Care Quality Commission, the government entity responsible for national quality assurance, acknowledged that is failed to respond to whistle blower reports of abuse and neglect. (The Care Quality Commission has been widely criticized in the media for "nourishing obscurity," not conducting a sufficient number of inspections, misreporting the number of inspections carried out to parliament, ignoring whistle blowers, and disbanding effective investigation teams.)

This lead to a national reduction of 35% people with ID living in hospitals by 2013. This had been done mostly by placement of people who were older and easier to manage (Glover et al. 2014). No data have been published as to whether the restraints or abuse have reduced or quality of life has improved due to these moves.

The Winterbourne scandal highlights a number of issues related to contemporary British services for people with Intellectual Disabilities related to restraint. First, even in small, private facilities there are services with high levels of abusive use of restraint. This echoes the finding that a minority of British community services continues to use restraint on a regular basis (Sturmey 2009). Second, there is insufficient oversight of restrictive behavior management practices from both responsible local and national government agencies and local service boards. This results in poor quality services, such as lack of client activity, choice and autonomy, lack of staff training, lack of FBA's and behavior support plans, lack of client skills training, and ambiguity over use and reporting of restraint and abuse in geographically dispersed services run by multiple agencies and monitored by different uncoordinated government entities. At least four surveys of British services (Deveau and McGill 2007; Murphy et al. 2001; McGill et al. 2009; Murphy et al. 2003) reported that British services for adults with Intellectual Disabilities often have policies or are "working on" policies, may have some approved form of personal restraints, and may have some form of staff training in place within the organization, but service quality was poor. For example, the most recent survey (Deveau and McGill 2007) found that only 54% of organizations who responded to their survey had a physical intervention policy that 27% of new staff had to wait for training, a quarter of organizations did not include any monitoring of physical interventions quality and of those using physical interventions, only a quarter reported using applied behavior analysis in any way. These data are very liberal. For example, the survey only asked if there was *any* quality assurance monitoring, but did not evaluate if it met any specific standards or was effective, neither did the survey validate the participants self-reports.

6.3.2.10 Áras Attracta Centre, Republic of Ireland

At the time of writing, newspapers began reporting another community scandal reminiscent of Winterbourne at Áras Attracta Centre, Republic of Ireland. Again, following funding cuts to community services, a whistle blower contacted the media. The media placed an undercover investigator into the home who recorded both verbal and physical abuse, such as slapping and forced feeding, and a female staff dragging a woman with Intellectual Disabilities across the floor like a rag doll or object. Some staff have been suspended and the matter is being investigated. The issue has received national coverage in the republic of Ireland where the government is responsible for oversight of these services.

6.3.2.11 Summary

Excessive and abuse use of restraint continues to this day both in institutional and community settings alike. Indeed, as government-run institutions have largely closed in many countries, the provision of community service raises special challenges. These include monitoring hundreds or something thousands of geographically dispersed service units run by a complex network of state, for profit and not for profit providers. Often such community service providers face challenges such as the temptations to make money of otherwise feather the nests of administrative staff and owners; cutting services while keeping clients safe during funding cuts; working with some clients who are highly challenging; having a largely untrained and often unsupervised workforce in geographically dispersed settings; limited availability of professional support and training; and lack of effective management systems to run current community services.

6.3.3 Nursing Homes

6.3.3.1 Leas Cross, Ireland

Following an unusually high number of deaths between 2002 and 2005 at Leas Cross nursing home, the Irish government set up an inquiry. The report (O'Neill 2006) found grossly inadequate documentation of all care from admission to discharge and death. This included "alarming" use of restraint, preventable injuries, poor restraint policy, a failure to comply with professional standards, failure to inform the coroner of deaths, cursory attempts to obtain or document consent, and almost no documentation of bed rails. There was little evidence of implementation of written policy or oversight of that policy and poor or no staff training and poor staff supervision. As noted in other such examples, the inquiry reported inadequate service funding at a time of rapid privatization of state services.

6.3.3.2 Deaths in Bedrails

The US Consumer Product Commission is widely concerned with product safety related to restraints including restraint devises in products for children, such as strollers, child seats, restraints in rides in amusement parks, and restraints in vehicles, such as car seat restraints among other products that involve restraints. Following complaints from families concerning deaths of older people in nursing homes restrained in bed rails the Consumer Product Safety Commission (2012). Their review identified 531 deaths from bed rails in the USA from 1985 to 2013. Ninety-three percent of deaths related to people being trapped in the rails and 7 % were due to falls. Eighty-three percent of victims were aged over 60 years, most (61 %) occurred at home and only 16 % occurred in nursing homes and the most common disabilities were cardiovascular diseases (15 %) and Alzheimer's disease (12 %).

6.4 Police and Restraint-Related Deaths

There have been a number of reports of deaths in restraint and seclusion during police arrests, especially involving people with mental illness, Intellectual Disabilities or autism, custody and during detention of immigrants, and when bouncers from bars or clubs restraint customers. For example, *The Guardian* reported that at least ten children and adults with autism had died in restraint in British police custody (Roberts 2013).

In the USA, Eric Garner died in New York allegedly from choke hold restraint by police after saying "I cannot breath" 11 times. The police attempted to arrest him for selling cigarettes on the street. Video of the incident was widely disseminated[3]. Many people believe that the choke hold was expressly forbidden by police policies. Subsequently, a grand jury failed to indict the officer resulting in worldwide protests concerning the restraint-related death and lack of legal protection. Four days earlier, Ronald Singleton, 45, died in restraint while was also detained by New York police on July 13, 2014.

6.5 Immigration Services

Jimmy Mubenga, a Nigerian national, died during physical restraint on board a plane at Heathrow airport during detention proceedings. Three guards working for G4S, a private for profit security company, restrained him for more than 30 min. During that time he cried out that he could not breathe and that he was going to die. The staff used an unapproved "head down" method of restraint with his hands

[3] https://www.youtube.com/watch?v=dj7czohj-3o

handcuffed behind his back and used racist language. This practice was known by staff as "carpet Karaoke" because the detainee was "made to sing to the carpet."

Four years later, the British Crown prosecution service had failed to prosecute anyone, even though an inquest had ruled his death to be unlawful. The Coroner was critical of the quality of the staff training given to these staff as it failed to provide training in the contexts in which they used restraint—in limited spaces on board planes—and the prohibitions against use of dangerous restraint were ineffective. In 2014, charges of manslaughter were finally brought against the three guards. During the trial the guards denied forcing him into a seat and pinning him down, although other witnesses did recall this. The guards were found not guilty in December 2014 (*G4S guards cleared over Jimmy Mubenga death* 2014).

In 2014, the British Home office's Independent Panel on Non-Compliance Management reported that detainees were escorted with force during, 13 %, 13 %, 11 %, 10 %, 10 %, and 6 % of removals during 2008, 2009, 2010, 2011, 2012, and 2013 respectively (Shaw 2014). These forcible escorts mostly occurred during the removal to a plane immediately before deportation or on the plane and staff from privately run security companies who had contract with the government to conduct the escorts. The Independent Panel on Non-Compliance Management made recommendations to replace the old system of restraints, approve certain forms of mechanical restraint, and to improve the quality of training escort staff receive.

Detention of immigrants in Australia has received considerable negative press over recent years. As part of these broad concerns several reports have evidenced prolonged and illegal detention and use of unnecessary mechanical and chemical restraints (Williams 1998).

6.6 Bouncers

In 2010, the BBC reported that bouncers must have mandatory training on restraint (Reed 2010). The BBC reported that about half of bouncers had been attacked in the previous year and approximately 90 % had been attacked in the previous 5 years. There had been at least ten deaths and severe injuries, such as broken necks, related to bouncers restraining members of the public. The exact number is probably much higher as there is no systematic data collection.

There is extensive press controversy surrounding these restraint-related deaths in similar kinds of contexts. No systematic data exist, however, other than data on escorts during detention, on the extent of application of restraint and restraint-related injuries and death.

6.7 Psychiatric Hospitals

Restraint-related deaths continue to this day in psychiatric hospitals. The death in four-point restraint of a Joshua Messier, psychiatric patient Bridgewater psychiatric hospital in 2009 near Boston, was caught on security camera[4] (Rezendes 2014a). The guards were ruled to have used an inappropriate form of restraint known colloquially as "suit casing" which involved compressing the man's chest on his knees. They were found to be inadequately trained. At first this death was ruled by the state medical examiner to be a homicide. The state attorney general subsequently declined to prosecute and three of the four guards continued to work at the facility. Subsequently, restraint use increased at the facility (Rezendes 2014b). Restraints were recently implicated in a total of three deaths (Rezendes 2014c) including one case of an individual restraint 23 h a day for 16 months. Following these deaths, the state awarded a contract to continue providing services to the same private corporation that had been running the facility while these restraint-related deaths occurred, perhaps in part because the facility superintendent was a member of the panel selecting state providers for that contract. Although the facility violated many state rules, the state imposed few fines and when it did, reduced many of them (Rezendes 2014c).

6.8 Families and Foster Parents

6.8.1 Parents Keep Child with Autism in Cages

Periodically the media reports that parents keep their children with disabilities in cages at home. This continues recently. For example, in Vancouver in 2011, two children with autism were found kept behind a "cage-like door" in a room with darkened windows by their two parents. The children did not attend school (Njus 2011). In 2013, the parents of a 6-year-old child with autism in Missouri were charged with keeping their child in a cage, in the basement, in filthy conditions. The child was found in its own urine and feces. The local newspaper alleged that they hid the cage from local service staff when they visited. Children were prevented from moving by installing the door knobs backwards. As of 2013, the parents were charged with endangering the welfare of a child (Held 2013). A similar report was published on July 12, 2014 in which parents kept their 11-year-old autistic son in a dog cage. The parents were Vietnamese immigrants and their son had limited communication and significant behavior problems, and it was unclear how long his parents had kept him there (Wagner 2014). His parents were charged with child endangerment and false imprisonment. In Wakemen, Ohio, police found 11 children

[4] http://www.bostonglobe.com/news/local/massachusetts/2014/02/15/bridgewater-state-hospital-surveillance-video-joshua-messier-restraint-and-death/VxHidCOaYM2KfVrB9ciw2J/story.html.

with various disabilities including autism kept in cages by two adults who were the adoptive or foster parents with the children. The children were removed to group homes and the adult charged with child endangerment *(Authorities Find 11 Children Locked in Cages, undated).*

These incidents are from a nonsystematic search of the World Wide Web and doubtless there are others that might be identified from a more systematic search of local and state newspapers. In such incidents it is worth asking why the parents resorted to such practices and what support, if any, they received from local educational and other services prior to the discovery.

6.9 Conclusions

These contemporary scandals are found in numerous different types of services and in different countries. They share several common features. First, oversight and regulation by external agencies was often lacking or deficient. This allowed services to drift into bad practice and for that bad practice to go undetected or, when that bad practice was evident local state agencies failed to respond to it. Indeed, in many cases local oversight agencies were ponderously slow to respond. They often avoided corrective actions by not fining service providers when they could have, maintaining administrators in positions of authority when they failed to take corrective action. They even implicitly rewarded poor performance by promoting staff who had restrained and killed clients and awarded contracts to service providers after restraint-related deaths. Second, often, only when problems became public, local agencies and sometimes unions often denied or minimized the problems by describing the incidents as isolated incidents or where there were clear problems with staff, describing them as isolated bad apples. Thus, by minimizing and apparently containing the problem, they were able to avoid taking system-wide action. Third, in many cases documentation of client care was often absent, incomplete, lost, and possibly hidden or destroyed by providers and/or state agencies. In some cases, state agencies did everything they could to not release documentation even when the person themselves of their legally authorized guardian requested such action. Again, by doing so, state agencies delay or avoid having to deal with difficult service reform. Fourth, staff training and performance was commonly an issue in these scandals. This was sometimes true at all levels of organizations. Often direct care staff did not know how to keep clients safe, how to prevent behavioral incidents that resulted in restrictive procedures, how to restrain safely, how to document, and how to recognize and respond to medical emergencies, etc. Fifth, supervisors and group home managers sometimes lacked basic management skills and sometimes used inappropriate methods with clients and their staff. In some incidents professional staff, including physicians, nurses, and psychologists, failed to take action when they should have or lacked the competencies to treat their clients effectively. Sixth, there were also examples of supervisors and/or state agencies engaging in retribution against whistle blowers. Such actions send a clear message that some organizations are more interested in maintaining good appearances and minimizing negative publicity and place this above the lives of the people they allegedly serve. Seventh, senior service managers and state officials often failed to institute and use basic oversight and data tracking systems, or when the information was indeed available failed to take appropriate action. Finally, government and legislative response to such scandals was often delayed by years and woefully inadequate when it arrived.

This chapter makes depressing reading. There are islands of excellence, some of which will be described in Chap. 11, but the evidence that restraint, seclusion, and restrictive behavioral procedures continues unabated with many vulnerable populations is clear. Individual clinicians and administrators, individual services, and sometimes even individual government agencies have reduced restraint and seclusion. Some are models of what can be done. Sadly, most of these positive examples represent reaction to outside pressure, such as changes in regulations combined with negative consequences, whistle blowers and media scandal, or are the result of quasi-heroic practitioners acting on their own, despite their supervisors and organization rather than because of them. There is evidence that despite all these attempts to regulate restraint and seclusion that restraint-related deaths continue. The most recent review of restraint-related deaths (Quip for Quality 2011) reported a further 61 deaths during the period 1999–2005. These deaths occurred in a wide range of people–people with disabilities, children and youth and seniors—in nursing homes, wilderness camps, group homes, private residences, and general and psychiatric hospitals.

Too few services take the initiative to reduce restraint. We have failed to learn from John Conolly. More accurately, most people cannot be bothered to learn from John Conolly.

Part II
Interventions

Previous chapters have described the nature, correlates, and extent of restrictive behavior management practices in various populations and contexts. The next section goes on to consider interventions to reduce restrictive behavior management practices. The two most commonly used ones are those based on applied behavior analysis and organizational interventions, although there are also a range of others interventions. Those based on applied behavior analysis are based on learning theory, principally operant conditioning. These treatments have mostly been researched with people with Intellectual Disabilities, although applied behavior analysis has been applied to a much wider range of problems and populations. Naturally, applied behavior analysis have been applied most commonly where there are few other treatment options, that is severe aggression and self-injurious behavior and aggression in people with severe and profound Intellectual Disabilities. On the other hand, organizational interventions have used a wide range of interventions—some assembled intuitively and some using the principles of applied behavior analysis. Organizational interventions often include goal setting, staff and family member education, feedback, and other components. These interventions attempt to address reduction in restraint, and PRN medications and have often been used in nursing homes and larger residential facilities, such as psychiatric hospitals and youth facilities, as well as dispersed community mental health and intellectual disability services.

Chapter 7
Applied Behavior Analysis: General Characteristics

The most prolific approach to understanding and treating behavioral problems that often result in restrictive behavior management practices is applied behavior analysis. Applied behavior analysis is derived from basic research on learning called experimental analysis of behavior. Experimental analysis of behavior seeks to understand the science of learning without regard to its applications. Hence, the experimental analysis of behavior often studies arbitrary responses, such as pecking and bar pressing, in organisms such as pigeons and rats in highly controlled environments, such as Skinner boxes, designed to control extraneous influences on behavior for the purposes of demonstrating clear experimental manipulation of behavior. In contrast, applied behavior analysis focuses on problems of social significance, such as education, pollution, and drug addiction in which the responses are of social importance, the intervention methods are socially valued, the change agents are typical other people in the natural environment, and issues such as generalization and maintenance of behavior are of prime importance, not after thoughts.

Although much applied behavior analysis research has been done with children with disabilities and typical children, it has also addressed the needs of a wide range of populations including older adults, youth with emotional disabilities and at risk for delinquency, and a wide range of psychiatric disorders (Sturmey 2007). Applied behavior analysis emphasizes the influence of the current environment on behavior and the lawful, functional relationship between behavior and the environment. Pre-intervention assessments, which identify these controlling variables, form the basis of subsequent interventions, which should focus on increasing appropriate behavior that serves the same function as the target behavior. The agents of change are natural caregivers—family members and carestaff—living and working in the target person's typical environment. This chapter describes the general characteristics of applied behavior analysis and how they are applied to understanding restrictive behavior management practices and related phenomena, such as self-restraint, shown by some individuals who self-injure.

Functional assessment and analysis are not only about the behavior of the person who is restrained but also about the person who administers restrictive behavior

P. Sturmey, *Reducing Restraint and Restrictive Behavior Management Practices*,
Autism and Child Psychopathology Series, DOI 10.1007/978-3-319-17569-0_7

management practices. Functional analysis should also determine which environmental variables influence the caregiver to apply or refrain from applying restraints and what variables influence if caregivers implement other preventative and treatment strategies. The next chapter takes the ideas of functional analysis described in this chapter and extends them to the development of function-based interventions to prevent the use of restrictive behavior management practices.

Functional assessment and analysis focus on variables in the current environment. These include antecedent stimuli and consequences and their relationship to behavior. Antecedents include immediate antecedents that in the past have been associated with predictable reinforcement or punishment; it is sometimes useful to think of them as like red and green traffic lights for behavior. A second kind of antecedents stimuli are more distant in time and account for the motivation of behavior. They are known as establishing operations. Establishing operations include reinforcer deprivation, reinforcer satiation, and aversive stimulation. Establishing operations have two effects on behavior. They change the reinforcing value of a consequence at a particular moment in time and also elicit behavior that has been reinforced in similar situation in the past. For example, when highly deprived of water, water temporarily becomes a much more reinforcing consequence—we pay more money and walk further to obtain a drink. Also, we emit behavior that in the past was reinforced by water, such as looking for water. Consequences include reinforcer that strengthen future behavior and punishes that weaken future behavior. "Positive reinforcer" refers to stimuli that are presented after the response and "negative reinforcers" refer to stimuli removed following a response. Reinforcers are only defined by their effects on behavior, not whether we believe someone "likes" them. Thus, food can function as a positive or negative reinforcer depending upon level of deprivation or satiation and could function as a positive punisher in some situations. Removal of aversive stimuli, such as noise or social demands may function as negative reinforcers. Likewise, "positive punishers" refer to stimuli presented after the behavior, and "negative punishers" refers to removal of stimuli that weaken the behavior. For example, presentation of painful stimuli and removal of positive stimuli often function as positive and negative punishers, respectively. The ratio of responses required to obtain the reinforcer or punisher is called a schedule of reinforcement.

Schedules of reinforcement and punishment for specific behavior do not operate in a vacuum. Even Skinner's pigeon in a Skinner box can choose to peck the disk for grain if it is hungry, take a walk, and ruffle its feathers or defecate to terminate discomfort. Thus, current behavior is the outcomes of the antecedents and consequences that influence many classes of behavior concurrently (Cooper et al. 2007; Skinner 1953).

7.1 Functions of Restraint

It is tempting to assume that restraint is an aversive stimulus that when applied contingent on aggression or self-injurious behavior functions as a positive punisher. Although there are many papers that have shown this, the functional analysis of restraint is more complex. Two common situations illustrate this. The first is the relatively brief and low-frequency application of a restraint contingent on aggression or self-injury. The second is the long-term use of restraint to prevent severe self-injurious behavior or life-threatening behavior problems, such as pica, in which the person is restrained most or almost all of the day.

In the first situation, the application of restraint may result in several kinds of consequences. These might include discomfort and pain directly from the restraints or when other people physically handle the client while applying the restraints and/or when attempting to ensure client safety. The application of restraints also limits movement and some behavior, which previously could be emitted, is no longer possible. This may result in the loss of potential reinforcers, for example, a client may no longer be able to access preferred stimuli, such as TV, or avoid non-preferred stimuli, such as requests or interactions with staff. Over time the application of restraint may also be paired with other consequences, which may change the consequent functions of the restraints. Thus, restraints may function as both positive punishers (Wallace et al. 1999) and negative reinforcers (Favell et al. 1978; Foxx and Dufrense 1984).

Restraints may also have other functions. Restraints may function as discriminative stimuli for a variety of behavior. The presentation of restraints, prior to their actual application, may occasion a variety of relevant behavior, such as attempts to escape the restraints or reductions in the target behavior or approaches. The presentation of restraints may also sometimes be paired with other relevant stimuli, such as verbal warning, which too may influence client behavior. Further, since restraints may involve lack of access to preferred stimuli, their application over time may, under certain circumstances, increase the reinforcing value of other stimuli, such as regaining access to preferred stimuli.

Some clients engage in both self-injurious behavior and self-restraint, such as sitting on their hands and wrapping their arms in their own or other people's clothing, and holding onto other people and/or objects. Often engaging in self-restraint appears to avoid self-injurious behavior and avoid other consequences, such as engaging in programmatic or interactional demands or restraint. Often interventions to reduce aggression and self-injurious behavior and restraint also attempt to reduce self-restraint, as it may interfere with treatment and reduces interaction.

Most empirical research has focused on the consequence functions of restraint and on the functions of self-restraint. There has been little empirical research on the discriminative stimulus and establishing operation functions of restraint.

7.1.1 Consequence Functions

Numerous papers have shown that contingent restraint may reduce aggression, self-injurious behavior, and a range of other maladaptive behavior. For example, Harris' (1996) review of restraint identified 25 treatment reports involving 32 studies with 73 participants with Intellectual Disabilities published between 1974 and 1994. He concluded that "...when personal restraint is applied contingently...it does result in significant reduction in the frequency of the target behaviour" (p. 117). This conclusion supports the possibility that restraint may function as a positive punisher.

Harris, however, noted that mechanisms other than positive punishment might also explain the efficacy of contingent restraint. When caregivers apply restraint, the person is unable to engage in much behavior, and restraint limits their access to positive and negative reinforcers. Thus, a restraint might also reduce behavior through timeout. Further, to the extent that restraint eliminated the reinforcer(s) maintaining the target behavior, restraint might also function as a form of extinction. These alternate explanations of the reductive effects of restraint may be distinguishable. First, if restraint functions as a positive punisher, there should be an immediate and rapid suppression of the target behavior and perhaps an increase in other responses (Cooper et al. 2007). Alternatively, if restraint is a form of extinction, then researchers should be able to observe behavior changes associated with extinction including: (a) behavior reducing more gradually, rather than immediate response suppression; (b) some of the so-called side effects of extinction, such as an extinction burst, the "emotional" side effects of extinction, such as aggression; and (c) increased response variability (Cooper et al. 2007). Although the literature has acknowledged these alternate explanations of the reductive effects of restraint, few studies have attempted to investigate them.

Two studies have evaluated a methodology to identify the positive punishment versus extinction effects of one form of restraint—response blocking. Lerman and Iwata (1996) argued that varying the schedule on which response are blocked would demonstrate the function of response blocking. For example, if one blocked every fourth response and if blocking functioned as a positive punisher, this would be an FR-4[1] punishment schedule. Alternatively, if blocking functioned as extinction by preventing the reinforcer maintaining the problem behavior, then the schedule would be an FR-1.3 positive reinforcement schedule. Thus, the positive punishment hypothesis predicts that richer schedules of blocking should be associated with immediate response suppression, and as the schedule is thinned, this affect might attenuate. Alternatively, if blocking functions as extinction, then thinning the schedule results in a progressively greater proportion of the responses being reinforced, and the response should increase initially until the schedule becomes so thin that responding gradually declines, a phenomenon known as "ratio strain."

Lerman and Iwata (1996) examined the effects of various schedules of response blocking on hand mouthing in Paul, a 32-year-old man with profound Intellectual Dis-

[1] A Fixed Ratio (FR) schedule of reinforcement or punishment is one in which the consequence is delivered every *n*th response.

abilities, living in an institutional setting. This experiment compared a no-intervention baseline, blocking each response, blocking every second, every third, or every fourth response. A functional analysis[2] (Iwata et al. 1982) indicated that automatic reinforcement maintained hand mouthing. During response blocking sessions, Paul sat in a chair with no interactions from other people and no materials available. The therapist sat behind Paul and blocked responses on the assigned schedule by placing her palm 2 cm in front of Paul's mouth, but the therapist did not permit Paul from attempting to hand mouth. In baseline, when there was no response blocking, Paul emitted approximately 0.5–4.5 responses/min. When the therapist implemented response blocking on an FR-1 schedule, hand mouthing reduced to near-zero levels immediately. Reintroduction of baseline resulted in a large increase in the rate of hand mouthing. In all subsequent blocking sessions, hand mouthing remained low, even on an FR-4 schedule. Lerman and Iwata (1992) interpreted these data as showing that response blocking functioned as a positive punisher.

Smith et al. (1999) reported contrasting results when they compared the effects of different schedule values of response blocking on eye poking in Louise, a 41-year-old woman with developmental disabilities and chronic eye poking. Smith et al. compared the effects of blocking each eye poke, half, two-thirds, or four-fifths of all responses. During baselines, Louise's rates of eye poking remained low and stable at approximately 1.1–1.6/min. The FR-1 schedule produced a gradual decrease in the rate of eye poking in which eye poking gradually reduced from approximately 1.5/min in early session to approximately 0.4–0.1/min in the very last sessions. During intermittent schedules, the mean rates of eye poking were 1.9 and 2.3/min when blocking every second and two-thirds of all responses. When the therapist blocked four-fifths of responses, the rate of eye poking was initially high (2.33/min) and gradually reduced to near-zero rates in the final session. Smith et al. argued that in this case, response blocking functioned as a sensory extinction procedure because (a) eye poking reduced gradually, rather than rapidly; (b) eye poking increased slightly during intermittent schedules of blocking; (c) there was evidence of extinction bursts during continuous blocking and blocking of four-fifths of responses; and (d) there was evidence of ratio strain, such as bursts of high rates of responding and breaks in responding, when the therapist blocked a large proportion of responses (Cooper et al. 2007). Thus, Smith et al. concluded that response blocking functioned as a form of sensory extinction.

In both of these studies response blocking reduced behavior, but it appears that response blocking did so by different mechanisms. In Lerman and Iwata (1996), response blocking appeared to function as a positive punisher, and in Smith et al., it appeared to function as extinction of a response maintained by an automatic reinforcement. Smith et al. noted that these finding has significant practical implications. Since punishment procedures can often be effective using intermittent schedules and sometimes on quite thin schedules (Lerman and Iwata 1996), treatment

[2] A functional analysis involves a systematic, experimental manipulation of the environment, whereas a functional assessment only described the current environment, but does not manipulate it.

integrity is of less concern, because if caregivers fail to consequate a response, there is probably little harm done. Similarly, the effort required by caregivers to implement the procedure effectively and safely can be relatively modest. In contrast, if response blocking is a form of sensory extinction, then caregivers have little room for error since any failure to apply response blocking might function as intermittent automatic positive reinforcement and may maintain or increase the target behavior. In this case, treatment integrity may be paramount and effortful, and perhaps such treatments routine caregivers cannot implement them effectively and safely.

7.1.2 Restraints Sometimes Increase Problem Behavior

A second function of restraints is that they may function as positive reinforcers. This may seem paradoxical since, at first sight, one may assume that restraints are aversive stimuli; however, it is not unusual to see some clients with Intellectual Disabilities who ask, point to, and approach their restraint devices, and there are many interventions using restraint that fail to reduce or even increase the target behavior. Hence, the possibility that restraint function as positive reinforcers is worthy of consideration.

Favell et al. (1978) reported three experiments evaluating whether restraint might function as a positive reinforcer. In the first two experiments, they treated self-injurious behavior in three children and adults with severe and profound Intellectual Disabilities. They had informally noted that these participants appeared to enjoy restraints in that they attempted to restrain themselves, appeared calm and happy in restraints, resisted their removal, and became agitated and unhappy when out of restraints. All participants had exhibited self-injurious behavior for many years, and multiple behavioral and other treatments had been ineffective resulting in the clients remaining restrained continuously or almost continuously.

One intervention will be used to illustrate this approach to treatment. Tim, aged 8 years, banged his head and slapped his face. He declined participation in programming and had remained in his bedroom for 2 months, and staff restrained his hands with wrist ties. His self-injurious behavior had resulted in opened sores and bruises, and he was in danger of brain damage from his self-injurious behavior. During the first ten treatment sessions staff said "Tim, get in bed" and restrained him on his bed for 3.5 min contingent upon 3 min of no self-injurious behavior. Staff did not interact with him during restraint. Treatment sessions were 10–42 min in duration. The experimenters used a reversal design. In the first baseline, Tim emitted self-injurious behavior between 30 and 100 % of intervals. During the first treatment phase, he emitted self-injurious behavior during almost no intervals. A brief two-session reversal phase resulted in self-injurious behavior being emitted during 100 % of intervals, and during the final treatment phase, he again emitted self-injurious behavior at near-zero levels. During that final treatment phase, the reinforcement interval was systematically increased from 3 min to 1 h over 14 sessions. The experimenters also faded the restraints by (a) releasing him when he tugged at the restraints so that restraints only lasted 30 s–2.5 min instead of 3.5 min and (b) only placing him on his bed without restraint during the last eight sessions. The experimenters ended contingent access to his bed by the end of 3 months. The experimenters found similar results with two other participants, although details of the treatment packages and restraint-fading procedures varied from person to person.

Further evidence that restraints may function as a positive reinforcer came from experiment 3, which evaluated whether contingent restraint could increase some arbitrary response—placing a marble in a hole in a box. Peg, one of the participants from the earlier experiments, participated. There were three conditions: baseline, intervention, and control. During baseline, the experimenter placed a marble in front of Peg and said her name. If Peg did not place the marble in the hole after 5 s, the experimenter removed the marble. The experimenter prompted Peg to put the marble in the hole during three trials of the first four baseline sessions. The therapist also touched Peg's wrists and arms continually in baseline sessions as a control for the effects of physical touch. Intervention sessions were the same as baseline except the therapist places arm splints on Peg's arms for 30 s after each correct response. After a correct response in the control condition, the experimenter delayed the next new trial by 30 s, but did not apply arm splints. This procedure controlled for the effects of delaying the new trial which was embedded within the intervention condition. During the first baseline, the mean proportion of correct responses was 7.9 % (range 0–33 %), and this increased to 93.7 % during the first treatment condition. Correct responses were consistently low during all the subsequent baseline a1l control conditions and were near 100 % in two subsequent intervention conditions.

The effectiveness of the two intervention experiments combined with the demonstration that contingent restraint increased some arbitrary response led Favell et al. to conclude that restraint did indeed function as a positive reinforcer. Subsequently, several other studies led to similar conclusions (Favell et al. 1981; Foxx and Dufrense 1984; Magee and Ellis 2001; Rooker and Roscoe 2005).

7.1.3 Antecedent Functions

The presence or removal of restraints may function as a discriminative stimulus for behavior. For example, in cases of chronic self-injury where the person is restrained more or less continuously, it is not uncommon to observe that when restrained, the person remains calm and does not attempt to self-injure. When attempts are made to remove the restraints or they are actually removed, then the person may become agitated and immediately begin to self-injure. Once the person sees that the restraints are being returned, they may begin to calm down and self-injure less, and the presence of the restraints may result in other behavior, such as reaching for the restraints. Thus, anecdotally, restraints appear to exert strong antecedent control over several relevant behaviors.

7.1.4 Summary

These studies discussed in the preceding section demonstrate the restraint may have a function as positive punishers, extinction of automatically reinforced responses, and as positive reinforcers. These findings have several implications. First, restraints have several functions, and one cannot assume that restraints are punishing stimuli. The application of restraints may have harmful effects in that they may reinforce the target behavior that intervention intends to reduce. Thus, clinicians must evaluate intervention programs using restraints and the emergency use of restraints cautiously. Thus, even when service providers rightly use restraint in an emergency to protect a client, peers, or caregivers from harm, this short-term plan must be supplemented by immediate and effective action to reduce the challenging behavior that resulted in these restrictive proactive, and to reduce the use of restraints. Second, understanding the functions of restraint and incorporating this information into treatment plans have important implications for the treatment design. For example, two studies on the different functions of response blocking had implications both for how response blocking might work and for which treatment plans might be practical in a real-world setting. Finally, research has focused on only a limited aspect of the functions of restraints, namely, the consequence functions of restraint. Other aspects of the functions of restraints, such as their establishing operation and discriminative stimuli functions may well be quite important. For example, restraint-fading procedures (see Chap. 9) are based on the assumptions that restraints act as discriminative stimuli for the absence of the target behavior and the absence of restraints function as discriminative stimuli for the target behavior; however, little research has focused on this. Similarly, it may be possible that time in restraint acts as an establishing operation for various relevant reinforcers. For example, if restraints are aversive stimuli, then time in restraint may be an important establishing operation in increasing the value of removal of restraint as a negative reinforcer. Such considerations might interact with treatment considerations, such as the appropriate duration of restraint and the use of Fixed or Variable Time schedules of reinforcement[3] in restraint (see below). Finally, the use of restraints involves consequences for both client and caregiver. Although authors have often noted that application of restraints may involve the termination of aversive client behavior and thus negatively reinforce staff application of restraints, little research has specifically demonstrated this and incorporated such considerations into case formulations and treatment plans.

---

[3] Fixed Time and Variable Time schedules of reinforcement are schedules of reinforcement in which the reinforcer is delivered based on the passage of time independently of the behavior. For example, a Fixed Time 1-min schedule involves delivering the reinforcer every minute, and a Variable Time 1 min involves delivering the reinforcer at various intervals that average out at 1 min.

7.2 Self-Restraint

7.2.1 Description and Definition

Fisher and Iwata (1996) described self-restraint as a "curious phenomenon" (p. 93) usually associated with self-injurious behavior, rather than aggression or other maladaptive behavior. Isley et al. (1991) noted three broad categories of self-restraint: (a) restriction of body parts using clothing, such as wrapping arms in a towel or wrapping arms inside a sweater; (b) movement restriction of one's own body parts, such as sitting on hands; and (c) using objects to restrict movement, such as holding cups or carrying a ball. Sometimes they appear to aggress toward others, but in fact they may only be trying to wrap their hands and arms in other people's clothes.

7.2.2 Functions of Self-Restraint

Intuitively, it appears that people self-restraint to prevent self-injuring. There are several lines of evidence supporting this hypothesis. For example, Powell et al. (1996) observed self-restraint in a sample of 99 adults with severe or profound Intellectual Disabilities and found that 46 % of them exhibited self-restraint. This association between self-restraint and self-injury supports the intuitive notion that people who self-restrain do so to avoid self-injuring. Other studies have found that between 10 and 50 % of people with developmental disabilities who self-injure also self-restrain (Oliver et al. 2003; Smith et al. 1992) including people with Cornelia de Lange syndrome (Hyman et al. 2002). Self-restraint is also more likely in individuals who self-injure and who do not have mechanical restraints. For example, Oliver et al. (2003) surveyed the prevalence of self-restraint in 88 individuals with Intellectual Disabilities, 41 of whom wore protective devices, such as gloves, splints, and helmets. They assessed self-restraint using *the Self-Restraint Questionnaire (SRQ),* a 23-item measure of specific forms of self-restraint in which informants rate each item on a 5-point scale as to the frequency of the self-restraint. Inter-rater agreement was variable and sometimes low (mean item inter-rater agreement = 0.49, range 0.04–0.89) and inter-observer agreement for four subscale scores was 0.87, 0.17, 0.72, and 0.61, perhaps in part reflecting the very low frequency of some items. Oliver et al. also reported two forms of validity. First, they demonstrated good convergent validity between direct observation of self-restraint and *the SRQ*. Agreement between the two methods was 89.6 % (range 64.2–100 %). They found that, whereas almost all individuals who did not self-restraint never self-injured, 100 % of those who self-restrained also self-injured. They also found other evidence of a negative correlation between self-restraint and self-injurious behavior. For example, only 58.5 % of those in protective devices self-injured, but 91.5 % of those without protective devices self-restrained. Those people with no protective devices rarely showed multiple forms of self-restraint. In contrast, those people without restraints often showed multiple forms of self-restraint. For example, less than 10 % of those with restraints showed 6 or more forms of self-restraint, whereas almost half of those without restraints exhibited 6 or more forms of self-restraint. These results in combination with other surveys confirm that self-restraint and restraint are often associated. Thus, a comprehensive functional analysis of self-injurious behavior should also address the relationship between restraint and self-restraint.

One useful way to think about self-restraint is as a form of self-control. Skinner (1953) described self-control as the effects of emitting one behavior (the controlling response) on another behavior (the controlled response) which describes a very broad class of behavior. For example, in that description, Skinner described several forms of self-restraint that many of us show. For example, we put our hands over our mouth or bite our tongue to stop saying something foolish, and we stick our hands in our pocket or fold our arms to prevent ourselves from fidgeting. These examples appear similar to the phenomenon of self-restraint in people with chronic self-injury: Perhaps they have learned self-restraint (a controlling response) to prevent self-injury (a controlled response). This is useful in that it suggests that intervention might be based on teaching self-control to people who self-injure, such as clasping hands or wearing acceptable mechanical restraints such as hats, glasses, and watches, to replace head slapping and reduce associated restraint. In other cases, where people already self-restrain in ways that are unacceptable because of continuing self-restraint, say through wrapping arms in clothes that prevents interacting with the environment and reinforces self-injury, then intervention might involve teaching better, safer, and more acceptable forms of self-restraint, such as those mentioned above.

7.2.3 Self-Restraint as Compulsive Behavior

An alternate perspective comes from King (1993) who suggested that self-restraint is an involuntary compulsion that is unrelated to environmental events, at least for some people. For some, he suggested that self-restraint is a form of compulsive resistance to ritualistic self-injurious behavior, analogous to resistance to ego dystonic compulsions in people with Obsessive Compulsive Disorder. Thus, setting events that increase anxiety might increase self-restraint, which then terminated the anxiety and self-injurious behavior. Thus, this theory has some similarities to the negative reinforcement hypothesis of self-restraint, where what is avoided is not only the self-injurious behavior but also intervening anxiety. Several empirical studies support this idea (Bodfish et al. 1995; Dykens and Kasari 1997). For example, Hyman et al. (2002) found a positive association between self-injurious behavior, self-restraint, and compulsions in people with Cornelia de Lange syndrome.

These studies offer some support to the compulsive hypothesis of self-restraint. Such ideas could be incorporated into the functional assessment and treatment of self-injury and associated restraint. For example, the possibility that avoidance or termination of anxiety might negatively reinforce self-restraint might be a useful idea to consider, especially if "anxiety" can be operationally measured and reliably observed. This theory has two weaknesses. First, assuming that self-restraint is not under environmental control might simply reflect and incomplete functional assessment/analysis. A second challenge is that it is difficult to apply the notion of ego dystonic self-restraint in people with severe cognitive impairments.

7.2.4 *Functional Analyses of Self-Restraint*

7.2.4.1 Hypotheses

When conducting functional analysis of this phenomenon, clinicians and researcher must describe and account for sometimes complex sequences of self-injurious behavior, self-restraint, restraint, and other behavior and events may occur which have implications for our understanding of restraints, self-injurious behavior, self-restraint, and treatment. For example, a person might show little self-injurious behavior and self-restraint while in mechanical restraints. Later, when taken out of mechanical restraint, they may show increases in self-injurious behavior and/or self-restraint. A person might also show multiple forms of self-restraint, such as holding other people's clothes, folding their arms, sitting on their hands, and entwining their limbs in their own clothes and furniture. A functional analysis/assessment should account for all of these phenomena.

Fisher and Iwata (1996) and Smith et al. (1992) proposed that four hypotheses might account for the maintenance of self-restraint and self-injurious behavior. First, self-restraint and self-injurious behavior might both be members of the same response class. That is, both self-injurious behavior and self-restraint might be controlled by the same establishing operations, discriminative stimuli, and consequences. For example, both self-injurious behavior and self-restraint might be more likely if task demands are presented more frequently, an establishing operation that both temporarily increases the value of escape from demands as a negative reinforcer and results in a higher rate of all forms of behavior that have previously been reinforced by escape from demands. They might both be more likely in the presence of discriminative stimuli that previously have differentially predicted the availability of escape from demands, such as the presence of certain tasks or people. Finally, both self-injurious behavior and self-restraint might be more likely if escape from demands is more likely after self-injurious behavior and self-restraint than at other times. Self-restraint might come to dominate the person's behavioral repertoire in part because self-restraint may be significantly less effortful than self-injurious behavior (Pace et al. 1986). A parallel analysis of self-injurious behavior and self-restraint could be made if both were maintained by positive reinforcers, such as attention. It might be more difficult to argue that when self-injurious behavior is maintained by sensory consequences, that self-restraint might also result in the same consequences (Fisher and Iwata 1996).

The second hypothesis is that self-injurious behavior and self-restraint might both be functionally independent of one another, that is, they may both be maintained by *different* consequences and controlled by different establishing operations and discriminative stimuli related to the two consequences for each response class. For example, self-injurious behavior might be reinforced by access to preferred materials, but self-restraint might be maintained by its attention or its sensory consequences. Fisher and Iwata (1996) noted that they had observed caregivers encourage clients who self-injure to self-restrain. This suggests the possibility that attention from caregivers might maintain self-restraint, independent of any function of the self-injurious behavior. Fisher and Iwata also noted that at that time they were unaware of any data to support this hypothesis. Both Peterson and Peterson (1968) and Smith et al. (1992) noted that some forms of self-restraint might result in sensory consequences, such as warmth and tactile stimulation when wrapping one's arms in a blanket. Again, these sensory consequences might be different from the consequences maintaining self-injurious behavior.

The third hypothesis is that self-restraint may function as a positive reinforcer for self-injurious behavior. Fisher and Iwata (1996) invoked the Premack (1963) principle, namely, that a high probability response may positively reinforce a low probability response. Thus, since some clients self-restraint for extensive periods of time and typically emit self-injurious behavior in relatively brief, bursts, then self-injurious behavior may be reinforced by access to self-restraint. They also went on to speculate that when a client who self-restraints for extensive periods of time is asked to engage in incompatible behavior, such as self-help and educational or vocational tasks, that as time progresses without self-restraint, this period of reinforcer deprivation increases the value of self-restraint as a positive reinforcer. Thus, when a client subsequently begins to emit self-injurious behavior and caregivers permit access to self-restraint, two things may occur: First, self-injurious behavior is now positively reinforced by access to self-restraint at a time when self-restraint is an especially powerful positive reinforcer. Second, the caregivers' behavior of stopping teaching and permitting or encouraging self-restraint is negatively reinforced by termination of the client's self-injurious behavior and reduction of effort associated with working with a challenging client.

The fourth hypothesis is that avoidance or termination of self-injurious behavior may negatively reinforce self-restraint. Here, Fisher and Iwata (1996) presented an interesting and subtle analysis of the possible relationship between self-injurious behavior and self-restraint. At first blush, it seems implausible that self-restraint would negatively reinforced self-injurious behavior by terminating the presumptive aversive consequences of self-injurious behavior (i.e., pain) since simply not emitting self-injurious behavior would result in such consequences without the effort of engaging in self-injurious behavior. Fisher and Iwata argued that self-injurious behavior might result in both favorable and unfavorable consequences, such as aversive stimulation after each self-injurious behavior and some positive consequences, such as attention for some self-injurious behavior responses. They went on to suggest that self-injurious behavior might be similar to approach–avoidance behavior which results in both favorable and aversive consequences.

This model permits an analysis of self-injurious behavior and self-restraint as being controlled by the independent variables that control the favorable and unfavorable consequences of self-injurious behavior. These include the relative schedule values, quality of the favorable consequence, aversiveness of the negative consequence, and prior exposure to deprivation and satiation for each consequence. Since these variables are likely to change over time, they may explain the variation in self-injurious behavior and self-restraint over time. For example, if self-injurious behavior has recently resulted in a painful injury, self-injurious behavior may be less frequent, and self-restraint may be more frequent than before. Likewise, if attention maintains self-injurious behavior, then recent variation in deprivation and satiation of attention may also shift responding between self-injurious behavior and self-restraint. Thus, if, for some individuals, the aversive consequences of self-injurious behavior exceed the positive consequences of self-injurious behavior, then self-restraint might develop and be maintained.

A second study that offers partial support for the negative reinforcement hypothesis comes from Forman et al. (2002) who conducted naturalistic observations of self-injurious behavior and self-restraint in a 26-year-old man with Down syndrome. They also observed environmental events such as staff attention, staff demands, and staff denials of access to possible reinforcers. They found no relationship between three self-injurious behavior topographies and environmental events; however, there was a clear relationship between self-restraint and mouth poking, but not face hitting. Specifically, mouth poking was much more probable immediately after self-restraint and thereafter its probability declined. Mouth poking was also increasingly likely before self-restraint. Forman et al. speculated that (a) termination of mouth poking may have negatively reinforced selfrestraint and (b) termination of self-restraint may have been an establishing operation which temporarily increased the reinforcing properties of escape from mouth poking.

It is possible that all four of these hypotheses might be true for different individuals reflecting idiosyncratic contingencies and learning histories. These individual differences in the functions of self-injurious behavior and self-restraint indicate the need for individual treatment strategies based on a functional analysis of each individual's self-injurious behavior and self-restraint (Smith et al. 1992). Part of the next chapter describe intervention studies related to self-injurious behavior and self-restraint below.

7.2.4.2 Empirical Evidence

There is a modest empirical literature that has tested these hypotheses. For example, one of the earliest studies to address this phenomenon comes from Silverman et al. (1984) who evaluated the effects of protective clothing on arm self-restraint and leg self-restraint in a 13-year-old, legally blind boy with profound Intellectual Disabilities who punched his eyes and chin and also kicked his leg and slammed his forearm against hard objects. There were three experimental conditions. In one condition, he did not wear any restraints. In the second condition, he wore a padded helmet. In the third condition, he wore both the helmet and padded slipper restraints. Additionally, within each 6-min session, there were three, 2-min sub-conditions which included (a) placing blocks in a can for 10 s of contingent music, (b) winding a radio for 30 s of music, and (c) standing or walking for 10 s of music.

When restraints were unavailable, the participant emitted self-injurious behavior consistently. When he wore the helmet, self-injurious behavior to his head and hitting the helmet were almost eliminated. Further, at least one arm was unrestrained with many more intervals in this condition than in either of the other two conditions, indicating a reduction in arm self-restraint. When he wore both the helmet and slipper restraints, leg self-restraint was reduced. During the experiment, a new form of self-injurious behavior emerged—injury to other body parts with his arm, such as slapping his legs. Self-injurious behavior occurred at almost zero levels during the no-restraint condition, but occurred most often in the two restraint conditions. During the course of the experiment, the participants also began manipulating materials appropriately while self-restraining by placing his arm through his pant leg and manipulating the radio or blocks. Finally, self-restraint was also a function of the three sub-conditions in that arm self-restraint was much less likely when he could access the radio and manipulate the blocks than when he was asked to stand and walk.

Silverman et al. concluded that these data were compatible with the hypothesis that avoidance of self-injurious behavior negatively reinforced self-restraint. That is, since (a) the helmet eliminated self-injurious behavior to his head and subsequently arm self-restraint decreased, (b) the slipper restraint eliminated self-injurious behavior to his legs and subsequently leg self-restraint decreased, and (c) the effects of restraint were specific to the form of self-restraint, then it was possible that self-restraint has been extinguished since it no longer resulted in the elimination of self-injurious behavior. Although other explanations for these data are possible, they are compatible with the hypothesis that self-restraint is negatively reinforced by avoidance of self-injurious behavior. For example, Smith et al. (1996) noted that in this study, if restraints were a conditioned reinforcer for self-injurious behavior, then, when restraints were continuously available in the two restraints conditions, this condition may have functioned as noncontingent reinforcement; hence, reduction in self-injurious behavior and self-restraint may have been due to elimination of the motivation to engage in self-injurious behavior and self-restraint. They also noted that self-injurious behavior and self-restraint both tended to occur in the same sessions, supporting the alternative hypothesis that both self-injurious behavior and self-restraints were members of the same response class. Thus, Smith et al. (1996) conducted the first experimental analysis of the functions of self-restraint.

In a second study, Smith et al. conducted modified functional analyses (Iwata et al. 1982) of both self-injurious behavior and self-restraint in five boys and men with profound Intellectual Disabilities aged 13–36 years living in an institutional setting. Illustrative examples of self-injurious behavior and self-restraint include Jerry, who bit his hands and wore rigid arm splints which made self-injurious behavior impossible, and Lonnie, who exhibited multiple forms of self-injurious behavior and self-restraint by entangling his arms in his own or other people's clothing, furniture, and holding and placing objects around his head and shoulders. Smith et al. exposed the participants to the four functional analysis conditions (attention, demand, alone, and play). They also included sub-conditions when restraint was either available or unavailable. For example, in Jerry's restraint available condition his arm tubes were freely available, and he could freely place them on or remove them. In the restrain unavailable condition, hid arm tubes were unavailable.

The results of these experiments varied from one participant to another and were complex. The interested reader should refer to the original paper for full details; this section will only describe some illustrative findings. When restraints were available, Jerry self-restrained continuously and never emitted self-injurious behavior. During the functional analysis conditions without restraints, Jerry emitted self-injurious behavior most often and consistently in the demand condition, indicating that avoidance and termination of demands negatively reinforced his self-injurious behavior. Since self-restraint occurred in all restraint available sessions, Smith et al. could not make any firm conclusions about the functions of Jerry's self-restraint, although some evidence pointed to the possibility that his avoidance of the aversive consequence of self-injurious behavior negatively reinforced his self-restraint.

Another participant, Bill, only experienced the restraint available condition since he self-restrained in his clothes; however, his results were more readily interpretable since he consistently showed more self-injurious behavior in the demand condition than all three other conditions suggesting that escape or avoidance of demands negatively reinforced self-injurious behavior. His data on self-restraint showed a large decrease in the number of intervals with self-restraint across all conditions; however, the number of intervals with self-restraint was consistently higher and reduced more slowly in the demand condition compared to all other conditions.

These results are compatible with the similar function hypothesis, namely that escape an avoidance of demands negatively reinforced both self-injurious behavior and self-restraint. Smith et al. concluded that the functions of self-restraint, like the functions of self-injurious behavior, are idiosyncratic and supported all of the hypotheses noted earlier. They noted that these results had some interesting implications for interventions to reduce both self-injurious behavior, associated restraint and self-restraint including identifying both indicated and contraindicated treatments. For example, if the function of self-injurious behavior and self-restraint are the same, it may be appropriate to promote self-restraint temporarily and then transfer stimulus control from transfer of stimulus control. (See the section on restraint fading in the next chapter).

Extensions of Smith et al.

Several subsequent empirical studies have confirmed and extended the findings of Smith et al.'s landmark study. Three studies have demonstrated that self-restraint may positively reinforce self-injurious behavior. For example, Smith et al. (1996) compared the rates of self-injurious behavior and self-restraint in Polly, a 32-year-old woman with profound Intellectual Disabilities who was blind due a history of chronic eye poking. Her self-injurious behavior included head hitting and hair pulling and her self-restraint included entangling her arms in her own clothing. During functional analysis conditions (Iwata et al. 1982), Polly self-restraint continuously except in the demand condition when she emitted self-injurious behavior when staff prompted her to engage in a task and subsequently could self-restrain. These data and staff interviews, that indicated that they often allowed self-restraint after Polly emitted severe self-injurious behavior, supported the conclusion that self-restraint positively reinforced self-injurious behavior. To test that hypothesis experimentally, Smith et al. compared three conditions: (a) noncontingent restraint, in which Polly was allowed to self-restrain and staff did not interact with her; (b) contingent restraint, in which the experimenter guided Polly's hands out of self-restraint and blocked all subsequent attempts to self-restraint; and (c) no restraint, in which the experimenter guided Polly's hands out of self-restraint and blocked all subsequent attempts at self-restraint and ignored self-injurious behavior.

Polly's rates of self-injurious behavior were zero in the noncontingent restraint condition. In contrast, during two contingent self-restraint phases her rates of self-injurious behavior systematically increased. Finally, in two no-restraint phases, her rates of self-injurious behavior systematically decreased to zero or near zero. Thus, Smith et al. concluded that self-restraint reinforced self-injurious behavior. They argued that (a) the noncontingent self-restraint condition functioned as a satiation condition, in which continuously available positive reinforcement abolished the motivation to self-injure; (b) the increase in self-injurious behavior during contingent self-restraint demonstrated that access to self-restraint positively reinforced self-injurious behavior; and (c) during no restraint, self-injurious behavior extinguished since the consequence maintaining it—access to self-restraint—was no longer available.

A study by Derby et al. (1996) also supported the hypothesis that self-restraint can positively reinforce self-injurious behavior. The participant was Mari, a 12-year-old girl with Tuberose Sclerosis, and profound Intellectual Disabilities. Her self-injurious behavior was severe and had resulted in two detached retinas of which only one had been successfully reattached giving her some residual vision in one eye. Due to the risk of permanent blindness, Mari wore arm splints that prevented self-injurious behavior to her face. Thus, the experimenters only permitted Mari to attempt or partially block self-injurious behavior and self-restraint. A functional analysis (Iwata et al. 1982) indicated that attention maintained Mari's self-injurious behavior. Therefore, the experimenters compared the effects of noncontingent attention, attention to self-injurious behavior, and attention to self-restraint in a reversal design. Noncontingent attention consistently resulted in low rates of self-injurious behavior and low self-restraint. When the experimenters attended to self-injurious behavior, but not self-restraint, rates of self-injurious behavior increased and self-restraint dramatically decreased. When experimenters attended to self-restraint, but not self-injurious behavior, self-restraint increased and self-injurious behavior remained at moderate rates. The authors concluded that the same positive reinforcer—attention—maintained both self-injurious behavior and self-restraint and that noncontingent attention was a viable and effective intervention strategy to safely maintain both low rates of self-injurious behavior and self-restraint.

Rooker and Roscoe (2005) reported similar data. In this study, a 5-year-old boy with autism and severe self-injurious behavior participated. His self-injurious behavior consisted of hitting his chin, and his self-restraint consisted of placing objects between his chin and shoulder. A functional analysis (Iwata et al. 1982) revealed that escape from demands reinforced George's self-injurious behavior. A stimulus preference assessment identified two objects as preferred items that he used for self-restraint. Subsequent experiments showed that when these items were available continuously George did not emit self-injurious behavior. When George did not have access to a preferred restraint object and self-injurious behavior resulted in access to preferred self-restraint items, his rates of self-injurious behavior increased reliably; however, when he had continuous access to self-restraint item and an additional self-restraint item was made available contingent upon self-injurious behavior, self-injurious behavior did not increase. Thus, these results supported the hypothesis that access to preferred self-restraint materials might positively reinforce self-injurious behavior.

Another recent study provided evidence that self-restraint was maintained by negative reinforcement in the form of escape from the aversive consequences of self-injurious behavior (pain). Fisher et al. (1996) compared the effects of blocking or not blocking self-injurious behavior on the rate of self-injurious behavior and self-restraint in Al, a 19-year-old man with severe Intellectual Disabilities and hearing loss. Fisher et al. were unable to identify the functions of Al' s self-injurious behavior because he self-restrained continuously during an attempted functional analysis. Self-restraint was made difficult by having Al wear tight-fitting clothing and prompting him to engage in tasks that were likely to interrupt self-restraint. They compared two conditions: (a) self-injurious behavior allowed, in which Al sat at a table and staff prompted him to fold laundry and in which staff did not block self-injurious behavior, and (b) self-injurious behavior blocked, which *was* the same as self-injurious behavior allowed, except staff placed his hand in front of Al's forearm to block any attempts at self-injurious behavior.

Rates of self-injurious behavior were strongly affected by blocking, which reduced self-injurious behavior from between 0 to approximately 60/min to zero or near-zero levels. Interestingly, self-restraint also varied, even though the experiment did not directly intervene with self-restraint. Self-restraint occurred for a much greater proportion of the sessions during which self-injurious behavior was allowed than during the session in which the experimenters blocked self-injurious behavior. These results are consistent with the hypothesis that avoidance of the aversive (painful) consequences of self-injurious behavior negatively reinforce self-restraint.

A final recent study that sheds light on the functions of self-restraint comes from Powers et al. (2007), which documented the emergence of self-restraint de novo during the initial application of physical restraints and which also identified other variables that might affect self-restraint. Gail, a 16-year-old with moderate Intellectual Disabilities, cerebral degenerative chorea, and who was nonambulatory, participated. Her self-injurious behavior was severe and had resulted in previous hospitalizations and placed her at risk for retinal detachment. During two brief baseline sessions without protective equipment, preferred items or any programmed consequences for self-injurious behavior, Gail emitted 103.3 self-injurious behavior per minute. During the next phase, the protective equipment (no toys) phase, the experimenters applied plastic arm splints that prevented self-injurious behavior to her eyes to protect her from potential blindness. During this phase, self-injurious behavior immediately fell to 0.3/min, but Gail began to self-restrain almost continuously by wrapping her fingers in the straps attached to her restraints. The third phase, protective equipment (with toys), was the same as the previous phase, but the experimenter also placed five preferred items that the experimenter has identified using a multiple stimulus preference assessment[4] (Fisher et al. 1997) on Gail's lap tray. If the items fell off her tray, the experimenter placed them back on her tray. During this phase, not only did self-injurious behavior remain at zero levels but self-restraint also fell to zero as Gail spent almost 100% of intervals interacting with the preferred items. The experimenters showed clear experimental control of self-injurious behavior, self-restraint, and interaction with items using a reversal design. This experiment showed a clear reciprocal relationship between self-restraint and the presence of preferred items that prompted item manipulation.

Fisher et al. reported that after this intervention they could then successfully conduct functional analyses of Gail's self-injurious behavior that demonstrated that automatic reinforcement maintained her self-injurious behavior. Based on these data and multiple preference assessments, they were then able to successfully fade the restraints.

This study nicely illustrated the complexity interventions for self-injurious behavior, which in this case included initially adding restraint to ensure Gail's safety, subsequently analyzing the functions of self-restraint, use of multiple preference assessments to reduce self-restraint, subsequent functional analyses of self-injurious behavior, restraint fading with use of concurrently available preferred stimuli which finally resulted in safe elimination of self-injurious behavior, self-restraint and mechanical restraint.

Taken together, these studies demonstrate that self-restraint may have at least four different functions and that the functions of self-restraint may be the same or different from the functions self-injurious behavior. The functional analysis of self-restraint and self-injurious behavior has important implications for identifying effective and deleterious interventions for self-injurious behavior and restraint reduction (Smith et al. 1996). When combined with other interventions, such as multiple preference assessments and restraint fading (Powers et al. 2007), the functional analysis of self-restraint and self-injurious behavior can result in safe elimination of both self-injurious behavior and restraints, although to date only one study has reported this (Powers et al. 2007).

---

[4] A multiple stimulus preference assessment is a systematic assessment of preferred items in which several items are presented in front of the person and they take one. The procedure is continued until all the items are selected or the person no longer takes an item. Preferred items may function as positive reinforcers.

7.2.5 Summary

Self-restraint, like self-injurious behavior and aggression and like personal and mechanical restraint, can serve several functions. It is tempting to assume that if task avoidance reinforces self-injurious behavior that it too reinforces self-restraint; the data reviewed above show that this may always not be the case. Self-restraint and physical and mechanical restraint may both complicate treatment of severe self-injurious behavior in a number of ways. Both self-restraint and physical and mechanical restraint may be necessary as a temporary measure to ensure client and caregiver safety; several papers noted that it might be appropriate to encourage and explicitly teach self-restraint during the early part of treatment. In other circumstances, the emergence of self-restraint during treatment of self-injurious behavior may be troublesome because it may require that treatment are modified fluidly and innovatively and inhibit accurate implementation of the treatment. For example, at several points during the course of treatment of self-injury in "Harry," Foxx and Dufrense (1984) encountered the emergence of self-restraint, including Harry placing his hands in his pants, in others' clothing, and self-restraining with objects such as glasses. Foxx and Dufrense hypothesized that removal of demands negatively reinforced Harry's self-injurious behavior and that access to restraints positively reinforced self-injurious behavior. Thus, Harry's treatment plan involved compliance training. The therapists reinforced compliance with access to restraints and used time out from his restraints as a consequence for self-injurious behavior. Harry's self-restraint inhibited treatment of his self-injurious behavior, because it made compliance training more difficult and effortful as it involved both removing his hands from self-restraint and prompting compliance. Further, removal of his hands from self-restraint sometimes occasioned self-injurious behavior resulting in time out from his restraints which Foxx and Dufrense presumed were positive reinforcers. The resulting treatment plan resulted in near elimination of self-injurious behavior, mechanical restraints, and self-restraint at 4.5-year follow-up. This chapter illustrates both the importance of simultaneously understanding the functions of self-injurious behavior, restraint, and self-restraint and the need for creative and flexible clinical treatment and persistence in such challenging cases.

7.3 Conclusions

Applied behavior analysis offers a useful perspective on understanding, assessing, and treating self-injury and self-restraint. By specifying the functions of the stimuli and behaviors of interest, we can identify important individual differences that determine effective and ineffective behavioral interventions. The next chapter goes on to consider behavioral interventions related to restraint.

Chapter 8
Applied Behavior Analysis Interventions

A wide range of applied behavior analysis interventions is available to reduce restraint safely and treat challenging behavior effectively. These interventions include: (a) effective treatment of the target behavior to obviate the use of restraint and seclusion; (b) modification of antecedent stimuli; (c) restraint fading; (d) schedule thinning; (d) differential reinforcement of other behavior[1] using restraint as a positive reinforcer; (e) empirical analysis of the least intrusive degree of restraint necessary to ensure client safety and maximize client participation; and (f) a variety of procedures to reduce the target behavior, self-restraint, and restraint simultaneously. Applied behavior analysis interventions can be distinguished from behavior modification interventions, such as differential reinforcement of other behavior using arbitrary reinforcers and punishment, because the former is characterized by a clear analysis and understanding of the functions of the target behavior and its relationship with the environment based on a pretreatment functional assessment. Applied behavior analysis interventions also teach alternative appropriate behavior to compete with the target behavior which serves the same function as the target behavior, that is, paying attention to treatment integrity, training caregivers, assessing and planning generalization, and maintenance (Cooper et al. 2007). The following sections review the use of applied behavior analysis for people with Intellectual Disabilities, children and adolescents, dental and medical procedures, and older adults.

[1] Differential reinforcement of other behavior refers to a group of treatments in which behavior other than the target behavior is reinforced. It is useful to distinguish between reinforcement of any other behavior (differential reinforcement of other behavior), differential reinforcement of some specific alternate behavior, differential reinforcement of physically incompatible behavior, etc.

P. Sturmey, *Reducing Restraint and Restrictive Behavior Management Practices*,
Autism and Child Psychopathology Series, DOI 10.1007/978-3-319-17569-0_8

8.1 Intellectual Disabilities

There are now over 200 meta-analyses supporting the use of applied behavior analysis for individuals with Intellectual Disabilities to teach skills that enhance independency and perceived dignity and worth, and to reduce challenging behavior (Sturmey 2014a, 2014b, 2014c). Economic analyses of these treatments also support their use (Sturmey 2014d). Several meta-analyses have repeatedly shown that basing interventions on pre-intervention functional assessments results in larger effect sizes than interventions that do not (Didden et al. 1997; Sturmey and Didden 2014), including in people with mild Intellectual Disabilities (Didden et al. 2006). Thus, there is an extensive evidence base for the use of applied behavior analysis, which can be used to prevent challenging behavior that results in restraint, seclusion, and other restrictive behavior management practices. The following sections review some of these procedures related to Intellectual Disabilities.

8.1.1 Effective Behavioral Intervention to Reduce Restraint

Gaskin et al. (2013) reported a systematic review and meta-analysis of interventions to reduce restraint in people with developmental disabilities. They identified 14 single-subject studies, all but one of which used behavioral methods, one used mindfulness (see Chap. 10), and one used organizational behavior methods to reduce restraint across an entire organization (see Chap. 11). Examples of interventions include multicomponent staff training to increase environmental modification, early redirection, safe response to aggression, and post-incident review; choosing preferred staff members; modification of client schedules to increase preferred activities, use of fixed time instead of response contingent release, etc.

The mean reduction in frequency was 79 % (13 participants, 7 studies) and 45 % in duration (10 participants, 6 studies). Effect sizes were similar whether restraint was used to manage aggression and agitation or self-injury. The authors concluded that restraint reduction was quite effective, although outcomes varied from individual to individual considerably. The subsequent sections of this chapter review specific behavioral intervention strategies to reduce restraint.

8.1.1.1 Adding Positive Procedures

In many of the examples reviewed in earlier chapters, service providers appear to have attempted to prevent problem behavior solely or almost solely by the use of restrictive procedures. Yet, it is well established that combining punishment with other positive procedures is likely to enhance the effectiveness of intervention. For example, combined interventions may result in faster response suppression and acquisition of new responses. One example of this approach that relates to restraint reduction comes from Thompson et al. (1999) who evaluated the effects of reinforcement of other behavior during punishment, including using brief manual restraints, on self-injurious behavior. Four adults aged 28–44 years who lived in an institutional setting and exhibited self-injurious behavior participated. Functional analyses (Iwata et al. 1982) identified the functions as automatic positive reinforcement for all participants. The authors conducted both reinforcement assessments to identify preferred leisure materials and punishment assessments to identify consequences for self-injurious behavior and alternate behavior. The authors used punishment assessments to identify the least intrusive consequence that reduced self-injurious behavior by at least 75 %. For example, in one participant, they observed that both a reprimand and restraining a client's hands in her lap produced the same degree of suppression as the verbal reprimand alone and hence used only the verbal reprimand. For three participants, the punishing consequence was either holding the client's hands in their lap for 15 s or having the client fold their arms in front of their chest for 15 s. In the no-reinforcement condition, participants had no access to leisure materials. In the reinforcement condition, leisure materials were continuously available. For one participant with visual impairments, materials that produced tactile and olfactory stimulation were attached to his vest, and therapists reinforced any 2-s instance of independent object manipulation. The experimenters alternated the two no-reinforcement and reinforcement conditions in a multielement design embedded within no-punishment and punishment phases. In the no-punishment phase, therapists did not apply restraints following self-injurious behavior. In the punishment phase, therapists removed the toys and applied the manual restraints. The experimenters used a multiple baseline design across four participants with a no-punishment baseline and a punishment intervention phase; for the first subject, they also implemented a reversal design comparing punishment and no punishment.

During the no-punishment baseline, differential reinforcement had no systematic effect on rates of self-injurious behavior for three of the four participants. In only one subject, differential reinforcement resulted in a large suppression of self-injurious behavior. The addition of punishment contingencies resulted in large decreases in self-injurious behavior for all four participants. When the authors compared the rates of self-injurious behavior during the punishment condition, the reinforcement sessions resulted in further reductions in self-injurious behavior. When Thompson et al. examined the rates of punishment in the no-reinforcement and reinforcement conditions, they found robust reductions in the rate at which punishment was applied during the reinforcement condition for all four participants. For example, the largest difference occurred for Ricky who experienced an average of 16 punishing consequences during reinforcement sessions and 56 punishing consequences in the no-reinforcement condition. Thus, punishment combined with reinforcement was more effective than punishment alone in terms of both response suppression and reduction in the need for restraints.

Such reductions in the use of punishment are not only ethically desirable but may also be more practical for caregivers. The authors suggested that noncontingently available reinforcing leisure materials may function as a disestablishing operation for self-injurious behavior by providing sensory stimulation that may have maintained self-injurious behavior. A second learning mechanism that might account for the effects of reinforcement and punishment is that when punishment was applied, therapists also removed leisure materials, which may have also functioned as time out. This study replicated many findings in basic research in the interaction between reinforcement and punishment (Azrin and Holtz 1966).

A second study that illustrates the effectiveness of applied behavior analysis to reduce restraint comes from Jensen et al. (2012), who evaluated the effects of a client working with a staff assigned to her by the unit manager with the client choosing her own preferred staff. Staff occupy an important place in the lives of many people with disabilities. People with disabilities often have strong and reliable preferences for staff members which can be assessed using direct, verbal, and pictorial preference assessment methods (Jerome and Sturmey 2008, 2014; Sturmey et al. 2003). Further, attention from preferred staff is a more powerful reinforcer than attention from non-preferred staff (Jerome and Sturmey 2008, 2014), and the reinforcing value of attention from non-preferred staff can be modified by pairing non-preferred staff with preferred stimuli (Jerome and Sturmey 2014). Thus, identifying and incorporating client preferences for staff members have important potential for treatment and quality of life.

Jensen et al. (2012) measured the number of minutes of restraint in a 28-year-old woman with autism, moderate Intellectual Disabilities, and other disabilities, who lived in a large residential setting. She had severe self-injury managed by mechanical restraints and psychotropic medication. During the year prior to intervention, she spent an average of 386 min per day in restraints (range 0–786 min). The experimenters compared the effects of two conditions on time in restraint. In the no-choice condition, the unit manager assigned staff to work with Carol. In the choice condition, Carol indicated a first- and second-choice staff by pointing to photographs of staff or naming staff. The photographs were then pinned publicly where Carol could see them. During baseline, the median number of minutes of restraint was 268 min per day. During the last 10 days of the experiment, the median number of minutes of restraint was 358 and 178 min per day during the no-choice and choice conditions, respectively. During a final choice only phase, the number of minutes of restraint dropped to a median of 55 min per day. Thus, giving Carol a choice of staff resulted in a large and stable decrease in restraint.

These two experiments illustrate that effective behavioral treatment can result in reduction in restraint.

8.1.1.2 Modification of Antecedent Stimuli

Luiselli (2009) noted that at least two types of antecedent conditions might be associated with challenging behavior that might result in the application of restraints. First, discriminative stimuli such as the presence of non-preferred staff or non-preferred tasks might occasion challenging behavior. For example, a client might reliably show high rates of aggression toward an untrained, unskilled staff when that staff consistently asked them to engage in novel, difficult tasks when sitting in a noisy, crowded workshop. Second, establishing operations, such as periods of deprivation or satiation of a reinforcer that maintains the challenging behavior, may influence whether or not a client is aggressive. For example, if attention positively reinforces a client's aggression, then aggression may be more likely if they have been left alone for an extensive period of time.

Several studies have shown that application of restraints is often associated with antecedent stimuli that are specific to each client. For example, Luiselli et al. (2003) identified the antecedents for restraints in four adolescents with acquired brain damage attending a community-based day school. They found that caregivers used restraints most commonly in classroom rather than residential settings and for in-seat work, rather than during activities involving mobility. Luiselli et al. (2005) analyzed the antecedents to restraint in 15 students with acquired brain damage and Intellectual Disabilities aged 9–21 years in a community-based school. They used a standard form to assess the location (e.g., classroom, group homes, etc.) and activity (e.g., seat work, meal, or snack). Average interobserver agreement was 99% for location and 89% for activity. Of 107 restraints, 19 occurred during classroom in-seat work. Finn and Sturmey (2009) made similar observations in a day program for adults with Intellectual Disabilities and mental health/behavioral challenges. They found that caregivers used restraints during transitions between activities and during in-seat work, but rarely due to staff prompting or a client not earning a reinforcer.

This information is potentially quite useful as part of a functional assessment that might inform a treatment plan to reduce both challenging behavior and restraint. Intervention strategies might include removing the antecedents, modifying the antecedents, or removing and fading the antecedents back in. Luiselli et al. (2000) illustrated how a therapist can incorporate modification of antecedent stimuli into treatment plans. Two adolescent boys with Intellectual Disabilities and pervasive developmental disabilities who were aggressive toward peers and staff participated. Existing treatment plans during baseline specified pleasurable consequences for the absence of aggression and physical restraint for unmanageable aggression. In the second intervention, rather than leaving it up to staff judgment, there was a specific criterion for the application of restraint. Both of these interventions resulted in continued use of restraint over a 7-month period ranging from approximately 0–35 applications per month for Glenn and 4–16 applications per month for Paul. The authors developed new support plans based on analysis of the antecedents associated with restraints. For example, Paul's new program involved giving him more novel tasks, reducing sedentary activities, increasing preferred activities with staff, and reducing proximity with peers. The new programs greatly reduced restraints. Glenn's restraints were approximately 0–2 per month. Paul's restraints were approximately 0–10 per month over a 14-month period and only 0–2 per month for the last 9 months of intervention.

Thus, these studies show that modification of antecedents associated with restraints resulted in a large reduction in restraints over an extensive and meaningful period of time. One limitation of this study was that it did not use a multiple baseline design for the introduction of the modified programs which the authors introduced both at the same time; hence, the authors could not confidently rule out potential confounding explanations for change.

Scatterplots

A scatterplot is a grid in which the x-axis represents the day of the week and the y-axis represents the time of day (Touchette et al. 1985). The occurrence of target behaviors and/or restraints can then be plotted on the grid either directly from observation or by transcribing case notes. Sometimes the resulting pattern suggests possible stimulus control of behavior. For example, Jensen et al. (2012) constructed a scatterplot of restraints for one participant. They found that restraints were especially high after change of shift around 2 p.m. and that their intervention was especially effective before 2 p.m., but only moderately so after 2 pm, thus subsequently enabling them to focus effort at high-risk situations. Similar scatterplot data on challenging behavior in people with Prader–Willi syndrome were reported by Maas et al. (2009).

A third application to the analysis of antecedent stimuli that influence restraints, this time related to brain injury, comes from Persel et al. (1977) who used a scatterplot as part of a battery of behavioral assessments to identify the functions of aggression in a 40-year-old man with brain injury and aggressive behavior. They observed from the scatterplot that almost half of all aggression and self-injury occurred before 11 a.m. This observation was again useful in directing the clinicians to analyze both what the triggers might be for target behaviors at high-risk situations and what activities might be correlated with the absence of restraints.

8.1.1.3 Evaluation and Recommendations

Assessing the antecedents to restraint has some positive features. It is often a very convenient and low-effort method of conducting a functional assessment, and clinicians can often do this from existing client records relatively quickly. The information from such analyses is relatively coarse grained, but it does direct the clinician where to look in order to conduct more refined analyses. As shown by Luiselli et al. (2000), it is possible to incorporate information on antecedents to restraint to develop intervention plans that can lead to reductions in restraint over extensive periods of time.

This literature has several limitations. First, the information gathered from such analyses is necessarily crude. For example, knowing that 90 % of a client's restraints occur during lunch does not identify what aspect of the environment might be relevant, although further descriptive assessments might clarify this. Even when clinicians have conducted such descriptive analyses, the resultant data are correlational and, hence, ambiguous. For example, suppose a clinician observes that restraints occur frequently during lunch when staff redirect a client away from stealing food from the other client's plates and that sometimes the client still steals small portions of food before being restrained. It might be tempting to conclude that intermittent food reinforcement maintains stealing and loss of positive reinforcement (food) provokes aggression; however, it is possible that the response chain of stealing followed by aggression is negatively reinforced by removal from a noisy crowded environment. A final limitation is that only one intervention study was found, and it did not use an experimental design. Like other studies of restraint reduction, it only reported restraint data, but did not report data on the target behavior or client and staff safety. Finally, most of this research was conducted by one group of researchers and hence awaits independent replication. Hence, the evidence based for this approach is weak.

The reader should note, however, that antecedent interventions to reduce restraint is but one specific application of antecedent interventions. This literature is both extensive and quite relevant. Despite these limitations, many practitioners will find this approach simple, efficient, and potentially effective.

8.1.2 Restraint Fading

Restraint fading refers to procedures in which an existing restraint exerts stimulus control over the target behavior, and one or more of the properties of that antecedent stimulus are gradually and progressively modified until the restraint is no longer present, or it is modified into some socially acceptable and typical stimulus. An example of such a stimulus control might be when a client almost never displays self-injurious behavior when wearing arm splints, but shows high rates of self-injurious behavior as soon as the splints are removed. It might be that in the past when arm splints were removed, access to restraints that functioned as positive reinforcers might be readily available, especially after high and intense bursts of self-injurious behavior. As time passes, the client experiences progressively greater reinforcer deprivation, increasing the likelihood of self-injurious behavior. Thus, the absence of restraints sets the occasion for the availability of reinforcement.

When splints are applied, the reinforcer (the splints) is continuously available and hence the client experiences reinforcer satiation, thereby greatly decreasing the motivation for self-injurious behavior. Usually, splints also greatly increase the response effort and sometimes make it nearly impossible to obtain reinforcement through self-injury. Examples of restraint fading include gradually reducing the number of stays in arm splints, gradually increasing the degree of movement available in a hinged arm splint, reducing the pressure in air splints, and gradual modification of clothing or restraint devices to approximate typical stimuli and then substituting typical stimuli, such as watches, jewelry, hair bands, or regular items of clothing. (See Ball et al. 1985; Foxx and Dufrense 1984; Oliver et al. 1998; Silverman et al. 1984 for various examples of restraint fading). Restraint fading has also been applied to treatment and elimination of thumb sucking in typically developing young children (van Houten and Rolider 1984; see below).

Restraint fading is similar to some other intervention procedures but can be distinguished from them, because gradual transfer of stimulus control characterizes restraint fading, but not other similar procedures. Thus, identifying acceptable clothing that is associated with no maladaptive behavior (Kerth et al. 2009; Silverman et al. 1984) is not restraint fading, because it does not involve progressive modification of existing stimuli that already exert stimulus control of the maladaptive behavior. It is also important to distinguish restraint fading from procedures using restraints as a positive reinforcer to shape progressively longer periods of time or progressively greater numbers of responses, since there procedures involve shaping of behavior, rather than gradual modification of antecedent stimuli. Restraint fading is based on the gradual transfer of stimulus control from the restraints to other antecedent stimuli.

Pace et al. (1986) reported one of the earliest examples of restraint fading for treatment of self-injurious behavior in people with Intellectual Disabilities. Jack, an 18-year-old with profound Intellectual Disabilities, participated in the first experiment. Jack had a 9-year history of ineffective treatment for self-injurious behavior including medication, a variety of behavioral interventions, and several forms of restraints. At the time of the study, Jack wore 47-cm rigid tubes on each arm that made biting his hand and flexing his arm impossible. In the baseline, the experimenter presented Jack with toys and permitted him to play alone, with the experimenter, or move around the room. The experimenter ignored self-injurious behavior and praised, and made physical contact contingent upon toy play. The experimenter chose toys that required arm movement to try and encourage Jack to remove the restraints. In the first treatment phase, the experimenter prompted Jack to remove restraints and reinforced the absence of restraints every minute. In the restraint-fading condition, the experimenter gradually reduced the length of the restraints from 47 to 5 cm over 22 days. When the restraints were only 5 cm long, they no longer restricted arm movement, and the experimenter covered them with fabric and faded them to tennis wristbands. The experimenters used a multiple baseline design across two settings.

In baseline, Jack engaged in high amounts of self-restraint and low-rated self-injurious behavior. When the experimenter removed restraints completely for a brief 2-min probe, Jack engaged in self-injurious behavior during 100% of intervals. Prompting and differential reinforcement resulted in a gradual reduction in self-restraint to near zero levels in one setting and rapid reduction in self-restraint in a second setting. Restraint fading, prompting, and reinforcement resulted in elimination of restraints without any increase in self-injurious behavior. Followup at 1, 6, 12, and 24 months revealed that Jack remained free of both self-injurious behavior and restraint, wore his wristbands, and continued to interact appropriately with toys.

Pace et al.'s second experiment evaluated a second form of restraint fading: fading air pressure in pneumatic splints. Bart, a 15-year-old teenager with profound Intellectual Disabilities, participated. He had been institutionalized when he was 1 week old and started severe ear scratching when he was 1 year old. He engaged in multiple forms of self-restraint, and caregivers used rigid elbow splints to prevent self-injurious behavior. Baseline was similar to the previous experiment. During air-splint fading, the experimenters substituted air splints for existing restraints. They then gradually reduced the pressure in the air splints over 63 days.

During baseline, Bart engaged in self-restraint almost continuously and rarely selfinjured or engaged in toy play. Once the experimenters introduced air splints, his self-injurious behavior remained at zero levels and toy play immediately emerged for most of the sessions. Subsequent fading of the air-splint pressure did not affect self-injurious behavior, toy play, or self-restraint. When the experimenters conducted a probe with splints removed, Bart engaged in high rates of self-restraint. After the experiment, the staff continued to use the faded air splints, but encountered many problems with their use and within a few weeks substituted mechanical restraints and faded them by shortening them and decreasing their angle from 180 to 115 °. The staff reported that both self-injurious behavior and self-restraint were possible, but Bart did not engage in them.

The study by Lerman et al. (1994) illustrates the degree of ingenuity and persistence needed in managing chronic self-injury and self-restraint. The participant was a 20-year-old man with profound Intellectual Disabilities who self-injured and self-restrained in his clothes. The study was in three phases. Because they were unable to fade his clothes, the authors taught him to self-restraint in a large towel around his neck. This was gradually faded over a number of days to sweatbands on his wrists, a headband, and finally a bandana. Although phase I left him with low rates of self-injury, he still self-injured when asked to do something. Therefore, phase II consisted of compliance training, for example, taking his hands out of self-restraint and taking a candy. Compliance training resulted in increased interaction with the environment without self-injury, although he showed minimal communication. Therefore, phase III consisted of teaching him to request items using signs. (Since the conventional signs were similar to his self-injury, the authors taught an individual sign to request items). Thus, complete management of self-injury and self-restraint required development of individual forms of restraint that could be faded and teaching skills to give the person access to alternate forms of reinforcement.

Fisher et al. (1997) also evaluated the effects of restraint fading. The three participants were Marty, a 20-year-old man with Down syndrome; Matt, an 8-year-old boy with profound Intellectual Disabilities; and Art, a 7-year-old boy with profound Intellectual Disabilities. During functional analyses, all three participants showed high and variable rates of self-injurious behavior across all conditions. Since all three participants exhibited hand-to-head self-injurious behavior, the experimenters introduced canvas arm sleeves. The canvas arm sleeves had four pockets and each pocket could hold either one, 2 mm thick or 5, 0.5 mm thin metal stays. The therapist could substitute thin metal stays for thick metal stays and progressively reduce the number of metal stays during restraint fading. The clients also wore a light stocking to reduce the possibility of skin breakdown.

The experiment consisted of three phases: A prefading analysis, restraint-fading, and a post-fading analysis. In the prefading analysis, the experimenters compared the rates of self-injurious behavior when the client had bare arms (no restraints), wore the restraints without restraints in the sleeves (flexible sleeves), and wore the restraints with rigid sleeves. During the prefading analysis sessions, the therapist ensured that preferred stimuli were present and modeled, and reinforced their use, but provided no consequences for self-injurious behavior. Restraint fading took place on the client's living unit. Fading consisted of gradually substituting thin for thick stays and gradually reducing the number of thin stays until none remained. The therapists faded restraints contingent upon predetermined reductions in self-injurious behavior and increased additional stays contingent upon increases in self-injurious behavior. The authors also evaluated additional procedures including the addition of contingent water mist (Marty), a trial of naltrexone (Matt), and a padded baseball cap (Matt). Once treatments were completed, the experimenters conducted the post-fading analyses which were similar to the prefading analyses.

During the prefading assessment, Marty exhibited high rates of self-injurious behavior during both the bare arms and flexible sleeve conditions and almost zero self-injurious behavior during the rigid sleeves conditions. During the initial sessions of restraint fading, Marty exhibited near-zero levels of self-injurious behavior, but once the number of stays was reduced to 14 thin stays, self-injurious behavior increased. Fisher et al. added contingent water mist that reduced self-injurious behavior. Returning to fading alone resulted in reemergence of self-injurious behavior. Thus, subsequent fading sessions included both restraint fading and contingent water mist that resulted in very low rates of self-injurious behavior. At post-fading analysis, Marty exhibited high rates of self-injurious behavior only during the bare arms condition, but not during the flexible sleeves condition. The results of prefading analyses, restraint fading, and post-fading analyses were broadly similar for Matt and Art. For Matt, an evaluation of several doses of naltrexone indicated that it was ineffective in reducing his self-injurious behavior. During the middle of restraint fading, Matt began to show a new form of self-injurious behavior, straight-arm self-injurious behavior. To treat this, Fisher et al. introduced a padded baseball cap, which was effective in reducing this new form of self-injurious behavior. Fisher et al. concluded that restraint fading was highly effective and safe for all three participants. Indeed, the experimenters could implement restraint fading relatively quickly—in only 48–65 days.

Oliver et al. (1998) reported two small *N* experiments with three participants, which also evaluated restraint fading. Dawn, a 25-year-old woman with profound Intellectual Disabilities and impaired hearing and vision who lived in a community hostel and attended a day center, participated in study 1. She restrained her arms by holding objects in each hand that restricted her arm movement and wrapped her arms in her clothes. If caregivers removed the restraints, she became distressed, attempted to retrieve them, and self-injured. Previous intervention using differential reinforcement of no self-injurious behavior with restraints and restraint fading had failed (Murphy et al. 1993).

Oliver et al. could not conduct a functional analysis because of Dawn's level of distress without her restraints and the high rates of intense head punching. Oliver et al. used a modular, hinged splint with two key features. First, they could adjust the angle of available movement from completely rigid to 120° (full arm movement). Second, since the splints were modular, they could modify components of the splints and modify them as part of fading. Dependent variables included direct observation of head and body punching, trapping arms, trapping hands, wrapping, positive and negative vocalization, engagement, and social contact. An interesting dependent variable was a restriction index where 1 represented constant restriction and no flexion, and 0 represented no restriction and continuous flexion. They calculated this by summing the proportion of time multiplied by the degree of flexion in each type of restraint and self-restraint. For example, "if Dawn was observed to be wearing both splints all the time at 50% flexion, trapping her arms for 25% of the time but no other forms of restraint were observed, then the restriction index for that session would be: ([100+(100×0.5)+25+0+0])/ 500=0.35" (p. 148). The restraint-fading procedure consisted of substituting new restraints for the old restraints. Over time, Oliver et al. increased the angle of flexion from 25 to 100% of the possible flexion in 25% increments. In brief experimental sessions, Oliver et al. compared the old restraint and new splint in multielement and reversal designs and progressively increased the degree of flexion with the new splint over several phases. They also conducted extended generalization sessions in the day program with a 17-month follow-up.

In the experimental phase, the addition of new restraints resulted in an immediate reduction in the restriction index compared to the old restraints. Self-injurious behavior occurred rarely or at zero levels during all observations. Self-restraint was somewhat more likely in the old restraint compared to the new splint. Both positive and negative vocalizations were rare during all experimental sessions, although during two sessions with the new splint negative vocalization occurred a great deal. Finally, during brief experimental sessions, engagement and social contact were lower with the new splint than with the old restraint. The increases in flexion with the new splint had no effect on behavior. During generalization sessions, the authors increased the degree of flexion to 100% over 52 days. Self-injurious behavior did not occur, self-restraint reduced greatly, and there were increases in positive vocalizations, engagement, and social contact.

To further evaluate the effects of restraint fading, Oliver et al. identified two participants with severe self-injurious behavior, no current program, and current straight-arm splints. Dean, a 32-year-old man with Down syndrome and severe Intellectual Disability who lived in a bungalow with eight other residents, and Sarah, a 29-year-old woman with severe Intellectual Disabilities (residence unspecified), participated in the second study. The studies took place in the participants' natural environments only and procedures and measures were broadly similar to those in study I. Again, the authors elected not to conduct functional analyses because of client distress and the severity of their self-injurious behavior.

Before the study, Dean's caregivers managed Dean's self-injurious behavior with cushions and an ice hockey helmet to protect him from injury and PRN diazepam. The authors then faded the restraints to 100% flexion and then faded the size of the splints. During baseline with the old restraints, Dean engaged in self-injurious behavior, and, following the addition of the new rigid splints, his self-injurious behavior was immediately reduced. During restraint fading, self-injurious behavior eventually remained at zero levels. Restraint fading resulted in a large decrease in the restriction index. There were periods of increased self-restraint, during 100% available flexion and removal of the upper section of the restraints, but by the end of the study self-restraint was zero. Positive and negative vocalizations were near zero in baseline and subsequently increased across all phases. Although negative vocalizations increased during 50 and 75% flexion, there was a mix of both positive and negative vocalization during subsequent phases; by the end of the study, there were more positive than negative vocalizations. Social contact and engagement increased during parts of the study, but by the end, they returned to baseline levels.

Intervention for Sarah was unsuccessful. Although the initial steps of restraint fading resulted in near-zero levels of self-injurious behavior, self-restraint continued to occur at moderate and variable levels. Addition of rigid restraints greatly decreased, but did not eliminate self-injurious behavior, and Sarah engaged in moderate self-restraint. When restraints were first faded to 25% flexion, self-injurious behavior reemerged and self-restraint increased, and so the authors reintroduced rigid restraints. Subsequently, when restraints were faded to 75% of flexion, staff had to block self-injurious behavior almost continuously, and so they reintroduced rigid restraints.

This study is interesting in a number of ways. Oliver et al. replicated earlier studies showing that restraint fading can be highly effective in treating self-injurious behavior and safely eliminating restraints. Their report of negative treatment effects was interesting and useful. First, one cannot assume that restraint fading will be effective for all participants. Second, in Sara's case, the new restraint was not completely effective even at 0% flexion. Thus, perhaps the particular form of restraint selection did not exert sufficiently strong stimulus control to make restraint fading as effective as in the other two cases. Further, the early continuation of both self-injurious behavior and self-restraint may have resulted in continued reinforcement of self-injurious behavior through access to self-restraint (cf. Smith et al.; 1996), thus making relapse more likely. Finally, the absence of a functional analysis is often associated with less effective interventions and perhaps that lack of information about the functions of self-injurious behavior made the development of a maximally effective intervention less likely.

This study has a number of significant strengths. In particular, study I was a true experiment, since it involved a multielement design, and also had impressive long-term follow-up and generalization from experimental to programmatic settings. Sara's data do contain a reversal design; however, Dean's data were an AB, nonexperimental case study, making inference of causality not possible.

Restraint fading is a robustly effective treatment strategy for eliminating restraint and self-injury in individuals with Intellectual Disability and severe, chronic self-injury. It may provide a useful model for other populations and contexts, such as fading out mechanical restraints in seniors.

8.1.3 Differential Reinforcement Using Access to Restraint Devices

The earlier section on functions of restraint noted that access to restraint materials can reinforce self-injurious behavior. Thus, several studies have evaluated the effectiveness of a various differential reinforcement schedule using access to restraint materials that appear to maintain the target behavior as a reinforcer for the absence of the target behavior or some other relevant response.

An earlier section described how Favell et al. (1978) used contingent access to restraints as a positive reinforcer in a differential reinforcement of other behavior schedule; however, this study also contained other procedures, including restraint fading. For example, in Tim's case, Favell et al. went on from restraining him on his bed to only allowing him to lie down on his bed. It is possible that other forms of restraint fading also occurred during this procedure involving reducing how much he restrained himself in his bedclothes. In additional, when Tim was away from his bed, caregivers gave Tim a string, which was described as a "preferred toy." Again, it is possible that this string functioned both as a positive reinforcer and, more interestingly, perhaps as a form of unobtrusive self-restraint. Favell et al.'s description of intervention for Peg also included both differential reinforcement of other behavior using restraints as a consequence and what appears to be restraint fading. Specifically, when the researcher first released one of Peg's wrists from restraint, the researcher stroked and gently squeezed her arm and then progressively reduced the pressure. This same procedure was then applied to releasing Peg's second arm from restraints. Thus, again, restraint fading was a component of this intervention.

After first demonstrating that access to restraint materials reinforced self-injurious behavior, Vollmer and Vondran (1998) went on to evaluate three variations of functional communication training and extinction of self-injurious behavior. Denise, a 29-year-old woman with severe Intellectual Disabilities, participated. Functional communication training consisted of the therapist reinforcing a brushing motion against her chest with access to the clothing item. Extinction involved not giving the jacket to Denise after she exhibited self-injurious behavior. Vollmer and Vondran evaluated the procedure with three different clothing items: the jacket that appeared to maintain self-injurious behavior, a shirt, and a cardigan. Treatment with the jacket and cardigan were effective, but treatment with the shirt was ineffective. Vollmer and Vondran noted some unique features of this study that might limit the generality of these findings. Notably, Denise did not exhibit self-injurious behavior when the jacket was absent from the room. This might be an atypical presentation of self-injurious behavior maintained by access to restraint material, since many such clients continue to exhibit self-injurious behavior at high rates in the absence of their restraint materials (Foxx and Dufrense 1984)

A highly influential training movie, *Harry, Behavioral treatment of self-abuse* (Foxx 1980), illustrates the role of management of restraint in treatment of chronic self-injury in a man with mild Intellectual Disabilities. The data were subsequently reported by Foxx and Dufrense (1984) with 10-year follow-up data (Foxx 1990). Harry exhibited severe self-injury, including smashing himself in the nose at high rates when out of restraint. He has been mechanically restrained for many years, which prevented self-injury, except when the restraints were removed for essential self-care, such as bathing. Foxx and Dufrense used the earlier information from Favell et al. (1978) indicating that mechanical restraints can function as positive reinforcers for self-injury. The movie illustrates the initial use of differential reinforcement for alternate behavior, such as counting, shaping up of progressively more complex and effortful behavior, such as counting longer, academic tasks, and increased social behavior and compliance, and time out from positive reinforcement (i.e., removal of the restraints) to reduce self-injury and increase adaptive behavior. As treatment progresses, different forms of restraint are substituted for each other. For example, plastic drinking glasses were substituted for arm splints, and eyeglasses were substituted for plastic drinking glasses. Finally, a general increase in the range of positive experiences, such as earning money at work, maintenance of work behavior with a token economy parent, and vocational training and increased community trips with family members, was used to maintain change over 10 years. The data showed elimination of self-injury and restraints, increases in many forms of adaptive behavior, and maintenance over own years.

The movie is fascinating in many respects. It shows a master clinician developing the program on the fly as Harry's behavior changes moment by moment. For example, as forms of self-restraint develop and new forms of noncompliance occur, Foxx identifies them and develops new ways to reinforce and shape appropriate behavior. In addition, certain aspects of the restraint fading are strange. Why did Harry accept forms of restraint that are physically different from each other, such as eyeglasses in place of holding plastic drinking cups? The answer is unclear.

8.1.4 Analysis of Least, Most Effective Safe Restraint

In some circumstances, it may be necessary to use restraint, at least temporarily, for example, when self-injurious behavior or aggression is very severe or during some intermediate step involving restraint fading. In these circumstances, therapists should use the least restrictive kind of restraint and maximize client interaction with the environment. This problem was noted by Rojahn et al. (1980) who conducted an observational study in which they found that continuous restraint prevented self-injury in three individuals but resulted in decreased interaction with their caregivers. Thus, developing less restrictive and effective methods of managing self-injury is an important part of management of restraints.

In some cases, instead of systematically fading a restraint, some have substituted one apparently less restrictive form of restraint for a more restrictive form of restraint. For example, Wurtele et al. (1984) made a protective mouth guard for a teenage boy with Lesch–Nyhan syndrome to reduce his self-biting and the use of gauze and bandage wrapping around the boy's thumbs and fingers to prevent finger biting. Substitution of the mouth guard for the gauze and wrapping resulted in a large reduction in self-biting and removal of the wrapping. This study was limited, in that it was a narrative case study without any reliable data or data on interaction with the environment.

One empirical approach to this is to evaluate differing degrees of restraint systematically and empirically. Wallace et al.'s (1999) study exemplifies this approach. They evaluated the effects of no sleeves, 0–25 thin metal stays, and 5 thick metal stays on the rate of self-injurious behavior and the number of trials in which the participants took a drink from a cup. The participants were two individuals with profound Intellectual Disabilities living in an institutional setting. Renee engaged in face hitting and has already experienced a failed restraint-fading program. Dana engaged in hand mouthing and had no prior exposure to restraint. Functional analyses indicated that the participants' self-injurious behavior was probably maintained by automatic positive reinforcement. Restraint analysis sessions were 5 min long, and the experimenters ensured that fluids were unavailable for 30 min prior to the first session. There were 3–9 sessions per day each separated by at least 5 min.

When Renee wore no sleeves and had up to 15 thin stays, she drank on almost all trials; and when she wore thick stays, she did not drink. When she wore no sleeve, she engaged in high rates of self-injurious behavior, and the rate of self-injurious behavior decreased dramatically upon the addition of the sleeves without stays. As the experimenter added more stays, she showed fewer self-injurious behaviors until at 20 stays she did not exhibit self-injurious behavior. Thus, she could drink independently and did not engage in self-injurious behavior when she wore 20 stays. For Dana, results were broadly similar, except for her the minimum number of stays that permitted high rates of independent drinking and no self-injurious behavior was 0 stays.

LeBlanc et al. (1997) conducted a similar study to determine the effects of restraints or no restraints with response blocking on rates of life-threatening pica in a 4-year-old girl with severe Intellectual Disabilities and pulmonary disease requiring continuous oxygen. She had undergone two hospitalizations to remove ingested objects from her stomach and esophagus. Her pica included ingesting strings, hair, and clothing. When left alone in her current restraints, she bit through and ate parts of her restraints and oxygen tube while in restraints. During restraints only, Mary wore canvas arm sleeves from shoulder to wrist, a foam helmet, and a face mask. The therapist blocked all attempts to remove them. During the no-restraint (blocking) condition, Mary wore no restraints, and the therapist blocked all pica attempts. The rate of therapist blocks was approximately equal in the first six sessions; however, thereafter the rate of therapist blocks increased to approximately four to ten per minute during restraints and reduced to less than one per minute for no restraint and blocking. Mary did not attempt pica during restraints; however, during the first three sessions with no restraints and blocking, she attempted pica approximately 1–3 times per min and thereafter only attempted pica less than approximately 0.5 per min; in the final restraint (and blocking) condition, she presented near-zero levels of pica. Since the no-restraint condition resulted in more toy play and fewer negative vocalization, a low rate of pica attempts without ingesting items, and relatively infrequent therapist blocking, her team decided that the no-restraint and blocking condition was the best option as an intermediate strategy before her team could develop a formal treatment plan. Her team subsequently conducted functional analyses of Mary's pica and developed a treatment plan that reduced her pica by 89% throughout the day.

Irvin et al. (1998) similarly evaluated the effects of different degrees of restraint on hand mouthing, engaging in leisure, and degree of elbow flexion in two women aged 25 and 41 years with profound Intellectual Disabilities living in an institutional setting. Both had experienced multiple failed behavior programs for hand mouthing. Caregivers used restraint which prevented injuries from hand mouthing, but restricted interaction with the environment. They used a neoprene elbow restraint with neoprene stays similar to canvas restraints with stays that caregivers could insert and remove. Functional analyses indicated that hand mouthing was probably maintained by positive automatic reinforcement for both women. In a preexperimental analysis, the authors selected an initial level of restraint. They then evaluated if the participants could pick up an item of food and if she engaged in self-injurious behavior for 20 % or fewer intervals. If the participant could pick up the food item and engaged in self-injurious behavior for fewer than 20 % of intervals, then the experimenter decreased the number of stays in the next session. Thus, they used four and two 5/16" stays for Debbie and Tammy, respectively.

Subsequently, Irvin et al. demonstrated that the selected degree of restraints were necessary to reduce hand mouthing to near-zero levels and permit manipulation of leisure materials. These results were maintained at 11- and 13-month follow-up for Tammy and Debbie, respectively; however, at follow-up, Tammy exhibited marked reductions in elbow flexion, indicating that restraints may have negatively impacted her adaptive behavior.

8.1.5 *Systematic Desensitization*

On a few occasions, individuals in chronic self-restraint appear anxious, fearful, and panicky when taken out of restraints. They may even verbalize their fears that they are going to harm themselves and ask for help. Thus, sometimes management of anxiety may be a part of intervention for chronic self-injury, restraint and self-restraint.

Bull and LaVeccio (1978) reported an interesting case report of treatment of self-injury and restraints in a nonambulatory 10-year-old boy with Lesch–Nyhan disease whose severe self-injury was managed by multiple restraints throughout the day and night. The boy also showed multiple forms of other maladaptive behavior. Noting that self-injury was often precipitated by removal of restraint devices, the authors used a treatment approach modeled after systematic desensitization. That is, they rank ordered how provocative removal of each item of clothing or restraint was. For instance, removal of a sock was unlikely to trigger self-injury, whereas removal of restraint devices was very likely to precipitate self-injury. Since it was difficult to induce relaxation in other ways, the authors used administration of nitrous oxide as a way to induce relaxation, which was incompatible with self-injury. They also noted that his self-injury was very manipulative, in that he did not self-injure when alone, but appeared to use it to obtain interaction from caregivers and tangible items. Therefore, the treatment package also included planned ignoring. The treatment was effective, although some self-injury and other behavior problems did occur during early sessions. Change was maintained using play therapy as a way to provide increased interaction. At follow-up, one and a half years later he was free of self-injury and acquired adaptive behavior, such as participation in education and independent ambulation.

8.1.5.1 Summary and Recommendations

These studies indicated that empirical analysis of the effects of varying degrees of restriction on maladaptive and adaptive behavior and participant safety can be performed, sometimes quite quickly. The results of these analyses can assist treatment teams in determining the least restrictive and effective degree of restraint needed and indicate the least restrictive starting point for subsequent intervention programs. As LeBlanc et al. (1997) indicated, such analyses are the starting and not the end point of intervention. Irvin et al.'s data indicate that long-term implementation of the least restrictive degree of restraint may still have negative effects on client adaptive behavior. Thus, careful and continuous monitoring and evaluation of restraints are required, even when an initial analysis has indicated that it was the least intrusive yet effective degree of restraint at the time of the initial assessment.

These methods have significant limitations. Several of the evaluations of the impact of restraint probably used highly reinforcing items, such as drinks after a 30-min period of no access to fluids. Thus, these analyses of the impact of restraint on adaptive behavior may be incomplete, since there may have been negative impacts on other adaptive behavior maintained by less powerful reinforcers (Wallace et al. 1999). A second limitation is that these evaluations are brief and, thus, only investigated short-term effects of restraint on behavior. Future research should also focus on the long-term effects of using the least restrictive, effective degree of restraint on behavior. Of course, the focus of clinical work should be on the reduction and safe elimination of restraints.

8.1.6 Interventions for Self-Injurious Behavior and Self-Restraint

Self-restraint is intimately involved in the functional analysis of self-injurious behavior and restraint (see above). Consequently, the treatment of self-injurious behavior and restraint reduction often requires simultaneous treatment of self-restraint from the beginning of treatment or as self-restraint emerges during treatment. (See the discussion of Foxx and Dufrense 1984, above for examples of treatment of emerging self-restraint during treatment of self-injury.)

Silverman et al. (1984) compared the effects of three different forms of mechanical restraint on self-injury and self-restraint in a 13-year-old boy with profound Intellectual Disabilities. His self-injury consisted of punching his face and body and slamming his body into objects resulting in bruising and other injuries. They compared self-injury and self-restraint during no protective equipment, a padded helmet alone, and a padded helmet and padded slippers. They found that the padded helmet alone eliminated self-injury to his head and some forms of self-restraint and that the addition of padded slippers eliminated self-injury to his leg and self-restraint involving his legs. Thus, careful analysis of different forms of mechanical restraint revealed differential effects on different forms of self-injury and self-restraint.

Powers et al. (2007) reported an analysis of self-injury and self-restraint in a nonambulatory 16-year-old girl with moderate Intellectual Disability and high rate of dangerous self-injury. Although the application of arm splints was effective in near elimination of self-injury, a new problem behavior emerged. Gail wrapped her hands in the straps of the restraints, thereby engaging in self-restraint and greatly reducing her opportunities to interact with the environment. Powers et al. showed that addition of five preferred items on her lap tray eliminated self-restraint, while keeping her safe from injuries.

An interesting example of a similar paper comes from Kerth et al. (2009), who reported a case study of functional analysis and treatment of self-injury and self-restraint in a 16-year-old boy diagnosed with autism, intermittent explosive disorder, and moderate/severe Intellectual Disabilities. He had been admitted to an in-patient unit because of the severity of his self-injury and was taking multiple psychotropic medication. When not engaged in self-injury, he would twist his arms in materials, such as straps, and pull his shirt over his head. They first conducted two experimental functional analyses that indicated that self-injury was probably positively reinforced by access to tangible items. In a subsequent analysis, they compared the rates of self-injury and self-restraint in two conditions—wearing or not wearing a hooded sweatshirt. They found that, even though he did not self-restraint when wearing the hooded sweatshirt his rates of self-injury fell by approximately half.

Management of restraint, self-restraint, and self-injury is a serious clinical challenge. As these chapters show, there are considerable idiosyncrasies in the presentation of self-injury, restraint, and self-restraint that sometimes require considerable ingenuity on the part of the clinician to identify the potentially independent functions and interrelations between these three groups of behavior. Safe elimination of restraint and management of self-restraint and self-injury may require: (a) contingency management using restraint equipment as a consequence to eliminate self-injury and build up adaptive behavior; (b) selection of the most effective and least restrictive form of restraint that permits interaction with the environment while maintaining client safety; and (c) careful design and modification of new restraint equipment.

8.1.6.1 Summary

There are a wide range of applied behavior analysis procedures to eliminate or reduce restraint in people with Intellectual Disabilities. This approach is supported by many individual small *N* experiments and a recent systematic review and meta-analysis (Gaskin et al. 2013). At this time, there is little evidence of alternate approaches being effective in doing so (although see Chap. 10 for some such evidence). Further, the evidence that interventions are based on functional assessments/analyses has frequently been noted. Thus, there is good evidence that applied behavior analytic interventions based on functional assessment/analyses should be the treatment of choice when intervening with individuals with Intellectual Disabilities to reduce restraint and other restrictive procedures.

8.2 Children and Adolescents

8.2.1 Young Children

Thumb sucking in young children can appear immature and stigmatizing and in some cases may result in dental problems. Historically, thumb sucking was seen as a sign or precursor of emotional disorders and hence worthy of restraint in some cases (Gillis 1996). Thus, there are a wide range of patented restraint devices, splints, and gloves to prevent thumb sucking through restraint, and at least one study has treated thumb sucking using restraint (Lewis et al. 1981).

An interesting early example of restraint fading comes from van Houten and Rolider (1984) who used restraints and restraint fading to reduce nocturnal thumb sucking and eliminate restraint in typically developing children. They reported four experiments with ten children aged 4–7 years, several of whom had been referred because they had or were at risk for periodontal problems, such as bite problems. In the first three experiments, the restraint-fading procedure consisted of having the child wear a boxing glove or heavy woolen restraint mitten on the hand that the child sucked his/her thumb. If this restraint eliminated thumb sucking, the authors substituted absorbent cotton around the thumb secured with an Elastoplast bandage, then only the Elastoplast, and finally no restraint. In the experiment, the two children exhibited thumb sucking between 0 and 100% of intervals. Addition of boxing gloves almost completely eliminated thumb sucking, and the children's parents successfully implemented restraint fading with no reemergence of thumb sucking which was maintained at 4-month follow-up.

Experiment 2 found that in three children positive reinforcement alone did not reduce thumb sucking, and replicated the effectiveness of restraint fading and maintenance up to 7 months. Experiment 3 evaluated the effects of the cotton restraint and reinforcement contingencies alone without the mitten. This experiment found that in three more children the cotton restraint, contingencies, and restraint fading were again effective in eliminating thumb sucking with maintenance at a 6-month follow-up.

Finally, experiment 4 evaluated whether the fading procedure was necessary. Two children participated. In this study, the experimenters used the cotton restraint but simply removed it after approximately 30 nights rather than fading it. The cotton restraint was again effective in eliminating thumb sucking. Abruptly eliminating the restraint for the first child resulted in no reemergence of thumb sucking; however, in the second child, thumb sucking reemerged approximately 2 weeks after the restraint was eliminated. Reintroduction of the restraint again eliminated thumb sucking, but a second abrupt removal again resulted in subsequent relapse. Thus, experiment 4's results were equivocal, in that abrupt removal of restraint did not result in relapse for one child, but for the second child abrupt removal of restraints reliably occasioned relapse. This study showed that restraint and restraint fading were effective in eliminating thumb sucking, that reinforcement contingencies alone were ineffective and that abrupt removal of restraints might be associated with relapse.

8.2.2 Residential Settings

Some studies of child and adolescent in-patient units have shown several different forms of effective behavioral interventions. For example, Greene et al. (2006) reported a remarkable reduction in restraint in a child and adolescent in-patient unit following the introduction of cognitive behavior therapy strategies to teach staff and children to solve the problem together. The study took place in a 13-bed locked unit for children aged 3–14 years selected because of extremely high rates of restraint. Before the program began, there were 281 episodes of restraint in 9 months, whereas after the program began this fell to only 1 restraint in 15 months.

Similar kinds of outcomes were reported by Dean et al. (2007) who evaluated the effects of a behavioral package of individual behavior plans, early reduction, staff training and reinforcement on child and adolescent aggression, and measures of restrictive behavior management practices. They also found that introduction of behavioral methods over a 6-month period reduced aggression, injuries, restraint, and duration of seclusion in a child and adolescent in-patient unit.

8.2.3 Summary

Applied behavior analysis can be effective in reducing restraints both for thumb sucking and for challenging behavior in adolescent in-patient units. Although applied behavior analysis has been used effectively to address a wide range of child and adolescent problems, the literature on elimination of restraint and seclusion is small and, thus, these promising results require replication.

8.3 Dental and Medical Treatment

Behavioral approaches to noncompliance and fear during dental treatment can be quite effective and often involve a treatment package including graded exposure, modeling, and reinforcement for compliance which can result in reductions in problem behavior, increased compliance, and successful completion of dental procedures in children who cannot have dental treatment completed (Allen and Stokes 1987). Reinforcement can include not only positive reinforcement for compliance in the form of presentation of stimuli such as stickers but also negative reinforcement in the form of brief contingent breaks from dental treatment.

As noted in chap. 1, dentists use a wide range of restrictive management practices, which are sometimes potentially dangerous, to manage behavior problems during dental treatment. Thus, it is interesting that O'Callaghan et al. (1987) reported changes in restraint use in five children aged 4–7 years referred because disruptive behavior made dental treatment both long and distressful to the children. Intervention consisted of a fixed time (noncontingent) schedule of negative reinforcement.

That is, at first, the child received a short break every 15 s of dental treatment. This interval was gradually stretched to break every 60 s. The treatment resulted in large reductions in the percentage of intervals with verbally and physically disruptive behavior. In four of five children, who were restrained during baseline, restraint was reduced to zero in two cases and reduced from eight to one instance in each of two other children.

In a subsequent randomized controlled trial, 151 children, 2–9-year old, were randomized to two conditions. Both groups received tell–show–do, praise, redirection or reprimands, and prizes during anesthesia, drilling, and restoration. The experimental group also received breaks on a fixed time schedule beginning at fixed time of 15 s, and the dentists thinned the scheduled as they deemed fit up to a fixed time of 5-min schedule. Dentists used restraint much less with children in the experimental group ($p<0.01$, small-to-medium effect size). When they compared the proportion of children who need any restraint, only 27 % of the experimental group but 45 % needed restraint in the control group ($p<0.05$).

Over a third of children with cancer undergoing venipuncture had to be restrained, causing great distress to children, family members, and staff alike (Jacobsen et al. 1990). Thus, Manne et al. (1990) conducted a unique study on restraint reduction in children undergoing medical treatment. Manne et al. (1990) attempted to reduce child and parent distress during venipuncture in children during invasive treatments for childhood cancer. To enter the study, children had to have participated in an earlier study of behavior during venipuncture, been restrained during baseline, and had to be accompanied by parents regularly for venipuncture. The authors approached 90 children, of whom 85 agreed to participate and 30 were restrained during baseline. Twenty-three completed the treatment, as six terminated the treatment and one died. After baseline observations, children were alternately assigned to either behavioral intervention or an attention control group. The authors observed venipuncture during three trials scheduled approximately 40–60 days apart. Behavioral intervention included having the child use a party blower with parent coaching, slow pacing of the child's breathing timed by the parent counting aloud, and positive reinforcement in the form of stickers, etc., for keeping the arm still during venipuncture and for using the party blower. A psychologist coached the parents in these strategies for 10 min before the first session and then faded themselves out over subsequent sessions. In the attention control condition, the psychologist instructed the parents to use whatever techniques they found helpful and provided support and reassurance to the parents for their attempts to reduce child distress. The intervention significantly reduced child behavioral distress, parental anxiety, and parent rating of child pain, but not child or nurse ratings of child pain.

During baseline, 100 % of all children were restrained. Restraint reduced in the control group 80 %, 80 % and 70 % in the attention-control group, but reduced to 53 %, 38 %, and 38 % during trials 1, 2, and 3, respectively. This difference was significant at trial 2 ($p<.05$). Thus, the behavioral intervention reduced restraint use by approximately half compared to an attention-control procedure.

8.3.1 Conclusion

There are at least three group-design experiments showing that behavioral interventions may be quite effective at reducing and eliminating restraint during dental and medical procedures for quite challenging problems.

8.4 Older Adults

Applied behavior analysis has been applied with older people, including older people with dementia for many years (Burgio and Burgio 1986). It has been used to provide pleasurable activities, extensively to remediate skill losses, and to conduct functional assessments and analyses of challenging behavior (Sturmey 2003; Trahan et al. 2011). Although there are applied behavior analytic studies reducing challenging behavior in older adults, no studies using applied behavior analysis to reduce restraints were found. Future studies are required to address this.

8.5 State of Behavioral Services

Despite the strong evidence for applied behavior (Sturmey 2007; Sturmey and Didden 2014), behavioral services are often not implemented, are of poor quality, and, when implemented, they lack essential elements and proper implementation. For example, as noted in Chap. 5, investigations by the US Department of Justice in the state institutions revealed poor quality of behavior plans, lack of professional competency, lack of implementation, and oversight. There is also substantial evidence that community services for people with disabilities are no better in this regard. For example, in Ontario's community and institutional services for adults with disabilities, Feldman et al. (2004) found that many restrictive procedures were conducted without written behavioral support plans and without training or oversight. In the UK, Emerson et al. (2000) surveyed behavior management strategies in a sample of 500 adults with disabilities and found that restrictive behavior management practices were common, but behavior support plans were often not even written. Just over half of the sample had "moderately serious" or "serious" challenging behavior in the preceding month with fully 44% of the sample with challenging behavior experiencing restraint, 35% sedation, 3% mechanical restraint but only 15% had any written behavior plan. More recently, Webber (2013) not only reported similar data from Australia but also found that even when plans were written many essential preventative strategies, such as use of reinforcement (!), clear goals, teaching replacement behaviors, communication strategies, and team coordination, were omitted. A related problem is that often behavior plans are too long and technical for staff to use (Singh et al. 2009; Vollmer et al. 1992), a problem that has been noted often in the past for other staff training materials (McGaw and Sturmey 1993; Sturmey 1990, 1993). For example, Adkins et al. (2002) found that most behavior plans they reviewed were written at college-level English for staff who had mostly graduated high school. They also found that more readable plans were correlated with a modest increase in positive client outcomes. When they trained practitioners to rewrite plans in a readable fashion, they found that this strategy enhanced treatment outcomes.

Similar problems exist in American schools. In a study of staff training in schools, Medley, Little Akin-Little (2008) reported that behavior plans in the control group were weak ($N=16$) or underdeveloped ($N=3$), and none were rated as adequate or superior, whereas in the schools that had received training in positive behavioral supports, the corresponding numbers were 9, 3, 6, and 3, respectively. Thus, in untrained school plans, almost all behavior plans were mostly inadequate, but even in trained school half of the behavior plans were also inadequate. This finding is important because other studies have found quality of written treatment plan in schools predicts treatment integrity quite strongly ($r=0.71$, $p<0.005$) (Lane et al. 2009).

It is notable that most of the literature relates to disabilities and to a lesser extent children. It does not, however, address other groups at risk for restrictive behavior management practices, such as nursing homes, psychiatric facilities, and youth facilities. This is another omission on the part of services, as many such people could benefit from behavior support plans which might also reduce reliance of restrictive behavior management practices in these populations.

These observations suggest a lack of oversight and support for the design and implementation of behavior support plans and lack of competency on the part of the few people who do write the plans. Consequently, in the absence of effective training and motivation to do otherwise or due to oversight, many services by default medicate, restrain, and restrict the movement of their clients.

8.6 Summary

Behavior analytic treatment related to restraint has focused on children and adults with Intellectual Disabilities and the use and fading of restraints in treating self-injury. Other applications of applied behavior analysis have included the use of non-contingent escape in dentistry, behavioral packages during venipuncture, and fading of mechanical restraints. These approaches are often highly effective, are based on a well-conducted functional assessment, and are designed and implemented properly. Unfortunately, many services fail to meet the minimum requirements for providing any behavior analytic services, let alone competent services.

Chapter 9
Other Approaches

The previous two chapters show that applied behavior analysis offers a useful way to understand restrictive behavior management practices and the reasons for their use and forms a useful basis for interventions to reduce their use either indirectly by reducing the target behaviors for which restrictive behavior management practices are used or directly, for example, through interventions to promote alternate effective strategies. In addition to applied behavior analysis, there is a wide range of other interventions that have varying degrees of empirical support that are commonly observed in service settings to attempt to reduce restrictive behavior management practices. These include staff training, mindfulness, legislation, advanced psychiatric directives, and aversive consequences. This chapter also reviews interventions to manage other restrictive behavior management practices such as seclusion, time-out, and as needed (PRN) psychotropic medication.

9.1 Restraint

9.1.1 Staff Training

For many researchers, the best evidence to identify effective treatments comes from randomized controlled trials in which a treatment is compared to no treatment, treatment as usual, or some placebo condition. Mohler et al. (2012) reported a Cochrane review of randomized controlled trials to reduce restraint in older people in long-term care. They included six cluster-randomized controlled trials which included various forms of staff education, and some also included subsequent consultation, guidance support, and access to free technical aids. The studies were of low quality and results were inconsistent. One good quality study found *increased* use of restraint after staff education in both the experimental and control groups, and four low quality studies found reduced use of restraint after staff education. The authors

P. Sturmey, *Reducing Restraint and Restrictive Behavior Management Practices*,
Autism and Child Psychopathology Series, DOI 10.1007/978-3-319-17569-0_9

concluded that there was insufficient evidence supporting the use of education to reduce restraint and the effective components of intervention were unclear.

Despite the practical and ethical concerns in conducting randomized controlled trials on restraint reduction, there are, surprisingly, more than a handful of randomized controlled trials evaluating interventions to reduce restraint and related procedures. This section reviews some of these randomized controlled trials, almost all of which were conducted in nursing home for older adults using some form of staff training intervention, although there were also randomized controlled trials on restraint reduction during dental procedures for children, children undergoing venipuncture, and psychiatric patients. The outcomes of these studies have been mixed, with some reporting positive outcomes and others negative outcomes.

9.1.1.1 Studies with Positive Outcomes

Several studies have reported that staff training is effective in decreasing restraints (Capezuti et al. 1998; Evans et al. 1997; Pellfolk et al. 2010; Ray et al. 1993; Rovner et al. 1996), and some that also measured falls have found no increase in falls when restraints were reduced (Capezuti et al. 1999). For example, Testad et al. (2005) randomly assigned four public nursing homes to either staff training or control conditions. The nursing homes were assigned to group after stratification for size and with the constraint that there were two homes per condition. There were 55 participants, mean age approximately 85 years in the experimental group, and 96 in the control group with mean age of 84 years. The groups did not differ on demographic variables or use of psychotropic medication, except that a larger proportion of the experimental group than the control group used antidepressant (41 vs. 23 %, $p<0.05$). Intervention included a manualized 6-h seminar on dementia, behavioral issues, decision making, and alternatives to restraint, and 1 h every month for 6 months of guidance, review of individual patients, and development of individual care plans. The control group received care as usual. The mean number (and range) of physical restraints was 3.3 (0–29) and 1.5 (0–10) for the experimental group and 3.1 (0–29) and 3.7 (0–25) for the control groups, respectively. The groups did not differ at baseline, but did so at follow-up ($p<0.017$). Notable was the 45 % reduction in the mean number of restraints per patient, but also the large reduction in the range of restraints in the experimental group indicating that those patients who had been restrained many times in baseline were restrained far fewer times at follow-up. The authors also assessed agitated behavior with a standardized rating scale, and there was no change in this measure in either group. Notable positive features of this study included data collection by an interviewer who was blind to participant assignment, relatively long period of intervention, and data collection and relatively cheap intervention after the staff training.

Huizing et al. (2006) also reported a cluster randomized controlled trials. In this study, they assigned five psychogeriatric nursing home wards from one nursing home to an educational intervention (three wards) or no treatment control group (two wards). One hundred sixty-seven residents with dementia participated. The educational program consisted of encouragement to adopt a philosophy of restraint-free care and familiarization with individualized care techniques presented at 2 months period in 5, 2-h presentations. The topics covered included decisionmaking process related to using restraint, alternatives to restraint, and discussion of real life situations with staff. Approximately one third of staff from each ward participated ($N=23$ staff) in three groups, and there was one final session from all staff in one group. Consultation involved staff support for 28 h per week, visiting each ward once per week, attending multidisciplinary meetings, and input on restraint use for individual residents. The experimenters collected data using questionnaires and direct observation during unannounced visits 1 month before and 1 month post intervention. The measures included the percentage of residents restrained during any part of a 24-h period, the number of restraints per resident, and the type of restraint used.

Pre- and post-data were available on 126 residents due to mortality and new admissions. The groups did not differ at baseline on demographic variables except the experimental group had more symptoms of depression. The proportion of residents restrained did not change in the experimental group (54 vs. 56 %) but significantly increased in the control group (56 vs. 70 %, $p<0.021$). Similarly, the mean number of restraints per resident did not change in the experimental group (1.44 vs. 1.57) but *increased* significantly in the control group (1.41 vs. 1.89, $p\leq0.05$). Analysis of the specific types of restraints indicated that the use of sleep suit restraints did not change in the experimental group (8 vs. 11 %), but significantly increased in the control group (22 vs. 39 %, $p<0.01$). The experimental group was at greatly reduced risk of restraint compared to the control group (Odds Ratio = 0.129, 95 % CI = 0.031–0.541).

A similar study comes from Kuske et al. (2009) who evaluated a nursing home staff training program in a three-arm cluster-randomized controlled design. They randomly selected six nursing homes from a list of ten homes with at least 90 residents and then selected 20 wards in which almost all residents had dementia. They randomized the six homes to the three conditions. Complete data were available from 210 residents from an initial pool of 321 residents. The residents' average age was 81 years and approximately three quarters were women. Of the 134 staff who entered the trial, 96 (72 %) completed sufficient sessions of staff training and completed data collection on all three occasions. The staff average was 44 years and 94 % were women. The intervention group received 13, 1-h sessions weekly in groups of up to 12 staff. A nurse-scientist delivered the training which included five modules that addressed knowledge of dementia, sensitization to residents with dementia, communication skills using lectures, videotapes, handouts, brain storming, and games. The second group received 13, 1-h sessions of relaxation training that a clinical psychologist delivered using progressive muscle relaxation, breathing techniques, and imagery. The control group was a wait list control that received no training. The authors collected data before and immediately after the intervention and at 6 months follow-up using resident charts to calculate the number of residents restrained in 4 weeks, the number of residents who had fallen, and the number of residents who had received regular and as-needed sedative drugs.

Training increased staff knowledge on a multiple-choice questionnaire in the experimental group, but not the relaxation or wait list control groups. Staff in the relaxation group, but not the experimental or control groups, reported fewer health complaints on a standard questionnaire measure of health. Thus, there were specific effects of intervention in both the experimental and relaxation, but not the control groups. Over the three data points, restraint did not change in the experimental group, but *increased* in both the relaxation ($p<0.001$) and control groups ($p=0.015$). The proportion of residents restrained in the relaxation group increased from 41% to approximately 52 and 58% after the training, and similar figures for the control group were 34% and approximately 37 and 42%. Thus, residents in the relaxation group experienced a large *increase* in restraints. The number of residents who fell decreased in the experimental group from 11 to 6 at 6 months follow-up and increased from 5 to 8 in the control group. There was no change in sedative medications in all three groups. Thus, staff training resulted in no increase in restraint, possible reduction in falls with no changes in sedative medication, whereas the relaxation group experienced a large increase in restraints, and the wait-list control group experienced a moderate increase in restraint.

A study of psychiatric wards in Switzerland comes from Abderhalden et al. (2008) who conducted a randomized controlled trials to reduce violence and coercive practices. They approached 86 wards in 32 psychiatric hospitals. Sixty-two declined to participate and five requested the intervention without the possibility of randomization. They randomly assigned the nine wards to either structured risk assessment or treatment as usual. Intervention group nurses completed a structured short-term risk assessment in which they rated six extra-personal maladaptive behaviors, such as verbal threats, and an overall rating of risk of imminent violence using a visual analog scale, within 3 days of admission. They carried out ratings twice daily, and the authors made recommendations for individual patients from a standard list of strategies, such as walk out doors in a group, relaxation, etc. The authors asked staff to record aggressive incidents and then rate the use of coercive strategies, such as forced injection of a psychotropic medication or mechanical restraint, for each incident. There was a larger decrease in severe incidents of aggression in the treatment (Relative Risk[1] = 0.59, 95% CI = 0.41–0.83) than the control group (Relative Risk = 0.85, 95% CI = 0.64–1.13) ($p<0.0001$). Attacks declined more in the treatment (41%) than control groups (7%) ($p<0.0001$), and the coercive measure decreased in the treatment group by 27%, but *increased* in the control group by 10% ($p<0.0001$). (Results for the six wards that selected the intervention without the possibility of randomization were even more positive.) A limit to the study was that there was evidence that randomization did not result in equivalent groups at baseline. (The intervention group patients appeared to have more severe aggression than the control group.)

[1] Relative Risk is the probability of an event occurring in an at-risk group compared to a comparison group.

9.1.1.2 Studies with Negative Outcomes

While it is tempting to assume that staff training must be associated with positive outcomes, that may not necessarily be the case. For example, staff training may be ineffective and wasteful or might cause harm to staff or residents by legitimizing the use of restrictive intervention procedures or might not provide sufficient training to allow the staff to conduct restrictive procedures safely. Evidence for such negative outcomes comes from Cole et al. (1994) who randomly assigned patients aged 75 years and older, admitted to the medical department of a primary acute care hospital and who had delirium within the first 24 h to either intervention or a treatment as usual control group. Intervention consisted of initial consultation by a geriatrician or geriatric psychiatrist within 24 h of referral and follow-up by a liaison nurse. The consultation included a diagnosis of the probable cause of the delirium and written treatment recommendations. The nursing intervention protocol included adjusting the sensory input of the environment, ensuring that orientation cues, such as a clock, were present, ensuring that familiar objects were present, that communication was appropriate to the patient, and that the patient was encouraged to move freely and engage in self-care and to avoid physical restraint. Although the intervention group had modestly better cognitive impairment, at 8 weeks follow-up 37 % of the intervention and 29 % of the control group required restraint, which was not a significant difference.

Mador et al. (2004) randomly assigned 77 eligible patients from a larger sample of 127 to either a behavioral advisory service or treatment as usual control. They were medical or surgical patients aged over 60 years referred because of behavioral issue not due to a primary psychiatric disorder. The behavioral advisory service group received a management plan which involved nonpharmacological interventions to manage problematic behavior, such as close supervision, minimizing restraint use, reducing risk of falls, communication skills, basic nursing care, behavioral strategies, such as music, and behavior modification, such as understanding behavioral triggers and ongoing support, and advice from an extended practice nurse. At day 1, 64 % of the intervention group and 68 % of the control group had more than one restraint on that day. At a median of 9 days follow-up, there was no difference between the groups in measures of agitation, sleep, use of antipsychotics, benzodiazepines, falling, and restraint. Thus, staff training was ineffective.

Kotynia-English et al. (2005) recruited 22 of 26 residential care facilities to participate in a randomized controlled trial of early psychiatric intervention for seniors whose average age was approximately 84 years. Early intervention included screening for psychiatric morbidity with measures of mental state, depression, and neuropsychiatry status. A multidisciplinary psychogeriatric team reviewed the patient and drew up a treatment plan for those participants with psychiatric disorders within 2 weeks. The team followed-up as needed usually up to 3 months. The control group received standard care. There were no significant differences in mental health measures between the groups, and just over 80 % continued to exhibit behavior problems in both groups. There were nonsignificant trends to reduce PRN medication (86 vs. 97 % in the experimental and control groups, respectively, $p = 0.071$), less increase in the use of psychotropic medication (74 vs. 68% in the experimental and control groups, respectively, $p=0.313$), and higher use of restraints in the intervention group (22 vs. 15% in the experimental and control groups, respectively, $p=0.599$). Although there was a statistically significant reduction in restrictive behavior management practices, the overall rate remained very high in the treatment group after the treatment.

Huizing et al. (2009) recruited 15 wards from 15 psychogeriatric nursing homes to participate in a randomized controlled trial of an educational intervention to reduce restraint use. Of the 432 residents who were selected, 371 participated at baseline and 241 participated at 8 months follow-up. The authors assigned the 15 wards to either treatment or control status. The intervention included five, 2-h educational session derived over a 2-month period, and a 90-min plenary a session for all staff and consultation with a registered nurse. The education intervention encouraged the staff to adopt a restraint-free philosophy and to familiarize themselves with individualized care techniques. Approximately one quarter to a third of staff from each ward attended, including the charge nurse. The authors selected staff who had key roles in the ward and who had different degrees of innovativeness. The nurse specialist followed up for up to 8 months after the intervention, made weekly ward visits, and advised nurses when staff made specific referrals. Eleven observers collected data on restraint use using direct observation. The definition of restraint was broad and included "any limitation on an individual's freedom of movement" (p. 1141) and also belts, chairs fixed to boards, infrared motion alarms, etc. During one baseline session of interobserver agreement, 2 of the 11 observers agreed 100% on identifying which residents had restraints. After the intervention, the proportion of residents restrained, the number of occasions residents were restrained during 1 day, and the mean number of restraints per resident *increased* both groups, but there was never any significant difference between the two groups at any time. Restraint use was high. For example, at 8 month follow-up, 64% of the experimental and 60% of the control groups were restrained.

9.1.2 A Note on Commercial Staff Training

There are now many companies and individuals providing training to the staff and family members on restrictive behavior management practices and their alternatives. Some training companies are large chain stores with branches across the state or even the world. Some state agencies also use in-house approved training courses or contract with outside training companies to provide such training. In some cases, there are certain forms of accreditation. For example, The British Institute of Learning Disabilities has an accreditation process for restraint training and maintains a register of approved providers of training as does The Institute of Conflict Management.

The duration, format, and content of such training courses vary widely. Some courses last only an hour or so and other courses last 1–2 weeks. Some courses have extensive coverage of preventative strategies and address applied behavior analysis approaches, such as functional behavioral assessment, skills training, modification of antecedents, and consequences, whereas others focus on training a large number of reactive strategies, such as physical holds, blocks, and different forms of mechanical restraint. Some training courses claim to use methods that would not cause pain, whereas others are up front that the methods they train do and *should* cause pain. Some training courses are offered as once off events, and other training companies offer ongoing consultation, training, and support. Courses also vary in the methods used for training. Some are predominantly information and discussion-based. Others include skills practice, perhaps in role play, and may or may not require some mastery criterion. Courses also vary in size from small groups in which individual attention to skills training is possible to large classes in which it is difficult to monitor any form of participation.

There is limited information available on the effectiveness of courses. For example, some courses have reported data on staff satisfaction with the course and often find that participants enjoy them and find them relevant and helpful (McDonell et al. 2008). Outcome data, for example, on reductions in client problems behavior, reductions in restrictive behavior management practices, promotion of acceptable less restrictive alternatives, and client and staff safety data are generally unavailable. Few papers have compared one form of training with another (see Lee et al. 2012, for an example).

Training staff in workshops presents special challenges for generalization. Namely, staff (may) acquire skills in the workshop under training conditions (a trainer role playing a client grabbing the staff member's clothes) and in the training setting (a large open space with little furniture), but must subsequently use those methods under other conditions (an actual client crying and throwing cups) in another setting (a crowded bedroom with little room to maneuver) 3 months later. Training using behavioral skills training to teach staff and parents basic teaching sills with children with disabilities produces generalization to similar people and material (Gianoumis and Sturmey 2012), but there are no data on staff training on restraints producing generalization of staff intervention skills. Several teaching strategies are likely to produce such generalization, such as multiple exemplar training and general case training (Stokes and Baer 1977), but to date these methods have not been used and evaluated during staff training and restraint.

Purchasers of such training products should be cautious when doing so. Hollins and Patterson (2009) have voiced concern that poor quality training can have negative impact on patient dignity, be humiliating, and harmful to patients. Companies that sell restraint training are selling something, and so claims made by company owners and practitioners may be biased, incomplete or inaccurate. In many cases, once off training events to large audiences may be ineffective or even harmful. (See Box 8.1). Let the buyer (and service user and their family members) beware!

Box 9.1 Harmful Staff Training
A school with some special education classes was concerned about liability issues, child and staff safety. The school purchased a 2-h staff training event from a local provider. The principal asked her secretary to find someone local and not too expensive. The staff training consisted of discussions of the causes of violence and video, prevention strategies, and video demonstrations of physical restraint methods. Staff had to complete a quiz to indicate mastery of the content and satisfaction with the training. No follow-up training was scheduled. The afternoon after the training, the principal told a special education teacher that she was now the "violence prevention coordinator" and was the lead teacher during any such incidents.

A few days later, there was an incident with a child with mild Intellectual Disabilities with a history of running away. (The school had not conducted functional behavior assessment, and there was no behavior support plan and no specific staff training for working with this child.) After pushing another child and scratching a staff member, the child ran out of the classroom and hid under a mobile classroom. The newly appointed violence prevention coordinator spent 45 min trying to persuade the child to come out. When the child did, the teacher attempted to use a physical restraint and a struggle ensued. The teacher was kicked in the eye detaching her retina. The teacher went on long-term disability. The child was excluded from the school. There were almost no winners, except for the training company that received payment for their training and had already added name of the school to the list of the satisfied customers.

9.1.3 Conclusions

The data on conventional approaches to staff training is very mixed: Sometimes it results in large and safe reductions in restraint, other times it is ineffective and sometimes it may result in increases in both restrictive behavior management practices and injuries. What accounts for these differences is unclear. Many of these studies have significant weaknesses related to treatment integrity, some of which are quite crude and others of which might be more subtle. Some studies did not report what proportion of staff attended the training or whether they attended key elements of the training. We might ask which staff member received treatment—the one who attended most sessions, but missed the key sessions on preventative strategies and subsequently used restraint more frequently than before the training, or the staff who attended one key session that enabled her to prevent behavioral incidents and never used restraint again? A more subtle aspect of treatment integrity goes beyond assessment delivering treatment by measuring mere attendance, self-report measures of satisfaction with training, or measure of knowledge, but rather measures delivery of training by change in staff behavior to some predetermined level of competence. For example, although a staff member might be present for all training sessions, they may learn nothing important that transfers to sufficient and meaningful change in their behavior at work.

These mixed outcomes of staff training interventions have important implications for services. Services cannot assume that providing training will help achieve the client outcomes that they hope for, rather that must include evaluation of the effects of training on those client outcomes after training has taken place. Additionally, organizations should plan to have systems of quality assurance to ensure that procedures that have been trained are in place, that problems are identified, and effective plans of action are in place when they identify such problems.

9.2 Mindfulness

The last 15 years has seen increased attention to mindfulness training to a wide range of mental health and other problems (Baer 2003; Singh et al. 2008). Marlatt and Kristeller (1999) defined mindfulness as "bringing one's complete attention to the present experience on a moment-to-moment basis" (p. 68). It derives from Eastern meditation practices, but also may be a part of contemporary psychotherapies, such as dialectical behavior therapy, acceptance and commitment therapy, and some forms of cognitive therapy (Baer 2003). Baer (2003) noted that mindfulness may overlap, but can be distinguished from relaxation training in that, although mindfulness may involve accepting observations of arousal and muscle tension relaxation, it does not necessarily do so, since it may involve nonjudgmental and accepting observations of arousal and muscle tension without relaxation.

There is now a growing literature on mindfulness related to both clients and staff and parents of people with disabilities (Chapman et al. 2013; Harper et al. 2013; Hwang and Kearney 2013) most notable by Singh and The Mindfulness Research Group (Singh et al. 2009) who have reported data on reduction of restraint and PRN medications in people with Intellectual Disabilities using the soles of the feet meditation (Singh et al. 2003). The soles of the feet meditation involves role play and practice to teach the person to recognize situational triggers for aggression. The therapist then guides the client through the soles of the feet meditation, which includes adopting a natural, nonaggressive posture, breathing naturally, imagining previous situations that made the person angry, shifting attentional focus to the soles of the feet, and focusing on moving the toes and feet until one is calm. Role play situations might include responding to someone who has offended you and responding to someone who pushes you around. Singh et al. (2003) used this procedure twice a day for 5 days in 3-min practice sessions.

A second mindfulness intervention is a 12, 2-hr-session mindfulness training program for staff (Singh et al. 2009) in which they learn the notion of mindfulness, practicing meditations on being in the moment, adopting a beginner's mind, being one with the individual client, nonjudgmental acceptance, letting go, loving kindness, problem solving, and practicing mindfulness outside the sessions. In the latter parts of the staff training and after training is completed, the instructor asks the staff to use mindfulness exercises in their daily work, but no further instructions are given after training is over.

Several studies have evaluated the effects of mindfulness on use of restrictive behavior management practices. For example, Singh et al. (2008) evaluated the effects of mindfulness training on aggressive behavior, restraints, PRN medications, staff and client injuries, and self-report measures of incidents and self-control. Six adults living in a forensic setting participated. One had mild Intellectual Disability. (The paper did not specify the level of Intellectual Disability for the others.) All had forensic histories of violence and/or sexual offences, such as sexual battery against a minor, pedophilia, incest and rape of a child. Based on a review of records, during the previous 12 months, they had each assaulted staff between 8 and 62 times and previous behavioral interventions were ineffective.

Therapists taught each client mindfulness skills during individual sessions. The client practiced mindfulness at least twice a day and had to practice mindfulness when incidents occurred that might have provoked aggressive behavior. Mindfulness training continued for up to 27 months. The authors reported that when they asked the participants to demonstrate the steps of mindfulness, all six could do so, but the authors did not to assess whether the participants used the skills on the unit on a daily basis. The experiment used a multiple baseline across participants design and took place over 34 months. Baselines were 3, 5, or 7 months long. Staff recorded data on incidents and aggressive behavior during morning and afternoon but not night shifts. Independent pairs of staff collected interobserver agreement data during 25 % of baseline and 15 % of intervention months. Interobserver agreement was 92 % (range 88–100 %).

There was a large reduction in the number of aggressive behaviors across all participants. Reduction in aggressive behavior only occurred after interventions, thus one may conclude that the intervention caused the reduction in aggressive behavior. During baseline, the number of incidents of aggression ranged from 0 to 4 per month. Impressively, all six participants' aggression was at zero for at least 6 months at the end of intervention and for one participant aggression had not occurred for 23 months. In baseline, the mean number of physical restraints ranged from 1.14 to 2.60 per month for each participant. After intervention, restraints were not used at all for any participant. Injuries to staff and peers occurred only during baseline and never occurred following intervention for all six peers.

This is an impressive study on a number of counts. First, the impact on aggressive behavior, restraints, and injuries was large, robust across all six clients and maintained over a very extensive period of time. Further, the participants were people that most would consider challenging and who had clinically significant levels of violence that resulted in severely restricting consequences for them. The study has at least two significant limitations. First, since the staff collected their own data, we cannot be sure of its accuracy. The study reported high interobserver agreement on the number of aggressive behaviors; however, the number of aggressive behaviors was low, and the authors reported overall levels of interobserver agreement, rather than occurrence interobserver agreement, thus, chance levels of agreement for this high level of interobserver agreement might account for high interobserver agreement. Second, as the authors themselves noted, they did not confirm if participants used mindfulness skills in the natural environment. Thus, it is unclear what the mechanism for change might be. For example, change might have occurred because staff reduced the number of triggers they presented to the clients, rather than through actual use of mindfulness skills when triggers occurred.

A second similar study comes from Singh et al. (2006) who evaluated the effects of training staff to use mindfulness skills in 15 group home staff who worked the first shift (7:30 a.m.–4:30 p.m.) in three groups homes. The residents were 18 adults aged 25–47 years all with severe or profound Intellectual Disability, 11 of whom had behavior plans for aggression and psychotropic medication for an Axis I mental health diagnosis. All clients had person-centered plans. The authors staggered staff training across the three group homes, so that there was a multiple baseline across settings design. When staff first began work, they participated in a 2-h training in behavior programming, and during the baseline of this study, they also participated in a 5-day training on behavior management. The training did not include any material on aversive contingencies. During mindfulness training, staff participated in a 5-day workshop that taught mindfulness principles and practiced medication and mindful-enhancing exercises. The main measure of aggression was "staff interventions for aggression" which the authors defined as "Staff interventions for aggression by the individual were recorded each time they occurred. The authors defined aggression as "an assault on another individual or staff member in any manner, to any intentional act against property that was meant to break, damage, or destroy it" (p. 549).

The mean numbers of staff interventions for aggression were 20.9, 18.4, and 13.1 per week during baseline, behavioral training, and mindfulness training, respectively. The data were stable during both baseline and behavioral training, and when mindfulness training began, there was a systematic decrease in staff interventions for aggression in each group home which occurred only when mindfulness training began. Data on restraint use were broadly similar. The mean number of restraints per week in each group home was 12.0 during baseline. During behavioral training, the mean number of restraints was 7.4 and 1.0 per week during baseline, behavioral training, and mindfulness training, respectively. Thus, behavioral training resulted in a moderate reduction in restraints; however, mindfulness training resulted in a large reduction in restraints, and by the end of the intervention, the staff did not use restraints at all.

As with the previous study, the large reduction in staff interventions for aggression and the elimination of restraints following mindfulness training is impressive, but the study has some significant limitations that weaken the conclusion that mindfulness caused the reduction in restraints. First, the authors did not report any interobserver agreement and, since the definition of aggression is not fully operationalized and staff collected the data themselves, it is not completely certain if the data on aggression are accurate. Further, the independent variable was complex and included many possible components. For example, the authors reported an increase in the number of client objectives mastered and increases in socially and physically integrated activities. Thus, it is unclear if we should ascribe these changes to simple Differential Reinforcement of Alternate Behavior, or whether the changes resulted from staff adopting mindfulness practices.

Singh et al. (2009) also reported a similar study in which they evaluated the effects of training staff in mindfulness practices. Twenty-three staff from four group homes participated in training. There were four group homes each with five people with Intellectual Disabilities. There were 1, 4, 12, and 2 residents with mild, moderate, severe, and profound Intellectual Disabilities, seven took psychotropic medication and two took antiepileptic medication. Nine has no psychiatric diagnosis and five, four, and two had diagnoses of psychosis, mood disorder, and autism, respectively. During orientation training, staff participated in training in behavior management which took place 2 years before the beginning of the present study. Again, this training did not include any material on aversive contingencies. Mindfulness training took place over 12 weeks and included weekly 2 h trainings similar to that described earlier. After mindfulness training, the authors requested the staff to use mindfulness practices, but they did not ask them to stop using any behavior management practices. The authors introduced training staggered across the morning and afternoon shifts to form a multiple baseline design across two groups of staff.

On the morning shift, the rates of incidents of aggression were 10.67, 10.1, and 6.67 per week during baseline, mindfulness training, and mindful practice, and on the afternoon shift, the corresponding figures were 8.60, 7.08, and 6.22 per week. There was evidence that there were fewer incidents of staff interaction that might lead to resident aggression, for example, the use of verbal redirection and the number of interactions that might lead to aggression reduced after the introduction of mindfulness practice. On the morning shift, the rate of physical restraints was 2.67, 2.00, and 0.20 per week, and on the afternoon shift, the rate of restraints was 2.60, 1.50, and 0.35 per week during baseline, mindfulness training, and mindfulness practice, respectively. Near the end of the mindfulness practice phase, the rates of restraint were zero or close to zero for 22–25 weeks. There was also a large reduction in injuries to both residents and staff following mindfulness practice. Like the previous mindfulness studies, these results are both promising and compromised. The outcomes, if accurate, are highly meaningful, but the data may be compromised for the same reasons described in the discussion of the previous studies.

A fourth study extended the use of mindfulness training to reduce restraint and PRN medication in people with mental illness. Singh et al. (2007) evaluated the effectiveness of soles of the feet meditation on aggression and also followed them up over a 4-year period into community settings. They reported data on PRN medication and restraint in one of the three men who showed large reduction in both restrictive procedures both during intervention and at follow-up. (The other participants did not have any of these procedures throughout the experiment.)

These four studies of mindfulness are intriguing. The outcomes reported—reductions in aggression, restraint, injuries, staff use of potentially unpleasant interactions, and increases in client learning objectives, socially and physically integrated activities—are impressive and very meaningful; however, the accuracy of these data is unclear. Future research should evaluate the outcomes of mindfulness using reliable data collected by independent observers. It is tempting to conclude that these changes were caused by staff adopting mindful practices. Such conclusions are tempting as mindfulness and the adoption of meditation practices are currently popular; its appeal to loving kind interactions as one of the vehicles of change appears to have high social validity in contrast to the apparently mechanistic/scientific language of contingencies and stimulus control. Such conclusions, however, are unwarranted at this time as there are other plausible and more parsimonious explanations of the effects of mindfulness interventions, which, if one subscribes to science's value on parsimonious over non-parsimonious explanations (Cooper et al. 2007), one should prefer.

9.3 Psychiatric Advanced Directives

An interesting approach to reducing restrictive behavior management practices in patients with psychiatric disorder comes from Swanson et al. (2008) who evaluated the effects of psychiatric advanced directives. Psychiatric advanced directives have two elements—advanced directives for when the person is mentally unwell and an appointed proxy decision maker. Swanson used a six-item checklist of coercive measures, such as being handcuffed and placed in seclusion. Using multivariate statistics to control for confounding variables, they found that the odds ratio of coercive measures for people with psychiatric advanced directives was 0.50 ($p<0.05$), meaning that after controlling for other factors, psychiatric advanced directives reduced the risk of subsequent coercive measures by 50%, although differences between the Psychiatric Advanced Directives and nonpsychiatric advanced directives group was no longer significant at 24 months follow-up.

9.4 Legislation

Following restraint-related deaths, politicians and administrators have often passed legislation or revise agency policies and advocates lobby for legislation to ban or restrict restraint. Family members, advocates and any organizations such as National Alliance on Mental Illness and TASH have also called for legislation to restrict or eliminate various forms of restrictive behavior management practices. Is this approach effective in reducing restrictive behavior management practices and ensuring client safety?

Surprisingly, given the frequency of this approach, there is little research evaluating it. Keski-Valkama et al. (2007), however, did evaluate the effects of legislation in Finland which was intended to reduce restraint and seclusion in psychiatric hospitals. They found that the number of restraints and seclusions reduced, but the number of patients also reduced. When the rate of restraints and seclusions were analyzed between 1990 and 2004, they found that the rate of restraint and seclusion remained the same, but that the duration of seclusion had *increased*. Thus, there was little support for the notion that legislation is as effective in reducing restraint and seclusion.

It is tempting to believe that passing legislation will fix things, but how many people break the speed limit and drive dangerously every day! In many circumstances, adequate legislation already exists. Thus, the problem may not be the lack of legislation but rather the lack of adequate implementation and oversight of existing adequate legislation. For example, in the USA, the *Individuals with Disabilities Education Act* and many state laws are quite prescriptive in requiring practices, such as functional behavioral assessments and positive behavior support plans, which likely would be highly effective in reducing restrictive behavior management practices. Unfortunately, such legislation is widely ignored by schools in the USA with little effective state or Federal oversight to correct this failure. Legislators and advocates might consider investing their time ensuring correct implementation of existing laws, rather than waiting for new laws to be passed, which services might also not implement.

9.5 Aversive Consequences

Behavior modification using aversive consequences was used more commonly in the 1960s through 1980s than today. Indeed, most contemporary ethical and professional standards call for the use of non-aversive interventions based on functional assessment and functional analysis involving environmental rearrangement, skills teaching, and positive reinforcement procedures. Thus, although there is consensus that these procedures should be used first, there is disagreement among practitioners and researchers as to whether aversive procedures should be used in any circumstances at all.

Several papers have evaluated the effects of aversive procedures as part of an effort to reduce or eliminate both chronic, life-threatening self-injurious behavior and restraints. For example, Duker and Seys (2000) evaluated the effects of contingent painful electric shock on reducing the reliance on mechanical restraint to control self-injury. Parents had consented to treatment, which had also been approved by a human rights committee. They compared the degree of mechanical restraint in a group of eight adults with severe/profound Intellectual Disability who received contingent shock with a matched group of individuals who received other active treatments, such as psychotropic medication, behavior analytic treatment, and gentle teaching. They measured the degree of mechanical restraint using the *Imposed Mechanical Restraint Inventory* (Duker and Seys 1997), a standardized measure of the extent, degree of intrusion, and duration of mechanical restraint. Duker and Seys (2000) administered the *Imposed Mechanical Restraint Inventory* on two occasions 3 years apart before and at follow-up after contingent shock. There was a large and statistically significant reduction in the degree of mechanical restraint in the treatment group only. The control group continued to be restrained to the same extent as baseline throughout the study.

A second study from Duker and Seys (1996) reported the long-term effects of contingent electrical shock on self-injurious behavior and restraints in 12 individuals with severe or profound Intellectual Disabilities with lifelong, life-threatening self-injurious behavior. Nine lived in residential facilities and three lived with their families. Previous treatments with extinction, Differential Reinforcement of Other Behavior, positive punishment using contingent water mist, functional movement training,[2] gentle teaching, and multiple pharmacological treatments had failed to reduce self-injurious behavior, and their parents and caregivers had requested contingent shock. This was not an experimental study, but reported pre – and follow-up data on rates of self-injurious behavior and restraint use at 2 to 47 months follow-up. The intervention consisted of three parts. In phase 1, the therapist gave parents and staff information about the treatment and all had to experience the shock personally. The therapist then removed or partially removed restraint and administered shock contingent upon each occurrence of self-injurious behavior during a 30–45 min session. If self-injurious behavior was not completely suppressed, there was a second session the same day or a couple of days later. If a participant exhibited multiple forms of self-injurious behavior, then the therapist treated each topography sequentially. If intervention in phase 1 suppressed self-injurious behavior, they proceeded to phase 2 in which a case manager with a master's degree in psychology was responsible for implementing the procedure in the natural environment. The procedure included contingent shock, differential reinforcement of other behavior and supervision and feedback to staff and family members implementing the procedure, and individual teaching of communication skills to the client. In phase 3, the program was handed over to family members and staff with reduced supervision. There were several individual modifications to the program which Duker and Seys describe in detail. Interobserver agreement on the use of restraint was 96 % and for self-injurious behavior was 93 %.

Of the 12 individuals who entered the program, seven had virtually no restraint and no or close to no self-injurious behavior at follow-up. Three other clients had intermittent responses to treatment that included reduced use of restraint, but continued shock to suppress self-injurious behavior. Treatment failed in two cases: The therapists discontinued the program and these clients remained in the restraints at follow-up. The procedure had negative side-effects for some participants, such as panic, extreme anxiety, and aggressive behavior for five participants, and freezing for a sixth participant, when they first experience the shock. The therapists managed these side-effects with relaxation.

Mudford et al. (1995) reported similar effects of contingent electric shock greatly reducing self-injurious behavior. They speculated that their participant's self-injurious behavior was maintained by access to restraints commented that the shock

[2] Functional movement training is a form of positive punishment in which the person is required, and if necessary, physically guided through appropriate forms of behavior. For example, Foxx (1977) taught eye contact to children with autism and/or Intellectual Disabilities who had not learned eye contact through simple positive reinforcement procedures to make eye contact using functional movement training. Functional movement training consisted of prompting the child to look up, look left, and look right if they did not look after a simple instruction to do so.

device, that the participant appeared to be calmer and happier when wearing the device, assisted in placing it on himself and its removal provoked tantrums; thus, the shock device appeared to have acquired some of the functions that mechanical restraint may have had. Williams et al. (1993) also reported elimination of self-injurious behavior and mechanical restraint in another individual following treatment with contingent electric shock, although this individual subsequently relapsed.

One practical problem with positive punishment is that this procedure might require caregivers to apply punishment contingent on each response and to follow relatively detailed treatment protocols (Duker and Seys 1996) which might render this intervention too difficult or effortful to implement accurately. One alternative is to use schedule thinning in which the proportion of responses that caregivers punish is gradually reduced perhaps resulting in both the suppression of the first behavior and reduction and perhaps elimination in the use of the restrictive procedure (Lerman et al. (1997). In this way, positive punishment procedures can be reduced and perhaps eliminated.

9.6 Seclusion and Time-Out

Seclusion and time-out, as noted earlier, are two procedures that may sometimes share common features, but can be distinguished. Seclusion usually involves placing a person in a locked seclusion room, sometimes for extensive periods of time, usually in response to intense violence that caregivers cannot otherwise manage safely. As such, it is a management technique aimed to ensure client and staff safety. Some sources have argued that its use might be "therapeutic," for example, by reducing stimulation and thereby allowing the person to regain control of their behavior; however, the precise mechanism by which seclusion might bring about some beneficial change is unclear. In contrast, time-out is short for "time-out from positive reinforcement," including the reinforcement maintaining the problem behavior as well as other reinforcement. There are many specific procedures that might constitute time-out from positive reinforcement, depending upon the functional assessment/analysis and specifics of the situation. Some of these forms of time-out might be quite socially acceptable, such as a person taking their own time-out by removing themselves from a reinforcing situation. Other forms might be more concerning, especially if the procedure might involve risk of injuries to clients and caregivers and if the form of time-out is demeaning. Locked room time-out is of special concern on both counts, even if it reduces a dangerous target behavior.

Few studies have addressed elimination of seclusion and locked room time-out. Indeed, several recent reviews have failed to identity randomized controlled trials of seclusion reduction (Sailas and Fenton 2000). Despite the neglect of this issue, at least two studies have attempted to address reduction of these procedures.

Iwata et al. (2009) reported a unique study in which they evaluated the effectives of time-out and systematically eliminated it in many cases. The study took place in a community residential service and day program for 90 adolescents and adults with

Intellectual Disabilities most of whom had also been diagnosed with Prader–Willi syndrome. When the study began, 50 of the clients had time-out and a variety of positive procedures in their treatment plans. Eleven clients who exhibited very-low-frequency, high-intensity aggressive behavior did not participate. Fifteen per cent engaged in aggression, 15 % engaged in property destruction and 70 % engaged in both. The researchers eliminated time-out for the remaining 39 staggered over 1 year, such that they eliminated time-out for 3–5 programs during any month. Time-out involved one of two procedures to remove attention. These were either exclusion time-out, in which caregivers removed the individual from the environment, or non-exclusory time-out, in which caregivers restricted the individual's activity within the setting, such as requiring them to remain sitting. Data were available for 34 of the 39 clients.

For 21 individuals (62 %) when treatment teams eliminated time-out target behaviors, either remained at the same frequency or reduced (and in some cases ceased) from 2.6/day to 1.4/day. For 13 individuals, target behavior increased from an average of 0.9/day to 1.3/day. For ten of these individuals, increases were modest or caregivers could readily manage the target behavior with modified program, such as the addition of noncontingent reinforcement, escape extinction, token economies, etc. Only in 3 of 39 clients was time-out reinstated because it was shown to be effective and judged to be warranted. Group data for the entire program showed that prior to these interventions, the frequency and duration of time-out increased dramatically over a 9-month period; this coincided with staff training on correct implementation of time-out and other aspects of the treatment plans. After implementation of the reduction program, restraint frequency and duration decreased to below baseline levels.

This study showed that, in this community setting at least, much of the time-out was unwarranted and sometimes resulted in increases in the target behavior. Evaluation of the effectiveness of the restrictive intervention, by first ensuring caregivers correctly implement it and then systematically eliminating the restrictive procedure might be an interesting model for practitioners to use, both for individuals and entire service setting. The reader should note that this study has several limitations. These included first the lack of interobserver agreement data on the target behavior, restraint use, and treatment integrity, and second the fact that this is a unique study that awaits replication.

A second study that addressed reduction of time-out through organization-wide interventions comes from Davidson et al. (1984). This study is discussed in Chap. 12 related to reduction of multiple restrictive procedures including time-out.

9.7 Inappropriate Psychotropic Medication

The use of psychotropic medications for behavior management remains highly controversial in many populations. This section will describe efforts to reduce two forms of inappropriate psychotropic medication: PRN medication and excessive routine psychotropic medication.

9.8 As Needed (PRN) Medication

PRN medications are widely used to manage challenging behavior in many populations. They come with several costs. First, their widespread or routine use suggests a failure to implement less restrictive behavior management strategies effectively. Second, they often come with negative side-effects such as sedation and impaired learning. Thus, in many cases they work, not by suppressing challenging behavior, but by suppressing all behavior including desirable, adaptive behavior. Thus, in some cases sedation may be dangerous, for example by placing people with multiple disabilities at increased risks for choking and aspiration and by placing seniors at risk for falls. The use of antipsychotic PRN medication places people who are already taking antipsychotic and other medications at risk for high doses of antipsychotic medication and inappropriate polypharmacy. Finally, PRN medication is also potentially expensive in terms of staff time to administer and review their use and the indirect costs involved in managing their interactions with other medications.

9.8.1 Psychiatric Services

Studies have also reduced the reliance on PRN medications in psychiatric services. For example, Donat (2003) extended an existing database on restrictive procedures to track PRN medication. He used a criterion of three or more PRNs in 1 week to trigger a review by the patient's clinical team using a checklist. The checklist prompted the team to review the manner in which PRN medication was used, whether its continued use was likely and whether a behavior plan was needed. If PRN medications continued to be used at the high rate of 3 consecutive weeks, then the matter was referred to the facility's human rights committee for further review. This procedure resulted in a 30 % reduction in the number of patients with high rates of PRN medication. A subsequent replication study reported a 40 % reduction in PRN medication over a 12-month period in a large psychiatric hospital (Donat 2006).

An interesting lesson can be learned from a failed attempt to reduce excessive psychotropic medication. Barnes et al. (2008) reported an attempt to reduce excessive psychotropic medication in a sample of over 3000 psychiatric in-patients in 218 wards in 32 hospitals over a 2-year period. At year 1, they audited the use of high dose and combined antipsychotic medication and found that about a third of the population had excessive medication. Intervention consisted of deriving three audit standards from the literature, such as typical and atypical antipsychotics and should not be prescribed unless switching from one class to another. Additionally, information was disseminated to sites that were encouraged to disseminate it to clinicians. There was no effect on excessive prescriptions of antipsychotic medications 1 year later. Why? In contrast to the work of Donat and other effective studies, two key elements were missing. First, the treatment was left undefined. By leaving it up to local sites as how and even whether to disseminate the information to practitioners, it is unclear either what the treatment was, or, whether or not it was delivered. Second, the intervention included no consequences for practitioner for excessive use of psychotropic medication. For example, effective interventions usually include programming practitioner effort for continued use of inappropriate psychotropic medication, such as additional review activity and implementation of staff training, whereas in this intervention there was no programmed consequences for practitioners continued excessive use of antipsychotic medication.

Other approaches to reduce PRN medication in psychiatric in-patient facilities include increasing patient activity on the ward. For example, Thomas et al. (2006) found that increasing patient activity decreased use of PRN medication by about half on one of two wards. The reasons for the differences across the wards were unclear but could have been due to issues of treatment integrity of choice and quality of activities offered.

9.8.2 Developmental Disabilities

Davidson et al. (1994) conducted a broad organizational intervention including target setting and feedback to reduce several forms of restrictive behavior management practices including PRN medication. This intervention was effective in reducing PRN medication. (See Chap. 12 below for a more detailed discussion of this study.)

A more recent study comes from Brooker et al. (2014). They evaluated the effects of training 12 staff in mindfulness supporting seven clients over an 8-week period in two group homes. When comparing the use of restrictive behavior management practice before and after training, they found that mindfulness training resulted in a reduction in a range of restrictive behavior management practices, including reductions in PRN medication and seclusions.

9.8.3 Other Populations

Although PRN medications are widely used in nursing homes with seniors (Baker et al. 2008), little attention has been paid in the research literature to the alternatives to PRN medication to manage agitation and aggressive behavior. One study (Dean et al. 2009) reported on decreasing the use of PRN medication in a locked youth facility but did not describe a specific program that might be responsible for this change in practice. Likewise, Hueffner et al. (2014) reported reduction in the use of several restrictive behavior management practices including PRN medications at an inpatient unit using a cognitive behavior therapy program, but it is unclear of the reduction was due to the program or other factors.

9.9 Routine Psychotropic Medications

Several studies have evaluated attempts to reduce psychotropic medications. These efforts include randomized controlled trials, reports of less formal attempts to reduce use of psychotropic medication in routine services, and feedback and consultation interventions to reduce excessive and inappropriate psychotropic medications.

Ahmed et al. (2000) reported a randomized controlled trials in which they randomized 36 people with Intellectual Disability to a no-treatment control of a systematic drug reduction program for individuals taking antipsychotic medication for behavioral issues (individuals taking antipsychotic medication for psychoses were excluded). In the experimental group, antipsychotic medication was reduced by 25 % per month over a month period. Thirty-three percent of the experimental group successfully completed a complete elimination of medication and 33 % experienced at least a 50 % reduction. Reduction in medication was associated with no increase in challenging behavior, a marginal increase in engagement, some (beneficial) weight loss and increase in dyskinesia for some. When comparing responders with nonresponders, service factors predicted nonresponse. Namely, those in the control group who were in more restrictive residences and whose staff were not well trained in behavior management were more likely to relapse indicating that quality of service is important in protecting clients from relapse. In a subsequent analysis of these data, Smith et al. (2002) demonstrated that individuals who were tapered off their antipsychotic medication were not more responsive to staff interaction after withdrawal.

There are several reports of successfully reducing psychotropic medication in people with Intellectual Disability in clinical practice (Branford 1996; Briggs 1989; Fielding et al. 1980; Jancar 1970; Leppler et al. 1994; Luchins Dojka and Hanrahan 1993; Wressell et al. 1990) suggesting that this can be done in routine clinical services as well as in randomized controlled trials. Reducing inappropriate medication may also have significant financial benefits (Ellenor and Frisk 1977; Kojima et al. 2012). For example, direct costs such as the costs of medication may be reduced, but indirect costs, such as the costs of medication administration, review and oversight, may also be reduced or eliminated.

9.10 Conclusions

A variety of approaches other than applied behavior analysis can be used to reduce a full range of restrictive behavior management practices, although the outcomes are quite varied and the literature is patchy when one looks at different populations. In the next two chapters, we move to look at organization-wide interventions to manage restrictive behavior management practices.

Chapter 10
Organizational Approaches: General Principles

Previous treatment chapters have dealt with interventions for individuals; however, often we are interested in reducing restrictive behavior management practices on a large scale—at the level of an individual program, such as a nursing home, at the level of an organization, at the state, and even national level. This issue has been commonly addressed in institutions for people with Intellectual Disabilities, nursing homes, youth facilities, and psychiatric facilities. More recent data on high rates of behavior management practices in some community settings for adults with disabilities (Sturmey 2009), and special and mainstream education settings and some youth services, indicate the need for service-wide reductions in behavior management practices in other services as well.

Earlier sections of this book have examined whether individual differences predict the use of restrictive behavior management practices. Commonly they do, but often to only a small degree (Sturmey 1999). Thus, although externalizing behavior, such as aggression and self-injury, often precipitates the use of restrictive behavior management practices, there remain large differences between one setting and another in their use of restrictive behavior management practices that are not accounted for by the types of service users they have. Rather, it seems that there is something about certain service settings that makes them much more likely to use restrictive behavior management practices. Thus, one rationale for organizational interventions to reduce restrictive behavior management practices is that there is something about the organization that needs to be changed to reduce restrictive behavior management practices. A second rationale for organizational interventions is that sometimes restrictive behavior management practices are used very frequently within certain parts of an organization or at certain times of the day or week. Thus, although it could be possible to reduce restrictive behavior management practices on a case-by-case basis, it might be more efficient to deal with it at an organizational level. For example, if services are highly crowded, noisy, and disorganized at a certain time of day and this is associated with high use of restrictive behavior management practices, it might be better to address the performance of the organization and its staff rather than the behavior of its service users, at least in the first instance.

P. Sturmey, *Reducing Restraint and Restrictive Behavior Management Practices*,
Autism and Child Psychopathology Series, DOI 10.1007/978-3-319-17569-0_10

10.1 Common Components of Organizational Interventions

10.1.1 Six Core Strategies

LeBel, Huckshorn, and Jacobs (2014) reviewed six core strategies that formed the basis of the National Association of State Mental Health Program Directors nation strategy to reduce and eliminate restraint. Although others have produced similar lists, we will use these six core strategies to consider organizational approaches to reduce restrictive behavior management practices, since they are the basis of some empirically evaluated training and have been disseminated to numerous sites.

10.1.1.1 Leadership Toward Organizational Change

The first element consists of direct involvement of the executive staff participating, defining and articulating the mission, establishing philosophies of care, values developing, and overseeing the plan. These guidelines focus on what leadership should do, but we should also consider what leadership should refrain from doing that can undermine services achieving the goal of restraint reduction. Statements or behavior from leadership that undermine the goal and indications of disinterest or interest in frivolous, non-client focused activities by organization leaders may all undermine restraint reduction.

Leadership and organizational plans often include multiple components, one of which is goal setting. Goals may be set for reduction in restraints for individual high-rate restraint clients, as well as program areas or entire organizations. For example, an organization might set a short-term goal that "We will reduce the number of incidents of restraints from 10 per month to 5 per month by 2/1/14." Such goals can then be adjusted toward eventual elimination of restraints over time such as "We will reduce the number of restraints to 0 for 3 consecutive months by 12/31/14."

A second common component is to analyze the use and pattern of restraints. Restraints are often concentrated in few high-risk clients, high-risk program areas, and high-risk times of the day. Analysis of the patterns of restraint (see Finn and Sturmey 2009, for example) in this manner can be helpful in directing an organization to focus its resources to certain program areas. A third common component is some form of staff training and support. This can include relatively simple information about the importance of restraint reduction, focusing on specific clients and times of the day, intervention strategies for specific clients, teaching on generic prevention strategies such as increasing adaptive behavior, prevention of challenging behavior that results in restraint use, and promoting staff use of alternate methods of managing challenges without the use of restraint. A fourth very common component is the use of feedback systems. Feedback may be given verbally, graphically, or in writing and may be given to individual staff, program areas, supervisors, and program administrators. Feedback may be more acceptable if it includes recognition of staff efforts and areas of progress and suggestions for specific strategies to use rather than general exhortations for change. Feedback can also vary in its frequency. It may be more useful to provide very frequent—weekly or even daily—feedback for individual high-risk cases early. If progress is made, the frequency can be reduced. Similarly, feedback to program areas and organizations might begin relatively frequently early in restraint reduction, but might proceed from weekly to monthly to quarterly feedback if restraint is reduced a great deal and an organization moved from an intervention to a maintenance phase. A fifth procedure that is used less frequently is to improve the quality of Applied Behavior Analysis services. For example, some interventions have required conducting functional assessments and analyses, development of behavior support plans (Williams and Grossett 2011), required behavioral consultation following restraint (Donat 2003, 2006), or use of behavioral skills training to improve program integrity. A final component is the use of some form of oversight committee which may analyze and review data, organize and provide consultation and support to challenging situations, set priorities, and provide feedback.

Leadership and organizational plans also involve other more informal components that are not always specifically recognized. For example, attempts to reduce restraint often highlight staff performance and organizational problems. These can include long-standing unresolved staff performance issues in individual carestaff, supervisors, professionals and administrators, and the lack of resources and poor quality services, all of which may contribute to inappropriate restraints use and lack of preventative interventions. Sometimes these problems may be resolved by improved training and supervision of the staff and redesigning their jobs and responsibilities. Sometimes they are only resolved through staff reassignment and other negative supervisory actions. A second group of staff performance and organizational problems relates to the oversight mechanism that an organization may use. An effective oversight mechanism requires accurate and up-to-date data systems and sufficient resources, skills, and motivation to use that information effectively. Thus, oversight committees may fail due to the lack of accurate data, failure to analyze and interpret data, failure to take action, or failure to evaluate their actions and subsequently take appropriate actions. Finally, the role of organization-wide restraint reduction can highlight the effectiveness and motivation of an organization's leadership. Research has not examined the exact role of an organization's leadership in restraint reduction. One might expect that organizational leaders who show commitment to the project show some ongoing involvement, provoke their staff to take action, and who refrain from cynicism, indifference, undermining restraint reduction or supporting restraint use might have better client outcomes than those leaders who do not engage in these actions.

10.1.1.2 Using Data to Inform Practice

LeBel et al. recommended using data with staff in a nonpunitive manner to analyze organizational problems by examining restraint use by unit, shift, day, and staff members. Use facility baselines, set goals, monitor the use of restraint and seclusion over time, and compare data across facilities. Setting up and using valid datasets are challenging for many facilities. (The section below recommends some basic measures of service use of restrictive behavior management practices.) Unfortunately, some organizational leaders and professionals lack basic numeracy to understand restraint data or feign misunderstanding to avoid taking effortful but effective action. For example, over an extended period of time, the number of persons using a service will vary. Obviously, the number of restrictive behavior management practices will vary depending upon how many people use the services. Hence, valid data require some correction to the raw number of restrictive behavior management practices used reflecting the change in the number of service users. This can be done by expressing the number of restrictive behavior management practices as a rate per 1000 service user days or as a percentage of service users experiencing the restrictive behavior management practice in question. Finally, the database should indicate a clear baseline. This should include at least three data points before intervention begins.

Table 10.1 illustrates such an approach. The data include not only the number of restraints each month but also the number of service users and number of service user days. If the data consisted only of the raw number of restraints, it would be difficult to interpret the reduction in the number of restraints in May and June, as it might be due to a decrease in the number of service users. Inspection of the percentage of service users restrained and the rate of restraint use per 1000 service user days clarify that (a) the increase in restraints in April is large when using the rate per service days and that (b) the reductions in frequency of restraints in May and June are also large as reflected in both the percentage of service users restraints and the rate of restraints per 1000 service user days.

A significant challenge for many clinicians and organizations is that over time the database grows and can become difficult to manage and interpret. For example, an organization may monitor restrictive behavior management practices over several years. When doing this, the organization may be unable to evaluate its efforts to do so, if it fails to compare the current data to the original baseline or if it fails to take a new baseline to evaluate a new intervention to further reduce restrains after an initial restraint reduction. A second aspect of this problem is that in order to reduce restrictive behavior management practices, organizations should monitor all forms of restrictive behavior management practices. This is important to ensure that one form of restrictive behavior management practices is not substituted for another. For example, sometimes, as personal restraints reduce, pro re nata (PRNs) and mechanical restraints may increase. Data in Table 10.2 illustrate how the original data in Table 10.1 can be extended to cover both a 15-month period and track different forms of restrictive behavior management practices in a way that permits evaluation of recent trends, comparison of current practices with baseline and to evaluate whether reduction of one restrictive behavior management practices results in an increase in another form of restrictive behavior management practices.

Table 10.1 Illustrative data on the rates of restraint over a 6-month period

	January 2010 (baseline)	*February 2010 (baseline)*	*March 2010 (baseline)*	April 2010	May 2010	June 2010
Number of restraints	*60*	*58*	*47*	78	35	27
Number of service users restrained	*14*	*17*	*15*	17	9	8
Average number of service users	*310*	*315*	*314*	309	304	299
Number of service user days	*9300*	*8820*	*9734*	9579	9429	8970
Percentage of service users restrained	*4.51 %*	*5.39 %*	*4.77 %*	5.50 %	2.96 %	2.67 %
Rate of restraint per 1000 service use days	*6.45/1000*	*6.57/1000*	*4.82/1000*	8.14/1000	3.71/1000	3.01/1000
Mean restraints per service user	*60/301 = 0.199*	*58/315 = 0.184*	*47/314 = 0.149*	78/309 = 0.252	35/304 = 0.155	27/299 = 0.090

Table 10.2 Illustrative data on the rates of personal restraint, mechanical restraint, and PRNs during a 3-month baseline and during the last 3 months of a 12-month intervention

	January 2010 (Baseline)	*February 2010 (Baseline)*	*March 2010 (Baseline)*	January 2011	February 2012	April 2012
Personal restraint (percentage restrained and rate per 1000 patient-days)	*4.51%* *6.45/1000*	*5.39%* *6.57/1000*	*4.77%* *4.82/1000*	0.52% 0.35/1000	0.47% 0.29/1000	0.62% 0.45/1000
Mechanical restraint (percentage restrained and total duration in hours)	*0.56%* *257 h*	*0.68%* *326 h*	*0.79%* *425 h*	0.23% 43 h	0.19% 39 h	0.23% 42 h
PRNs (percentage restrained and rate per 1000 patient-days)	*1.5%* *2.14/1000*	*2.3%* *2.80/1000*	*1.9%* *1.91/1000*	0.2% 0.13/1000	0.0% 0/1000	0.1% 0.07/1000

Cheating With Restraint Data

"Restraints are down 17%!!!" announced a state director, but what does that mean? Are 17% fewer persons restrained this month compared to last month (or last year?) Does it refer to all restraints or only personal restraints? Does it refer to frequency or duration of restraints? (When I contacted the state agency that posted this information online, no one could tell me what the numbers meant, but the state director had recently resigned.)

Some organizations prefer to avoid embarrassment and work related to managing restrictive behavior management practices and behave in a way that indicates that appearances are more important that substantively achieving client outcomes. One way to do this is to cheat with restraint data to make it appear that there is no problem to address. Box 10.1 contains a list of the author's experiences illustrating

Box 10.1 How to Cheat with Restraint Data

1. *Deny that restraints occur.* I walked into a special education classroom with a program administrator. I observed a new staff member on the floor with her legs over the child's legs and her arms wrapped around the child preventing him from moving. I asked the program director "When did we start using restraint here?" and she replied looking around the room in every direction but at what was happening 18 in. from her feet, "We do not use restraint in this school. So I asked, isn't that staff restraining that boy?" to which she replied "Where?"

Upon seeing two teenagers tied to their wheelchairs in a community agency, my curiosity aroused, I asked the program director why they were tied to their wheelchair. Visibly embarrassed, she stated this was a physical therapy program. My curiosity aroused still further, I asked, so what happens when you untie the guys. "Oh please don't do that, they will bite their fingers off."When I reviewed their charts, there was no physical consult relating to positioning, no functional behavior assessment, and no behavior support plans, but there were liberal doses of ineffective yet potentially dangerous psychotropic medication.

2. *Cover up restraint use.* "We do not use restraint in my organization" proudly boasted an executive director, so I was surprised when I saw many children and adults held down on the floor. When I asked the now embarrassed executive director what this was, she hurriedly explained that although this *appeared* to be restraint the state did not define it as restraint as they were only required to return data on restraints that lasted 5 min or longer. To make sure they never had any "official" restraints they trained all staff to only hold service users for 4 min and 59 s, let go, and then reapply restraints to control self-injurious behavior.

3. *Use the word magic.* Services often use euphemisms to hide and deny restraint use. Seclusion rooms are often referred to as "calming rooms," "the blue room," etc. When asked if they seclude clients they deny it. But when challenged as to why a client is in the blue room screaming to be let out with the staff holding the door shut, they explain that this is not seclusion as the door is not shut. Sometimes physical restraints are given positive-sounding names, such as "physical supports" or "lap lizards," but if they impede clients moving they are just physical restraints.

"We don't restraint clients, we give them medicine" the doctoral pharmacologist pompously announced. "Besides, they ask for their medicine, so how could it be restraint?" Twenty minutes later, a client can barely move or even talk because they are so sedated and drooling so profusely.

4. *Do not look for restraints—You might not find them.* A professional at a workshop told me—apparently sincerely—that they did not use restraints anywhere in their services. I was surprised since they served several hundred clients. After a break, I asked the professional to come and talk to the direct care staff I had been talking to. One identified a women tied to her bed every night because of self-injury, and another described how all the clients of a day habilitation program were routinely escorted off the buses on leashes to stop them running into traffic. A third described how they routinely jammed one client into the corner with furniture to stop him running away and keeping him safe. The professional seemed genuinely concerned that all this restraint had been going on for years even though she had worked in this city for over 10 years. She returned to her office to do therapy with an individual client.

how organizations cheat with restraint data and thereby cheat their clients out of services indicating how these organizations do not actually commit to their expressed values. The way an individual or organization uses and presents restraint data is a real test of the values of the individual or organization.

Managing, using, and interpreting large datasets, such as those generated by organizations trying to reduce restrictive behavior management practices, is genuinely difficult in a number of ways. First, the data must be accurate. This requires both accurate and complete data entry at the time the restrictive behavior management practices is used and accurate data entry and maintenance of a database. Often the initial incident is difficult to document for direct carestaff because of both ineffective or absent training to do so and because the documentation is made unnecessarily burdensome. For example, sometimes restraint forms are too long, require narratives instead of checking boxes, and have to be signed by multiple persons often causing them to be lost or taking an inordinate amount of time to be entered in a database. Further, sometimes carestaff are required to fill out multiple forms for each incident, such as a restraint form, an Antecedent Behavior Consequence[1] form, one or more injury forms, and referral forms. Simplification of such procedures is essential if data are to be useful.

Data entry, management, and analysis can also be challenging. The advent of readily available databases, search functions, and graphs can be helpful. Larger organizations may need staff dedicated to this function. Such databases should be useful for generating reports such as scatterplots and breakdowns of restrictive behavior management practices by relevant variables, such as program units, days of the week, and time of the day or combinations of such variables.

Another challenge when working with large databases is that it can be difficult to interpret trends in the data. For example, small changes from one time period to another may represent random variation in stable data or the beginning of an undesirable increasing trend. It may not always be clear what the relevant baseline might be as details get lost over time. For example, in Table 10.3, the number of persons restrained and the total hours of mechanical restraint fell considerably from the 2-month baseline to the second month of intervention (October). Thereafter, there is no reduction in the percentage of persons restrained and the number of hours of

Table 10.3 Illustrative data on the use of mechanical restraints on one unit over a 6-month period

	July 2012 (baseline)	*August 2012 (baseline)*	September 2012	October 2012	November 2012	December 2012
Number (and percentage) of residents restraints	*5 (25 %)*	*7 (35 %)*	4 (20 %)	4(20 %)	4 (20 %)	4 (20 %)
Total hours of restraint	*271 h*	*252 h*	197 h	159 h	163 h	175 h

[1] An Antecedent—Behavior—Consequence form is a grid to record a behavior of interest, its antecedents and consequences (Bijou, Peterson & Ault, 1968). It is commonly used as part of a Functional Behavioral Assessment.

restraint remains substantially below the baseline, but is gradually trending upward. It is often tempting in such a situation to decide to "wait and see" as things are significantly better than baseline, but it might be better to revise the program in some way. One possibility is that the program was quite effective for a number of easier clients, but there remain four challenging clients or situations that have not yet been managed effectively.

10.1.1.3 Workforce Development

Lebel et al.'s third component is staff training, development, and human resource activities to create an environment that minimizes conflict and staff training that results in desirable client outcomes. This can be achieved by effective staff training, supervision, and job evaluation.

Staff and family members sometimes use restraint because they cannot do anything else—they may have no other relevant, effective response in their repertoire. Thus, a key component in reduction of restrictive behavior management practices is giving the staff other strategies they can use to prevent the problem behavior that results in restrictive behavior management practices and redirection strategies they can use in place of restraint. In some programs, this is done very informally and intuitively, by asking the staff to brainstorm other strategies they might use with high-risk clients or providing the staff with less coercive methods of preventing harm to other clients and staff, such as the use of cushions or padding program areas. In other cases, working with caregivers is more technological, such as training staff to correctly use interaction skills, prompting, reinforcement, choice making, and providing preferred activities to prevent precursor behaviors and target behaviors that results in restrictive behavior management practices. Similarly, staff may benefit from specific skills training on how to redirect clients engaging in precursor behavior, such as pacing, ruminating, and threatening and back to adaptive behavior, so that restrictive behavior management practices are unnecessary as the target behaviors do not occur.

Most organizations profess to train their staff well, but often need improvement in both the methods used and the coverage of staff training. Often staff training is presented in classes where the information is presented verbally or in written format, perhaps with videos to supplement a predominantly verbal presentation. It is well established that such methods are often ineffective as they do not give staff the opportunity to practice and receive feedback in key skills. A second challenge related to staff training is ensuring that all staff are trained and up to date with training. Sometimes, the managers are unaware of this issue because they lack the information and other times the managers see maintaining staff training as something to make a show during surveys or as part of responding to a crisis, rather than as a routine, good practice. The use of tracking and feedback systems is often helpful for the supervisors and managers. For large organizations, such datasets can be challenging to use efficiently and effectively. Table 10.4 illustrates such an approach.

Table 10.4 An example of a tracking system to ensure all staff remain up to date in training related to restrictive behavior management practices. The second row refers to training in generic prevention and restraint strategies required before working on the unit and annually thereafter. The third row refers to the training on current written behavior management plans for all the residents on the unit. The fourth row refers to whether or not the program is in compliance with the goals of maintaining 90 % of staff trained on prevention and restraint and all current plans. The tracking system also illustrates that greater difficulty in achieving compliance for staff training in behavior plans earlier on and thus was useful in prompting supervisors and professionals to invest greater resources in staff training in that area

	January 2013 (baseline)	February 2013	March 2013	April 2013	May 2013	June 2013
Staff trained in prevention and restraint	*8/10 80 %*	10/11 91 %	7/9 81 %	9/9 100 %	9/11 81 %	10/11 91 %
Staff current on all behavior plans	*5/10 50 %*	7/11 63 %	6/9 67 %	9/9 100 %	10/11 91 %	10/11 91 %
In compliance? (90 % target for both)	*No*	No	No	Yes	No	Yes

Specific Restraint and Seclusion Tools

Lebel et al.'s fourth component is the use of specific technologies, such as identifying high-risk clients and program areas, training in specific prevention and treatment strategies. It also includes environmental redesign, such as removing irritating stimuli and replacing them with a more pleasant soothing environment. Many such issues were discussed in the preceding section relating to staff and family member training.

10.1.1.4 Peer Roles in Patient Settings

Lebel's et al.'s intervention package was derived in the context of mental health services and uses peers as models and intervention agents because they have experienced many relevant problems and are more plausible models than the professional and treatment staff. In other contexts, such as services for children and adolescents, peers may be highly useful in modeling alternate behaviors, problem solving and self-management. This component has not been researched extensively.

10.1.1.5 Rigorous Debriefing

Lebel et al. include debriefing after behavioral incidents, and debriefing services have two purposes. First, it can review how service providers may have done things better—a kind of ad hoc training and feedback opportunity. Second, it can provide emotional support to both clients and staff, if the experience of restraint of seclusion was traumatic for either or both (Jones and Kroese 2006). Lebel et al. strongly recommend participation in medical staff in debriefing. (The practicality and relevance of this might vary from one context to another.) Again, there is little research on the value of debriefing in the reduction of RRBPs and there may be important differences in how debriefing is conducted that determines its effectiveness both in training staff and providing them with emotional support.

10.2 Conclusion

The work of Lebel et al. provides a useful framework to consider the elements that go into developing an organization-wide intervention for the reduction of restrictive behavior management practices. As noted elsewhere in this volume, restrictive behavior management practices are used in many different contexts, and hence this approach should be subject to considerable individualization according to the context in which an organization attempts to reduce restrictive behavior management practices. For example, the tracking sheets used in the preceding sections do not always make distinctions that may be important to certain contexts. Some organizations will wish to break down restraint use into more specific categories. For example, a residential service for adults with Intellectual Disabilities might prefer to break down personal restraints into cross-chest restraints, which might be viewed as the most dangerous, and break out holding someone's hands down separately as such a personal restraint would not be as dangerous as a cross-chest restraint. Likewise, in some nursing homes, distinguishing between bedrails, lap trays, modified chairs, strait jackets, etc. might be important, even though all are mechanical restraints. Each organization may have to tailor its approach to data collection to its own context, regulations, and goals. Other services may wish to track restraint use for new admissions to a service separately from other service users.

The data tracking systems described here are insufficient by themselves for administrators and clinicians to take effective action in many circumstances. For example, the meaning of the changes in restraint use in Table 10.3 is unclear. The gradually increasing rates of restraint involving four clients in the last few months raise many simple but important questions such as are these the same four people for all three months? Is the restraint stable among these people or is it variable among each person? Do these people have treatment plans?, etc. These more specific questions can be answered by follow-up with professional staff and family and developing, implementing, and evaluating specific plans to address these issues.

One of the main motivations for reducing and tracking restrictive behavior management practices is managing injuries. Whereas counting number or duration of restraints is relatively straightforward, measuring injuries is more problematic. Although it is relatively easy to compile reports that count frequency of injuries, developing a valid database and using it well is difficult. One problem is that the number of injuries may mean very little. For example, many people would feel that ten incidents of small scratches are much less serious than one near-life threatening injury. A further problem is that sometimes serious or near-life threatening injuries almost occur, but are prevented by good luck, but are still quite serious, such as when a staff member blocks a potentially very serious fall, but since no injury occurred, nothing may be documented. At this time, there is no good system of integrating injury data into a single numerical composite that allows services to track either an individual's or services injuries over time. At this time, practitioners must use good skills and judgment in evaluating client injury data alongside data on restrictive behavior management practices.

Chapter 11
Organizational Interventions: The Evidence

11.1 Literature Reviews

There have been numerous literature reviews of reducing restrictive behavior management practices, almost all of which have focused on restraints rather than other forms of restrictive behavior management practices. Most reviews of restraint have addressed specific populations. For example, many reviews have addressed restraint in nursing homes, especially in the late 1990s, reflecting the interest in restraints after the *Omnibus Reconciliation Act* regulations were revised (Bahrani and Snowden 2012; Cohen and Kruschwitz 1977; Cotter 2005; Evans et al. 2002; Quinn 1994; Sailas and Fenton 2000; Scheib et al. 1996; Wang and Moyle 2005), and some have addressed medication reduction (Richter et al. 2012). Other reviews have addressed psychiatric in-patients (Busch and Shore 2000), people with Intellectual Disability (ID) and autism (Harris 1996; Luiselli 2009; Maton and Boisjoli 2009; Newton 2009), child and adolescent services (Allen 2000; Delaney 2005; Delaney et al. 2001), critical care nursing (Martin 2002; Wilson 1996), and acute care nursing (Evans et al. 2002; Martin 2002; Sullivan-Marx et al. 1996) and multiple populations (Scanlan 2010). Some reviews were systematic reviews, for example, of specific intervention approaches, such as education (Meyer et al. 2012). (See below for separate discussion of systematic reviews and meta-analyses.) Finally, other reviews have focused on other restrictive behavior management practices such as seclusion (Busch and Shore 2000; Gaskin et al. 2007; Johnson et al. 2010; Sailas and Fenton 2000; Soloff and Gutheil 1988) and psychotropic medication, including pro re nata (PRN) psychotropic medication (Richter et al. 2012; Table 11.1).

Many of these reviews concur on several points including the desirability of reducing restrictive behavior management practices, the lack of data showing that such procedures improve client and staff safety, and the possibility of large reductions in restrictive behavior management practices through organizational interventions. An exception to this generalization was the review by Fisher's (1994) review of restraints and seclusion in psychiatry. Fisher concluded that restraint and seclu-

P. Sturmey, *Reducing Restraint and Restrictive Behavior Management Practices*,
Autism and Child Psychopathology Series, DOI 10.1007/978-3-319-17569-0_11

Table 11.1 Literature reviews of organizational interventions

Reference	Populations and settings	Summary
Quinn (1994)	Seniors	Identified three broad components to restraint reduction: (a) changing attitudes and beliefs, (b) patient assessments, and (c) avoid problems leading to restraint use. Noted that attitudes toward restraints with seniors were changing and that alternatives to restraints were being considered
Fisher (1994)	Psychiatry	Reviewed the literature from 1972 to 1994 on both restraint and seclusion. Concluded that: (1) restraint and seclusion were effective in decreasing injury and decreasing agitation, (2) it is nearly impossible to eliminate restraint and seclusion, (3) restraint and seclusion are harmful to patients, (4) restraint use is determined primarily by local administrative practices rather than clinical variables, (5) training can safely reduce restraint and seclusion, and (6) studies comparing different training programs would be useful
Harris (1996)	Children and adults with Intellectual Disabilities	Reviewed physical restraints. Distinguished three types of restraints: personal restraints (holding), mechanical restraints, and the person restraining themselves. Harris concluded that: (a) there are many mechanisms that go on during restraint that contribute to their (in)effectiveness, (b) the mechanisms that operate during contingent and noncontingent restraint are different from one another, (c) both contingent and noncontingent restraint can be effective, especially when noncontingent restraint is faded and when caregivers are involved in administration of contingent restraint, (d) the behavior of restraining oneself is reinforced whether by reinforcement from the restraint procedure itself or by escape from aversive consequences of self-injury, (e) staff behavior of applying restraints is negatively reinforced, for example, by termination of aversive client behavior, and (f) there is risk of staff and client injury, especially from emergency restraint
Wilson (1996)	Critical care nursing	Noted the movement to reduce restraint with the elderly, and reviewed the implications of this for nursing in critical care. The decision for nurses to use restraint is a serious decision and should be evaluated carefully. Alternatives should be considered and subject to cost-benefit analysis
Sullivan-Marx and Strumpf (1996)	Acute care	Empirical evidence shows that restraints have negative effects, including potentially serious negative effects, on safety and dignity. This should inform policy and professional ethics. Literature on restraint in the elderly can inform practice in acute care. Concluded that critical care nursing should embrace restraint-free care
Schieb et al. (1996)	Elderly	Estimated that up to 30 % of the seniors will be restrained in acute, rehabilitation, and long-term care. Restraints can be abused and have negative client outcomes and are expensive. There are alternate strategies. Restraints are incompatible with professional practice. Facilities should work toward eliminating restraints and should be managed by the entire treatment team
Castle (1998)	Elderly nursing homes	Reviewed efforts to reduce restraints following the nearing *Nursing Home Reform Act* (1988) including rationale, epidemiology, and changes in the national rate of restraint since the act. Rate of restraint fell from 41 to 21 % and the percentage of restraint-free facilities increased from 3.0 to 7.4 % from 1989 to 1996

Table 11.1 (continued)

Reference	Populations and settings	Summary
Allen (2000)	Children and adolescents	Based on a review of the literature from 1987 to 1998, the authors found that the staff had positive attitudes toward the use of restraint and seclusion with children and adolescents
Delaney et al. (2001)	Child and adolescent in-patient units	Derived guidelines for restraint reduction in child and adolescent units from nursing home and adult mental health literature. Several studies reported large reductions in restraints.
Martin (2002)	Acute and critical care	Reviewed regulatory standards and ethics. They found that the reduction of restraint is complex and involves liability issues for the staff. Restraint can be reduced by engaging leadership, understanding the meaning of patient behavior, a team approach, and involving the family are components of restraint reduction.
Wang and Moyle (2005)	Dementia	Reviewed literature between 1992 and 2003 and identified 42 papers. No evidence that restraints protect from injuries. Recommended involvement from state and federal government and leading organizations
Cotter (2005)	Seniors and nursing homes	Literature review which reviewed risks of restraints and interventions to reduce restraint use. Despite increased regulation to reduce restraint use, seniors continued to die from strangulation, asphyxiation, or cardiac arrest in restraint, for example, from bedrail entrapment. Restraints are used to reduce pacing, disorientation, and agitation. Physical restraints should be eliminated because of the harmful effects on seniors. Provides evidence that both organizational and individual interventions can reduce restraint
Delaney (2006)	Child and adolescent in-patient units	Reviewed organizational interventions, interventions to reduce aggression, and interventions to reduce PRN medications, update of preceding review (Delaney 2001). Found accumulating evidence from case studies of individual services to support evidence to support organizational interventions, but not aggression–reduction interventions
Gaskin et al. (2007)	Psychiatry	Reviewed literature on seclusion reduction. Multi-component packages including state administrative support, state policy, staff training and support, treatment planning, increasing staffing levels, pharmacological interventions, and patient participation can be effective
Luiselli (2009)	Intellectual Disabilities community services	Reviewed effects of antecedent manipulations and fixed time release criterion on reducing restraints. Concluded that both procedures can reduce restraint. Recommended future research focuses on long-term outcomes and adoption of evidence-based practices
Ranier (2014)	Alcohol withdrawal patients	Reviewed the use of restraints for people undergoing alcohol withdrawal. Considered alternatives to restraint for this population

PRN pro re nata

sion were effective in reducing injuries and that some restraint and seclusion was inevitable. Some systematic reviews, however, have noted the lack of experiments or the poor quality of experimental evidence supporting this conclusion, at least until recently (see discussion of systematic reviews below).

11.2 Empirical Case Studies

There are a very large number of papers reporting the reductions of restrictive behavior management practices—mostly restraints—using either pre–post designs or long-term time series data. Table 11.2 summarizes a sample of some of these studies. One striking observation of these studies is that they have been conducted in a full range of settings and populations, and large reductions in restrictive behavior management practices have commonly been reported over relatively short periods of time both at the level of individual units, hospitals, and statewide organizations. Thus, some studies have reported reductions in restrictive behavior management practices of 90 % or greater. Further, there are several reports of larger scale restraint reduction at the level of statewide interventions, which take place over a number of years with follow-up data as long as 10 years. Most interventions are packages and commonly include several of the elements described by Lebel et al. (2014) in the section above. Thus, goal setting, policy revision, and staff training in alternatives to restrictive behavior management practices and feedback on the amount of restrictive behavior management practices were elements used in many studies. Only a minority of studies reported data on indirect effects, such as safety data and changes in nontargeted forms of restrictive practices. In general, such reports have been positive, but Godfrey et al.'s (2014) report of increase in psychotropic medication following reduction in physical restraints is a worrying example of negative side effects of such potential programs.

These studies collectively have two limitations. First, an important aspect of reducing restrictive behavior management practices is the magnitude and speed of reduction; interventions that reduce restrictive behavior management practices more quickly provide greater benefits to clients, such as increased personal freedom, reduced stigmatization, and reduced exposure to harm and are also more efficient as more rapid reduction might cost less per unit of change than other, slower programs. Most of these papers only reported a percentage of change in restrictive behavior management practices over baseline, but such data are difficult to interpret as they often report data over different periods of time. For example, a 50 % reduction in restrictive behavior management practices over a year is a slower reduction in than a 25 % reduction in 3 months. Although the rate of reduction may be a useful metric in the first part of an organizational intervention to reduce restrictive behavior management practices, highly effective studies with long follow-ups may have a low average overall rate of restraint reduction because of the long period of time over which the data are reported. Experiments that directly compare the rate of reduction between different groups allow direct comparison of both the absolute

Table 11.2 A selection of empirical case studies reducing restraint, seclusion, and related procedures

Reference	Population and setting	Interventions time period	Outcome
Davidson et al. (1994)	Children and adults with Intellectual Disabilities in a large institution. The average numbers of residents ranged from 883.5 to 630.6 during the first and third years, most of whom had profound Intellectual Disabilities and were aged between 3 months and 98 years	Package of facility administrator setting goals, instructions and feedback to staff on number of hours of seclusion, number of hours of restraint, and percentage of residents taking psychotropic medications over a 3-year period. They used a multiple baseline design across three restrictive procedures	During baseline, there were 1231.75 h of seclusion per month. After feedback, there was a large reduction—approximately two thirds after 4 months and this reduced to 2 h per month by the end of the 3-year period for a 99 % reduction over 32 months. During baseline, there were 16,165.50 h of restraint per month in baseline, and at the end of the study there were only 1971 for an 88 % reduction over 32 months. In baseline, 36 % of the residents received psychotropic medication, which fell to 20 % of residents at the end of the study for a 44 % reduction. Rates of staff injuries were stable throughout this period of time
Dunbar et al. (1996)	16 nursing homes	Educational program which consisted of a 2-day workshop, telephone and quarterly on-site consultations, regional meetings, a newsletter, and written and audio–visual materials. Study was conducted over 2 years	"90 % reduction" in restraints but details of data collection not provided
Siegler et al. (1997); Capezuti et al. (2002)	$N = 446$ seniors in 16 nursing homes	Evaluated the effects of the 1987 *Omnibus Reconciliation Act* regulations limiting restraints on psychotropic medication prescriptions. Data were collected pre-intervention and 6 month post intervention. Capezuti et al. reported analysis of nighttime bedrails	Restraints decreased and there was no increase in psychotropic medication in homes that reduced restraints. Of those taken off restraints, only 2 % were started on neuroleptics. Benzodiazepine use also declined in the control home (18–11 %, $p < 0.014$). *Omnibus Reconciliation Act* regulations also decreased the proportion of residents with inappropriate neuroleptics from 21.3 to 14.6 % in all homes and from 39.9 to 8 % in the control home. At the same time, there was an increase in the use of bilateral bedrails from 58.7 to 64.1 % averaged across all three groups ($p = 0.021$) with no subsequent reduction in nighttime falls or injuries

Table 11.2 (continued)

Reference	Population and setting	Interventions time period	Outcome
Allen et al. (1997)	Adults with Intellectual Disabilities in a six-bedded residential institutional treatment unit	Evaluated the impact of a new training course on the use of restrictive behavior management which included: (a) understanding aggressive incidents, (b) primary prevention by modifying or removing environmental triggers, (c) secondary prevention by early redirection and diffusion of precursor behaviors, (d) reactive strategies such as self-defense and minimal physical restraint methods, and (e) post-incident support of clients and staff. Teaching methods included role-play and direct skill practice. Took place over a 5-year period	There was a modest decrease in major behavioral incidents, and rates of seclusion and restraint remained low, and there was a large reduction in the percentage of major behavioral incidents managed with restraint and PRN medication. Overall, there were 62 and 86 % reductions in physical restraint and emergency medication, respectively, during major behavioral incidents and a 75 % decline in staff and a 72 % reduction in client injuries
Neufeld et al. (1999) Study B	$N=2076$ in 16 nursing homes	Data taken 3 months before and 3 months after intervention	Physical restraint reduced from 41 to 4 % of the residents for a 90 % reduction. Serious injuries were reduced from 7.5 to 4.4 %, ($p<0.0004$), and combined moderate and serious injuries also fell ($p<0.0033$)
Mayhew et al. (1999)	Veterans facility	Used an interdisciplinary task force, changed restraint policy, and conducted staff training over a 2-year period	28 % reduction (but details of data collection lacking)
Sundel et al. (1994)	$N=170$ seniors in a nursing home; 182 staff	Staff training	Restraints reduced from 1.56 to 0.67% restraints per resident (−57 %) and the proportion of residents restrained reduced from 68 to 37 %
Levine et al. (1995)	A 816-bed nursing home	Policy modification and staff training over 3 years	Reduced restraint from 39 to 4 %, prevalence reduced from 20 to 4 %. No changes in accident rate

Table 11.2 (continued)

Reference	Population and setting	Interventions time period	Outcome
Donat (1998)	Psychiatric/institution	Developed a data system to identify high-risk patients. Used peer review and oversight committee to develop behavioral interventions and alternative less restrictive procedures	In a sample of 53 high-risk patients, restraint/seclusion was used 18.8 h per month during the 6 months before implementation. This fell to 7.2 h per month (−62 %) following intervention ($p<0.01$). Further, there was an increasing trend in restraint/seclusion use before the intervention, and after the intervention there was a decreasing trend. Similar interventions to reduce PRN medications resulted in reduction from 20.8 to 14.5 individuals per week during the 20 weeks before intervention to the 20 weeks after the intervention (−30 %, $p<0.01$) and from 5.7 to 2.9 per week (−49 %, $p<0.01$) from 10 weeks before intervention to 20 weeks after intervention in a second setting
Sullivan-Marx et al. (1999)	Mean age 84 years Three nonprofit, religious, affiliated nursing homes	Compared three forms of intervention (staff education, staff education plus consultation, and a no treatment control)	Of the 201 originally restrained, 135 were still restrained at the end of the program
Sturmey and McGlynn (2002) study one	Developmental disabilities/institution	A plan was presented to the facility's board and included goals for 25 and 50 % restraint reduction by specific dates. Interventions included (a) targeting homes with high rates of restraint by working with treatment teams on those homes using individualized training, and (b) a month of classes for direct care and other facility staff on restraint reduction from psychology staff, which stressed empathy with clients, current facility treatment practices, alternatives to restraint, and role-play of redirection methods. Took place over 7 months	There was a 23 % reduction in the number of people with programmatic personal restraints from 35 to 27 people and a 59 % reduction in the number of personal restraints from 99 to 41 incidents. There was a 63 % increase in the number of emergency personal restraints from 11 to 18 people and an 11 % increase in the number of incidents from 26 to 56. The number of people with mechanical restraints fell from 62 to 27 for a 57 % reduction and the number of incidents fell from 4216 to 160 for a 62 % reduction. The number of people who had emergency mechanical restraints fell from 9 to 5 people for a 45 % reduction. The number of people receiving psychopharmacology remained stable

Table 11.2 (continued)

Reference	Population and setting	Interventions time period	Outcome
Sturmey and McGlynn (2002) study two	Developmental disabilities/institution	An analysis of restraint use showed that only 60/310 residents accounted for 100 % in one quarter and only 18 residents accounted for 90 % of all restraint use. These 18 residents and 4 subsequent admissions, all of whom were adults with ID, were entered into a multi-component program over 6 months which included: (a) simplification of data collection, (b) verbal and graphical feedback to staff and supervisors, (c) posted graphs of restraint use, (d) use of restraint for hand mouthing was changed so that restraint was contingent upon skin breakdown and not hand mouthing, (e) additional monthly supervision and review for challenging cases by a PhD psychologist which was subsequently faded to quarterly and 6-monthly supervision, and (f) more frequent modification of the current behavior support plans and monitoring of implementation	There was a median reduction in restraint of − 72 % (range + 62 % to − 100 %). Two clients were now restraint free, 6 had at least a 90 % reduction and 6 had at least a 75 % reduction. Two residents had large increases in restraints (+ 50 % and + 75 %). Restraint reductions at 3 years were larger (median = − 95 % range + 213 % to − 100 %), although again two clients had large increases in restraint
Donat (2002)	Psychiatric/institutions, see Donat (1998)	Tightened criteria for peer review used in the preceding study to three applications or 12 h in 7 days, and then two applications or 8 h in 7 days	Restraint/seclusion fell from 1199 to 507 h per month (− 57 %) during the 12 months before and after the first program revision and to 256 h per month over 12 months representing a 51 % reduction over the preceding phase (all p's < 0.01)

Table 11.2 (continued)

Reference	Population and setting	Interventions time period	Outcome
Fisher (2003)	A large psychiatric hospital	Evaluated an organization-wide intervention involving administrative endorsement, client participation, culture change, staff training, data analysis, and individualized treatment plans. Conducted over a 2-year period	There was a 67 % reduction over 2 years in combined seclusion and restraint
Lebel et al. (2004)	State mental health agency	Child and adolescent units. Data analysis, quality improvement, regulatory oversight, and technical assistance over a 22-month period	For child units, restraints reduced from 84 to 23/1000 days (−73 %), for adolescent units from 72 to 34/1000 days (−47 %), and for mixed child/adolescent units from 73 to 30/1000 days (−59 %)
Jonikas et al. (2004)	Three psychiatric units in a university psychiatric hospital. $N=1910$ adult psychiatric patients and $N=227$ adolescent patients	Intervention included patient interviews to identify triggers and staff training. Reported quarterly restraint data over a 30-month period	Restraints decreased 99 % in the adult units and 98 % in the adolescents units 6 months after training compared to baseline ($p<0.01$)
Yeh et al. (2004)	37 novice nurses in an intensive care unit	Training on correct use of restraints presented in a 4-h class presented live to the day staff and via videotape to the night staff	Nurses reported using restraints less after training
McCue et al. (2004)	A 135-bed psychiatric residential service	Developed a 6-component program that included (a) identification of high-rate clients and development of individual treatment plans, (b) patient education, (c) staff education, (d) a crisis intervention team, (e) daily review of all restraints, and (f) a staff incentive program. Compared restraint and client assault, suicide, and self-injury data from 3 years before to 2 years after intervention	The rate of restraints reduced from 8.0 to 3.7 per 1000 patient-days ($p<0.0001$) with no increase in assault suicide or self-injury

Table 11.2 (continued)

Reference	Population and setting	Interventions time period	Outcome
Smalls (2004)	316 individuals with Intellectual Disabilities in a large institution; majority of the adults with profound disabilities	Intervention included staff training, increasing the requirements for authorization of restraints, 18 months	There was a 94 % reduction in restraints ($p<0.05$), psychotropic medication fell by 29 % and polypharmacy fell by 55 % (p's<0.05). Injuries also decreased
Lebel and Goldstein (2005)	One adolescent in-patient unit	Compared data 1 year before and 1 year after intervention. (Details of restraint program not provided in this chapter)	Number of episodes of restraint and seclusion fell from 3991 to 373 (−91 %). Associated costs from US$ 1446,740 to US$ 117,036 (−92 %). "Sick time, staff turnover and replacement costs, workers' compensation, injuries to adolescents and staff, and recidivism decreased" and patient adaptive behavior improved
Smith et al. (2005)	Psychiatric in-patients/psychiatric hospitals in Pennsylvania	General state reform on policies, staff training, and oversight of restraint. Data were collected between 1990 and 2000 for restraints and seclusion and 1998 and 2000 for injuries of staff in state hospitals in the Pennsylvania state psychiatric hospital system	Restraints were reduced from 4.2 to 0.3 episodes per 1000 patient-days, seclusion duration from 10.8 to 1.3 h, rate of restraint from 3.5 to 1.2 episodes per 1000 patient-days, and restraint duration from 11.9 to 1.9 h. The rate of staff injuries did not change
Miller et al. (2006)	Two private child and adolescent psychiatric units ($N=102$ residents and 85 staff)	A restraint reduction committee devised and oversaw a plan which included leadership, staff training and supervision, maintenance of training, documentation and clinical analysis, clinical case review, and program supervision. Milieu modification took place at high-risk times and data analysis. This took place over a 2-year 9-month period	Overall, a 59 % reduction ($p<0.0001$) over the entire study and a 56 % and 42 % reduction at sites 1 and 2

Table 11.2 (continued)

Reference	Population and setting	Interventions time period	Outcome
Ryan et al. (2007)	K–12 special day school for 316 students of whom 42 participated	Staff training included an initial training in Crisis Prevention Institute's (CPI) nonviolent crisis intervention training (a commercial training package), which included both informational presentations and role-play. Additionally, there was a 1-h twice a month training on de-escalation training techniques. Approximately, two thirds of the staff reported receiving 5–12 training during the year. There was also a school-wide behavior management plan to encourage the least restrictive use of seclusion and restraint. Data were collected 1 year before training and during 1 year of staff training	In year 1, there were 25 students restrained/secluded 439 times (range 1–43 per child), and during the year of training, 21students were restrained/secluded 266 times (−39 %) (range 1–66 per student). The number of students with 10 or more seclusion in 1 year reduced from 10 to 4 students in years 1 and 2, respectively. The mean duration of seclusion was 13 and 15 min in each year. Personal restraints fell from 68 to 56 per year (−18 %) and mechanical restraints were used only once in each year
Hellerstein et al. (2007)	Three units with 58 beds in a state psychiatric hospital. Data collected 20 months before and 67 months after intervention	Intervention package included (1) decreasing restraint/seclusion time from 4 to 2 h before new orders were required, (2) training staff to identify risk patients and use early intervention, and (3) assessed patient preferences for dealing with agitation with a questionnaire	Mean number of patients restrained fell from 0.35 ± 0.6 to 0.32 ± 0.5 patients/month; mean hours of restraint fell from 1.7 ± 5.2 to 1.0 ± 2.4 h/month; mean number of patients secluded decreased from 3.1 ± 1.4 to 1.0 ± 1.1 patients/month; and mean hours of seclusion decreased from 41.6 ± 52 to 2.7 ± 4.5 h/month. Elopements and fights decreased
Brockhardt et al. (2011); Madan et al. (2014)	95 beds over 5 units in a state psychiatric hospital over an initial 3.5 years with a 10-year follow-up	Intervention included trauma-informed care training, rules and language changes in policy, patient involvement, and changes to the physical environment	Restraint and seclusion fell to 82.3 % reduction and this change was maintained at 10-year follow-up

Table 11.2 (continued)

Reference	Population and setting	Interventions time period	Outcome
Ashcraft et al. (2008)	Two psychiatric crisis centers with 40 admissions per day of both voluntary and involuntary admissions and 95 staff. Intervention took place over 15 months	Interventions included (a) the program director informed that the program goals were now restraint and seclusion elimination, (b) program and policy revision to ensure services were driven by service values not inflexible rules, (c) four 3-h staff training presentations scheduled over 4 weeks that included participation of the executive director that emphasized values and moving from staff control to patient autonomy, and (d) debriefing and feedback following restraint and seclusion. The study took place over 58 months	The larger unit achieved zero seclusion and zero restraint in 10 and 31 months, respectively, and the smaller unit did so in 2 and 15 months, respectively
Sanders (2009)	Developmental disabilities/special education and community residential	Following appointment of a new service direct, evaluated an action plan, management support, staff training and monitoring. Participants were approximately 75 children and 43 adults in a day school and residential program for autism, Intellectual Disabilities, and psychiatric and behavioral disabilities. The study took place over 4 years	Between 2005 and 2008, rates of restraints fell from 10.33 to 0.06 per 50,000 client-days (−99.4 %), employee injuries from clients fell from 1.12 to 0.70 per 50,000 client-days (−37.7 % 2), and employee lost time costs fell from US$ 171,754.80 to US$ 13,254.56 per year from 2004 to 2008, respectively

Table 11.2 (continued)

Reference	Population and setting	Interventions time period	Outcome
Williams et al. (2009)	Developmental disabilities/specialized pica treatment unit in an institution over a 9-year period	There were four components: (1) A survey identified individuals who displayed pica which identified 41 individuals of which 9 had undergone surgery despite repeated administrative actions and restrictive management practices. (2) There were two trainings: One for staff who rarely observed pica, and one for those who commonly worked with these clients. (3) A facility-wide procedure to safely dispose of all rubber gloves, including spot checks to ensure staff compliance and behavior plans based on functional assessments. (4) The creation of a pica-safe environment free of items that could be ingested, enhanced staff, supervised walks, avoidance of the most dangerous area, written procedures for disposal of rubber gloves, and other dangerous items publically posted for all staff and visitors, and regular staff training and supervision related to pica and pica-free classrooms were used for training	After 9 years of the program, 26 clients remained in the restrictive pica program, six were in less restrictive settings, 8 were in less restrictive pica-safe settings and one had died but their death was not pica-related. 16 clients were still on restrictive programs that had not been safely eliminated. During the 9 years prior to the program, there have been nine surgeries, and during the nine years of the program there has been only one pica-related surgery in one client who was not on a pica-free restrictive home
Damen (2009)	Nonprofit child and adolescent/residential agency for children with emotional and behavioral problems	Evaluated the effects of a policy change on restraint use between January 2000 and December 2003. Used an AB time series design using data from 22 months before and 26 months after a policy change	There was a reduction in the rate of physical restraints from an average of 1.5 per child per month to approximately 0.5 restraints per resident per month for a reduction of approximately 70%

Table 11.2 (continued)

Reference	Population and setting	Interventions time period	Outcome
Iwata et al. (2009)	Developmental disabilities (Prader–Willi syndrome service)/community residential service	Evaluated systematic evaluation of elimination of time-out in a community residential and day program for adolescents and adults with developmental disabilities, most of who had Prader–Willi syndrome ($N=50$). Eleven were excluded from the program because of the severity of their aggression. For some, removal of time-out did not increase aggression, and for others alternate management strategies were effective	Elimination of restraint resulted in no change in the target behavior in 21 (62 %) individuals and in 13 (38 %) individuals; there was an increase in target behavior that was effectively managed by less restrictive procedures for 10 individuals. Only three individuals required continued use of time-out. Approximately, 80 % of the reduction occurred during the first 6 months. Elimination of time-out was relatively quick and effective for many individuals
Barton et al. (2009)	Individuals aged over 14 years with mental illnesses, mostly admitted from emergency departments. Setting was a 26-bed behavioral unit for individual aged over 14 years	Staff training based on trauma informed and person-centered care; and action plan with time lines over 18 months, leadership supported goal of 100 % elimination rather than reduction of restraint, and the seclusion room (which had not been used) was converted to a patient comfort room. Took place over 2 years	Restraints reduced from 19 per year in the year 2001–2002 to 0 restraints in 2007–2008. Unplanned reduction in PRN medication from 0.87 to 0.68 doses per patient-days. (−22 %). (Note these doses remained high after the program)
Williams and Grossett (2011)	925 persons with developmental disabilities in an institution. Most with severe/profound Intellectual Disabilities	Evaluated a three-component program that includes: (a) tracking priority clients with frequent self-injurious behavior, physical aggression, or high rates of mechanical restraint, (b) using behavior data monitoring and feedback, and (c) organizational contingencies	Mechanical restraints decreased by almost 80 % from 0.54 per month to 0.11 per day. Use of behavior intervention plans increased from 54 to 124

Table 11.2 (continued)

Reference	Population and setting	Interventions time period	Outcome
Gulpers et al. (2011); Gulpers et al. (2013)	26 wards in 13 Dutch nursing homes for seniors	The four-component EXBELT intervention included policy change, staff education, nurse consultation, and alternatives to restraints. Used an 8-month quasi-experimental design, collecting data at baseline at 4- and 8-months. Took place over 17 months	Belt restraint use decreased by 50 % decrease in belt use (odds ratio = 0.48, 95 % confidence interval = 0.28–0.81; $p = 0.005$) without other restraints increasing, and no increase in psychoactive drugs, falls, and fall-related injuries. At a 2-year follow-up, there was a 65 % decrease in the experimental and a 3 % decrease in the control group use of belt restraints ($p < 0.001$). The percentage of people in any restraint was 75 and 60 % in the control and experimental groups, respectively ($p = 0.03$), which was also reflected in the reduction in various specific types of restraints
Amata et al. (2012)	Two acute strokes and brain injury rehabilitation units ($N = 16$ and 18 beds) which were part of a 732-bed hospital	Evaluated a four-component program that included administration education and consultation feedback over 12 months	Restraints fell from 217 to 153 h and from 1054 to 883 h per 100 patient-days on the stroke and brain injury units, respectively. Falls reduced from 11 to 6 and from 9.1 to 3.3 per 1000 patient-days on the stroke and brain injury units, respectively (−64 %)
Allen et al. (2012)	Adults with Intellectual Disabilities. 3- and 8-bedded admission units in a long stay facility for adults with ID and challenging behavior	Trained staff in positive behavioral support with objective of restraint reduction, individual behavior plans periodic service reviews. Staff received acceptance and commitment therapy to meet their emotional needs. Study took place over 7 years	Physical interventions fell from 110 to 28 episodes per year from year 1 to year 7 (−74 %)

Table 11.2 (continued)

Reference	Population and setting	Interventions time period	Outcome
Leoni et al. (2013)	Large Italian institutional setting for 407 mostly adults with Intellectual Disabilities	As part of a broad organizational reform using organizational behavior management principles, restraint reduction was targeted using staff training, environmental improvement, and many local projects. Study took place between 2005 and 2011	Restraints reduced from 167 per month before intervention to 90 per month in year 1 and thereafter from 2 to 1 per month for years 2–6
Konetzka et al. (2014)	Seniors in nursing homes in six states	Intervention was state reporting of physical restraints. Sample included 809,645 residents with severe cognitive impairment and 4258 nursing homes between 1999 and 2008	Restraints declined most in nursing homes required to report physical restraint compared to those that did not (−8.3 % vs. −3.3 %, $p<0.001$). This was associated with increased use of antipsychotics (4.5 % vs. 2.9 %, $p<0.001$)
Wieman et al. (2014)	$N=43$ psychiatric facilities	Used six core strategies over 4 years. Tracked implementation in all facilities using a treatment integrity checklist	Reductions in restraint and seclusion varied a great deal from facility to facility. Those that continued to implement or that had implemented all elements of the six core strategies were more likely to reduce restraint and seclusion that those facilities that had never attempted to do so or that had stopped implementation. Most facilities reduced, but eight had no change and four had increased in restraint and seclusion
Godfrey et al. (2014)	Two units of a 398-bed psychiatric facility. $N=216$ psychiatric patients	Used crisis intervention training, pyramidal training, and a treatment integrity oversight committee to reduce mechanical restraint. Study took place over approximately 3 years	Restraints were reduced by 98 and 100 % on each unit and one unit remained restraint free for 559 days

ID Intellectual Disabilities, *PRN* pro re nata

change in RRMPs and the rate of change. (See below for a detailed discussion of experiments.) A second limitation is that, although there are examples of large-scale interventions in typical community settings, there is a preponderance of studies in institutional settings, such as developmental disability centers, and psychiatric and other large hospitals, but relatively few studies of community services that are geographically dispersed and organizationally complex.

11.2.1 Two Examples

To illustrate the variety of approaches to organizational interventions to reduce restrictive behavior management practices, we will consider two examples in some details. The examples will include a study of community services for children and adults with developmental disabilities that includes data on staff safety and a series of papers by Donat in psychiatric settings demonstrating how progressive modification of a program to reduce restrictive behavior management practices can be implemented and refined over time.

11.2.1.1 Community Services for Children and Adults with Intellectual Disabilities and Autism

A unique study of restraint reduction comes from Sanders (2009) who also reported data on workman's compensation for restraint-related injuries. The study took place in a community agency with 21 group homes and 2 day schools. There were 118 children and adults aged from 7 to 68 years of whom approximately one quarter were identified with profound ID. There were also approximately 250 staff members of whom approximately three quarters were direct care staff. Intervention took place over a 4-year period and included four components: (1) a "reported-on-the-street" staff member solicited staff views of restraint use; (2) a 2-h in-service that included both PowerPoint presentation and modeling and rehearsal of less restrictive alternatives to restraint, such as the use of pillows and/or shields to prevent restraint and injuries to clients and staff; (3) increased physical presence of supervisors and management including during the early stages of behavioral escalation; and (4) an oversight system that included both post-incident analysis and training and a review committee of senior managers, which met monthly.

The rates of restraints fell from 10.33 to 0.06 restraints per 50,000 adjusted client-days over 4 years (a 99.4 % reduction) and employee injuries from clients *fell* from 1.12 to 0.70 per 50,000 adjusted client-days over the same time period (a reduction of 37.7 %). Impressively, employee costs for lost time fell from US$ 171,754.80 to US$ 13,254.56 (a 93 % reduction). Thus, large reductions in restraint can be achieved in contemporary community agencies with simultaneous *reductions* in staff injuries and costs.

11.2.1.2 Donat's Studies

An interesting series of studies of restraint reduction in psychiatric settings comes from Donat (1998, 2002, 2003). These studies are interesting because not only do they demonstrate reductions in restraint but also provide some analysis of individual components of intervention packages. Donat (1998) evaluated an administrative procedure to reduce restraint and seclusion use in an in-patient psychiatric hospital following concern from the facility's human rights committee and external reviewers that restraint was used excessively. First, a data system was developed to identify all patients who had been restrained over 72 h or more than six times in the preceding month. Second, a peer review and oversight committee was set up that evaluated adequacy of functional assessment, treatment integrity, consideration of less restrictive alternative strategies, and that the unit psychologist signs the treatment plan. In a sample of 53 high-risk patients, restraint/seclusion was used 18.8 h per month during the 6 months before implementation. This fell to 7.2 h per month (−62 %) following intervention ($p<0.01$). Further, there was an increasing trend in restraint/seclusion use before the intervention, and after intervention there was a decreasing trend.

Subsequently, Donat (2002) reported two refinements of these procedures as the preceding intervention, although effective for the high-risk participants, did not lead to a large reduction in restraint facility wide. The next phase was an evaluation of tightening up the review criterion used in the preceding study to three applications or 12 h in 7 days, and then two applications or 8 h in 7 days. The first change resulted in a 58 % reduction in restraint/seclusion use from 1199 h to 507 h per month for the 12 months before and after the introduction of the program. The further tightening of the criterion resulted in a further reduction in restraint/seclusion use to 256 h per month over 12 months representing a 51 % reduction over the preceding phase (all p's <0.01).

The next two interventions addressed excessive use of PRN medication. Prior to intervention, PRN medication required only one, and no oversight was in place. Intervention included inclusion of PRN medication use in the database, and a required team meeting review if there were three or more PRN's occurred in 1 week with a check to ensure that the team met. Both the team psychologist and psychiatrist had to sign the review. If PRN medication continued over the criterion for 3 consecutive weeks, the facility peer review committee reviewed the case. This intervention results in a 30 % reduction in PRN use from an average of 20.8 to 14.5 individuals per week during the 20 weeks before intervention to the 20 weeks after the intervention ($p<0.01$). These results were replicated using the same procedure in a high-restraint-use ward. In this setting, the procedure resulted in a 49 % reduction in restraint use from 5.7 to 2.9 per week ($p<0.01$) from 10 weeks before intervention to 20 weeks after intervention. In a subsequent analysis of these data using multiple regression analysis, Donat (2003) demonstrated that the only predictor of restraint reduction was the changing criterion for review and administrative and clinical review of cases ($p<0.01$). Other variables such as staff to patient ratio, different types of committee membership, and quality measures of behavior plans did not predict reductions in restraint.

This series of papers is remarkable because of the long period of time over which the research was conducted and the large sample of participants. Even more importantly, these papers demonstrated that only one component of the review procedure predicted reduction of restraint/seclusion, namely more conservative criteria for external peer review resulted in larger restraint reduction than more liberal criteria

11.3 Systematic Reviews

As noted above, most studies on the reduction of restrictive behavior management practices are nonexperimental case studies. Such studies are very useful in that they show the kinds of interventions that may work and the magnitude and speed of change that may be achieved in a variety of populations and settings; however, because they are not experiments, they cannot exclude the possibility that the change occurred due to confounding factors, such as general improvements in services and general trends to reduce the use of restrictive behavior management practices that occur from time to time. Hence, well-designed and -conducted experiments perform an essential role in demonstrating causality. Over the last 10 years, researchers have conducted several randomized controlled trials and at least 13 systematic reviews, but no meta-analyses of interventions to reduce restrictive behavior management practices (see Table 11.3). In this section, we describe one illustrative experiment and then consider several systematic reviews and meta-analyses of interventions to reduce restrictive behavior management practices.

Testad et al. (2005) reported a several randomized controlled trial to evaluate a staff training and follow-up intervention in nursing homes. Four nursing homes participated. The authors randomly assigned them stratified based on size to either intervention or treatment as usual. There were 55 participants in the intervention and 96 in the control groups. The groups did not differ on demographic and medical variables at baseline or post-training. Intervention consisted of (a) a 6-h, one-day manualized training for all staff covering dementia, problem behavior, decision making, and alternatives to restraint and (b) guidance was given 1 h a month based on data collection and reviews of individual patients linked to the content of the initial workshop. The mean number of restraints per patient per week fell from 3.3 to 1.5 per week in the intervention group and increased from 3.1 to 3.7 per week in the control group. After training, the difference between the groups was statistically significant ($p<0.017$), but staff ratings of agitation was slightly higher in the experimental than the control group ($p<0.017$). The authors concluded that the intervention was effective and that the increase in agitation in the experimental group was tolerable.

Table 11.3 summarizes 13 systematic reviews of interventions which have reviewed interventions to reduce restrictive behavior management practices. These systematic reviews were published from 2000 up to the present day, but the majority

Table 11.3 A summary of systematic reviews and meta-analyses of restraint and seclusion reduction

Reference	Populations and settings	Method	Findings
Sailas and Fenton (2000)	Serious mental illness. Papers included for review related mostly to nursing homes	Cochrane review initially conducted in 2000 and updated in 2012, but new data not yet synthesized	There were no several randomized controlled trials that met inclusion criteria and data could not be synthesized
Evans et al. (2002)	Acute and residential settings	Systematic search for studies reducing restraint	A systematic search identified 16 studies of which one was a several randomized controlled trial. Three were in acute and 13 in residential settings. Evidence from both pre–post designs and one several randomized controlled trial supported the conclusion that restraints can be reduced effectively and safely in residential care. There is little evidence related to evidence-based practices in acute care
Nelstrop et al. (2006)	Adult psychiatric settings and emergency departments and management of violence	Systematic review	Found no experiments and could not conduct a systematic review or meta-analysis
Gaskin et al. (2007)	Psychiatric facilities	Systematic review papers "during the past 20 years"	Did not identify any experiments
De Hert et al. (2009)	Child and adolescents only	Systematically searched databases over preceding 10 years	Identified four studies that attempted to reduce restraint. Concluded that efforts to reduce the most restrictive practices were highly effective. The mean reduction in restraint was 93 % with a 54 % reduction in restraint duration. Average outcomes for less restrictive forms of restraint were near zero, but varied widely from a 97 % reduction to a 71 % increase. (One study reported an increase in the use of a padded seclusion room in lieu of what was described as "other more restrictive measures.") Excluding this outlier study, resulted in a 75 % reduction in seclusion episodes and a 32 % reduction in seclusion duration
Mohler et al. (2012)	Long-term geriatric care	Cochrane systematic review conducted in 2009	Identified six cluster randomized controlled trials of educational interventions combined with consultation (two studies), support, and technical aids (one study). Studies were generally of low quality. Results were inconsistent with one good-quality study documenting an increase in restraint, four low-quality studies finding reduced restraint in the treatment groups, and one study finding no decrease in the experimental group but increase in the control group. Concluded that there was insufficient evidence of effectiveness of restraint reduction programs in nursing homes

Table 11.3 (continued)

Reference	Populations and settings	Method	Findings
Scanlan (2010)	Psychiatric settings including children, adolescents, adults, and seniors	Systematic literature review	Used a systematic review to identify 29 empirical papers evaluating 23 specific restraint reduction programs. The seven key strategies in restraint reduction were: (a) policy change/leadership, (b) external review/debriefing, (c) data use, (d) training, (e) consumer/family involvement, (f) increase in staff ratio/crisis response teams, and (g) program change. Focused on program elements rather than outcome data
Stewart et al. (2010)	In-patient psychiatric units	Systematic literature review	Common intervention components include policy revision, changes in staffing levels, staff training, review procedures, improved crisis management, and changes in medication practices. Identified only one experiment that showed that occupational therapy did not decrease restraint. Thus, they concluded that there was little experimental evidence supporting restraint reduction
Richter et al. (2012)	Care homes	Cochrane review of medication reduction in seniors	Identified four cluster randomized control trials evaluating packages of educational and other interventions. Overall study quality was moderate with one high-quality study. Studies reported reductions in the number of patients with antipsychotic medications and the number of days with antipsychotic medications. The authors concluded that there is evidence that interventions can reduce use of antipsychotic medications, although this is based on a small number of studies
Bahrani and Snowden (2012)	Dementia-related symptoms in nursing homes patients	Systematic search of any intervention, but not specifically restraint and seclusion	Most studies related to psychopharmacology. Only identified two studies addressing restraint reduction with mixed outcomes. Made no general conclusion concerning restraint reduction due to small number of studies and contradictory results
Nazir et al. (2013)	Interdisciplinary reviews in nursing homes	Systematic search using Cochrane collaboration tools	Identified 27 several randomized controlled trials of which two targeted restraint reduction. One produced reductions and the second did not. Did not make any specific recommendations regarding restraint

was published after 2009. They have all focused on specific populations and/or specific settings such as psychiatric care/severe mental illness (Gaskin et al. 2007; Johnson 2010; Nelstrop et al. 2006; Sailas and Fenton 2000; Scanalan et al. 2010), seniors/nursing homes (Bahrani and Snowden 2012; Sailas and Fenton 2000; Mohler et al. 2012; Nazir et al. 2013; Richter et al. 2012), children and adolescents (De Hert et al. 2009; Scanlan et al. 2010), acute care (Evans et al. 2002), residential settings (Evans et al. 2002), and emergency departments (Nelstrop et al. 2006). It is worth noting that, although there are several narrative reviews of restraints that address restraint reduction in people with ID there were no systematic reviews, perhaps reflecting the absence of several randomized controlled trials in this area. These systematic reviews have asked different kinds of questions and varied in the breadth of their focus. For example, some have asked highly specific questions such as whether there are interventions to reduce psychotropic medications in care homes for seniors (Richter et al. 2012), whereas others have asked broader questions, such as whether there are evidence-based practices to reduce restraint in psychiatric settings (Gaskin et al. 2007; Johnson 2010; Nelstrop et al. 2006; Sailas and Fenton 2000; Scanalan et al. 2010).

These systematic reviews have reached quite different conclusions, ranging from the conclusion that there is no experimental evidence so no conclusions can be made (Gaskin et al. 2007; Nelson et al. 2006; Sailas and Fenton 2000; Scanlan 2010; Stewart et al. 2010), there is very little experimental evidence so no firm conclusions can be made (Evans et al. 2002; Johnson 2010), there is indeed experimental evidence but it is of poor quality and quantity, and although interventions seem promising, no firm conclusion can be reached (Bahrani and Snowden 2012; Mohler et al. 2012; Richter et al. 2012), and, finally, there are experimental interventions and interventions are effective, but outcomes are quite variable (De Hart et al. 2009). What accounts for these disparate conclusions? There are two simple explanations. First, there was only one experiment published before 2002 (Evans et al. 1997) and so systematic reviews before approximately 2007 indeed had little experimental evidence to consider. Second, when some systematic reviews focused on narrow questions, there may be no evidence related to a particular population, setting, or outcome measure. Thus, only broadly systematic reviews published in the last 5 years had more than two experiments to consider, and thus it is these systematic reviews that cautiously conclude that there are evidence-based practices in this area (Mohler et al. 2012; Nazir et al. 2013; Richter et al. 2012). These conclusions are tempered by the limitations of these studies which, among other limitations, include small sample sizes, lack of data on treatment integrity, lack of replication, and lack of data on safety in some trials.

11.4 Conclusions

There are now a very large number of empirical case studies of organizational interventions from many populations and settings, which often demonstrate large and sometimes rapid reductions in restraints, seclusion, and PRN medication. These organizational interventions usually have several or sometimes all of the multiple components outlines by Lebel et al. (2014). When studies report data on other outcomes, there is consistent evidence that reduction in restrictive behavior management practices is associated with *improved* safety and *reduced* costs. There is, however, evidence that in some circumstances reduction in one form of restrictive behavior management practices is accompanied by substitution of other forms of restrictive behavior management practices. Such relatively positive conclusions must be tempered by the possibility that publication bias may account for the relative uniformity of these positive outcomes; it may be that some organizations may have considerable difficulty in implementing such interventions for many reasons. Another significant challenge for implementing organizational interventions is defining the intervention clearly and maintaining its integrity over time. Despite these caveats, it seems reasonable to conclude that in many circumstances, motivated, competent clinicians and administrators can produce large reductions in restrictive behavior management practices at the organizational level, including large organizations, and can, if they persist and are not distracted by other events, maintain these reductions over many years.

Chapter 12
The Way Forward

Children in cages, adults with disabilities corralled under furniture in group homes, children with their mouths taped shut by their teachers, our senior citizens sedated so they fall and can no longer walk safely, adolescents and psychiatric patients locked in secluded rooms in the false name of treatment—we continue to use such practices too widely and in too many circumstances. We now know that in most cases such practices are dangerous and expensive, and are incompatible with most human right values, many code of professional conduct, and laws. Many humane, safe, respectful, and effective alternative strategies exist.

Many motivated individuals with little or no formal knowledge of behavioral sciences have been quite effective in safely reducing and eliminating restraint for nearly 200 years. Yet, if specialized technical and professional knowledge and skills are often not necessary, why do many good people not safely reduce restrictive procedures?

Restrictive procedures are mostly used to reduce or eliminate behavior in vulnerable populations which is aversive to caregivers—aggression, tantrums, threats, and self-injury in people with disabilities, children and adolescents and psychiatric patients and inconvenient or worrying wandering in vulnerable seniors. Applying restrictive procedures not only terminates aversive behavior, thereby negatively reinforcing caregiver use of restrictive behavior management practice, but also gives the opportunity to not have to interact with a difficult person for some time. Parents and other family members often do this when they put their overactive children in playpens or other acceptable restraint devices when they want to prepare a meal, do important work, and check the phone. Thus, it appears that the termination or reduction in intensity of these aversive behaviors is important in maintaining the use of restrictive procedures in many different contexts.

This is not the whole story. Caregivers with no effective alternative behavior—untrained care staff and professionals, isolated families who have challenging children, and inadequate services—often have a history of using similar procedures in other circumstances. Many of us learn to use similar procedures when we stand between two children who are fighting and lead one of them away or strap chil-

P. Sturmey, *Reducing Restraint and Restrictive Behavior Management Practices*,
Autism and Child Psychopathology Series, DOI 10.1007/978-3-319-17569-0_12

dren in strollers or car seats (for their own good, as we say). The use of restrictive procedure is made more likely by modeling from other caregivers and media, it is sometimes legitimatized through behavior management training courses, and it is implicitly and sometimes explicitly endorsed by some administrators, professionals, and supervisors. Services and professional training fail to provide effective training in less restrictive alternatives. When behavioral problems are construed as signs of underlying mental illness, drug companies market easy-to-administer sedating medication sold as humane treatment for illnesses for which the person had no responsibility. Nurses, physicians, and other professionals legitimize the use of psychotropic medication and their own professional role by making diagnoses and recommending psychotropic medication. In such circumstances, it is hardly surprising that caregivers implement restrictive behavior management practices that relieve caregivers from distress and discomfort.

Some people do not want to try to do anything else. Trying something new means getting out of the office, letting go of current practices which are ineffective, and recognizing them as such which is never comfortable. Some people—perhaps through lack of experience, rigidity, or insecurity—truly believe that their current inappropriate practices are, in fact, acceptable or even the best possible practice. Reducing restrictive behavior management practices means changing what we do. This is inconvenient and requires sustained effort.

Some people do not know what else to do. Sometimes people have truly tried everything they know to do and have perhaps reasonably given up trying, perhaps after months or years of trying.

Some people reasonably find restraints and other restrictive behavior management practices to be a highly satisfactory solution to a difficult problem. I have seen a number of parents of children with severe disabilities and self-injury who are firm advocates for physical restraints because the restraints protected their children from severe injuries when no other options existed. Staff, including professional staff, often concur with such decisions. Unfortunately, such use of restraint is an easy way out in the short-term but with long-term costs for the person restrained. It usually prevents injury to the person restrained in the short term, but prevents subsequent treatment of the problem behavior that resulted in restraint, as there is no longer any motivation to fix that problem.

A somewhat similar situation exists when caregivers seek the false Holy Grail of psychotropic medication to fix some severe problem behavior that resulted in restrictive behavior management practices. The solution is relatively low effort—waiting for an appointment and talking about the problem—and takes much responsibility off caregivers as they wait—often in vain for years—for the right new medication, dose, or combination. If a fix is found through psychotropic medication, it is often found through general suppression of all behavior, including desirable behavior, and may impede learning, interaction with the environment, and result in potentially serious and even life-threatening medical conditions in the long term. Again, although the problem behavior may be suppressed, in many cases no real treatment had been delivered.

Passionate advocates, frustrated administrators, righteous professionals, and angry family members calling for changes in laws and regulation may be no more than white knights and cockerels on dung heaps in their ineffective calls for changes in rules and laws that, by themselves, make little or no difference to daily practice. Often there are already well-crafted and potentially effective rules and laws, but they are neither implemented nor overseen effectively; failure to implement another rule or law is not the way forward and calling for new laws sometimes appears to be no more than just another form of avoidance of more effortful solutions.

12.1 Tend Your Own Garden

There are some things caregivers and administrators can do. "We must cultivate our own garden" wrote Voltaire in *Candide*. Practitioners and administrators should choose something important and do it well. Safely reducing and eliminating restrictive behavior management practices could be one of those things. One of the conclusions to this book is that safely reducing restrictive behavior management practices is not that difficult in the sense it often does not require a high level of behavioral technology, such as that described in the chapters on applied behavior analysis. Such sophistication may make for better interventions generally and may make an important difference in difficult cases, such as chronic self-injury and self-restraint and life-threatening pica, but these are relatively rare conditions. Most restrictive behavior management practices relate to aggression, tantrums, acting out in several populations, and wandering in seniors. Motivated people can solve many such problems intuitively, or more systematically using some of the data analysis tools described in Chap. 9, *Organizational Interventions*.

Some people are motivated to reduce restrictive behavior management practices but do not know what to do. If you do not know what to do, go ask someone who does. You can search online for alternatives to restraints. If you are a professional, you can find training in strategies such as positive behavior support and applied behavior analysis, or seek training and supervision in alternatives to restraints. If you are an administrator and are unsure what to do, you can bring in consultants and professional organizations to change both your own and your staff's behavior and skill set. Some family members too do not know what to do, but are disadvantaged because they do not know of alternatives, where to look for information, and by unresponsive service systems that they cannot influence. Like professionals, they too can seek knowledge and help from other parents, parent support groups, and professional organizations.

12.2 Last Word

If you really want to reduce restrictive behavior management practices, you can often do it. It is easier than you think. It requires adopting some of the practices described in this book, commitment to our clients and values, and considerable sustained efforts. John Connolly could do it 200 years ago. If we want to do it today, we can.

References

Abderhalden, C., Needham, I., Dassen, T., Halfens, R., Haug, H. J., & Fischer, J. E. (2008). Structured risk assessment and violence in acute psychiatric wards: Randomised controlled trial. *The British Journal of Psychiatry, 193,* 44–50.

Adkins, A. D., Singh, N. N., McKeegan, G. F., Lanier, A. E., & Oswald, D. P. (2002). Behavior treatment programs, readability, and treatment outcomes. *Research in Developmental Disabilities, 23,* 253–265.

Ahmed, Z., Fraser, W., Kerr, M. P., Kiernan, C., Emerson, E., Robertson, J., & Thomas, J., et al. (2000). Reducing antipsychotic medication in people with a learning disability. *The British Journal of Psychiatry, 176,* 42–46.

Alderman, N., Knight, C., & Henman, C. (2002). Aggressive behaviour observed within a neurobehavioural rehabilitation service: Utility of the OAS-MNR in clinical audit and applied research. *Brain Injury, 16,* 469–489.

Allen, J. J. (2000). Seclusion and restraint of children: A literature review. *Journal of Child and Adolescent Psychiatric Nursing, 13,* 159–167.

Allen, D. (2002). *Responding to challenging behaviour in persons with intellectual disabilities.* Kidderminster: BILD.

Allen, D. (2009). *Ethical approaches to physical interventions. Volume II: Changing the agenda.* Kidderminster: BILD.

Allen, D., Cornick, M., Jefferson, A., & Mills, R. (1996). *A policy framework to guide the use of physical interventions (restraint) with adults and children with learning disability and/or autism*. Kidderminster: BILD.

Allen, D., Hawkins, S., & Cooper, V. (2006). Parents' use of physical interventions in the management of their children's severe challenging behaviour. *Journal of applied Research in Intellectual Disabilities, 19,* 356–363.

Allen, D., Kaye, N., Horwood, S., Gray, D., & Mine, S. (2012). The impact of a whole organizational approach to to positive behavioural support on the use of physical interventions. *International Journal of Positive Support, 2,* 26–30.

Allen, D., Lowe, K., Brophy, S., & Moore, K. (2009). Predictors of restrictive reactive strategy use in people with challenging behaviour. *Journal of Applied Research in Intellectual Disabilities, 22,* 159–168.

Allen, D., McDonald, L., Dunn, C., & Doyle, T. (1997). Changing care staff approaches to the prevention and management of aggressive behaviour in a residential treatment unit for persons with mental retardation and challenging behaviour. *Research in Developmental Disabilities, 18,* 101–112.

Allen, K. D., Stanely, R. T., & McPherson, K. (1990). Evaluation of behavior management technology dissemination in pediatric dentistry. *Pediatric Dentistry, 12,* 79–82.

Allen, K. D., & Stokes, T. F. (1987). Use of escape and reward in the management of young children during dental treatment. *Journal of Applied Behavior Analysis, 20,* 381–390.

P. Sturmey, *Reducing Restraint and Restrictive Behavior Management Practices,* Autism and Child Psychopathology Series, DOI 10.1007/978-3-319-17569-0

Alty, A., & Mason, T. (1994). *Seclusion and mental health: A break with the past*. New York: Springer.

Amaral, D., Rodgers, S. J., Baron-Cohen, S., Bourgeron, T., Caffo, E., Fombonne, E., et al. (2011). Letter to the editor. Against "Le Packing": A consensus statement. *Journal of the American Academy of Child and Adolescent Psychiatry, 50,* 191–192.

Amato, S., Salter, J. P., & Mion, L. C. (2006). Physical restraint reduction in the acute rehabilitation setting: A quality improvement study. *Rehabilitation Nursing, 31,* 235–241.

American Association on Intellectual and Developmental Disabilities and The Arc. (2010). http://aaidd.org/news-policy/policy/position-statements/behavioral-supports#.U_d5-6Pp-So, downloaded 12/17/14.

American Association on Intellectual and Developmental Disabilities. (2012). Aversive procedures. http://aaidd.org/newspolicy/policy/position-statements/aversive-procedures#.U_eAdqPp-So, downloaded 12/17/14.

Amnesty International. (2009). Jailed without justice. Immigration detention in the USA. http://www.amnestyusa.org/pdfs/JailedWithoutJustice.pdf, downloaded 12/17/14.

Anderson, L. T., & Ernst, M. (1980). Self-injury in Lesch-Nyhan disease. *Journal of Autism and Developmental Disorders, 24,* 67–81.

Applied Behavior Analysis International. (2010). Restraints and seclusion, 2010. Downloaded from https://www.abainternational.org/about-us/policies-and-positions/restraint-and-seclusion,-2010.aspx 12.15.14.

Ashcraft, L., & Anthony, W. (2008). Eliminating seclusion and restraint in recovery-oriented crisis services. *Psychiatric Services, 59,* 1198–1202.

Association for Behavior Analysis International. (1989a). Right to effective treatment. https://www.abainternational.org/abai/policies-and-positions/right-to-effective-behavioral-treatment,-1989.aspx, downloaded 12//17/14.

Association for Behavior Analysis International. (1989b). Right to effective education. https://www.abainternational.org/abai/policies-and-positions/students-rights-to-effective-education,-1990.aspx, downloaded 12//17/14.

Asthana, A. (2006). School faces court battle over restraint of girl, six. Guardian, November 11, 2006. http://www.theguardian.com/uk/2006/nov/12/schools.education, downloaded 12/28/14.

Azrin, N. H., & Holz, W. C. (1966). Punishment. In W. K. Honig (Ed.), *Operant behavior: Areas of research and application* (pp. 380–447). New York: Appleton-Century-Crofts.

Baer, R. A. (2003). Mindfulness training as a clinical intervention: A conceptual and empirical review. *Clinical psychology: Science and practice, 10,* 125–143.

Baker, J. A., Lovell, K., & Harris, N. (2008). A best-evidence synthesis review of the administration of psychotropic pro re nata (PRN) medication in in-patient mental health settings. *Journal of Clinical Nursing, 17,* 1122–1131.

Ball, T. S., Datta, P. S., Rios, M., & Constantine, C. (1985). Flexible arm splints in the control of a Lesch-Nyhan victim's finger biting and a profoundly retarded client's finger sucking. *Journal of Autism and Development Disorders, 15,* 177–184.

Barker, K. (2006a). Prolonged hospital stays for disabled are criticized in D.C. http://www.washingtonpost.com/wpdyn/content/article/2006/02/25/AR2006022501290.htrnl, downloaded 12/20/14.

Barker, K. (2006b). Group home. Death of Disabled Ward Detailed. http://www.washingtonpost.com/wpdyn/content/article/2006/06/15/AR2006061501754.html, downloaded 12/20/14.

Barksby & Harper. 2011. BILD

Barnett, R. J., Stirling, C., & Pandyan, A. D. (2012). A review of the scientific literature related to the adverse impact of physical restraint: Gaining a clearer understanding of the physiological factors involved in cases of restraint-related death. *Medicine Science and the Law, 52,* 137–142.

Barton, S. A., Johnson, R., & Price, L. V. (2008). Achieving restraint-free on an inpatient behavioral health unit. *Journal of Psychosocial Nursing, 47,* 35–40.

Beer, M. D., Pereira, S. M., & Paton, C. (2001). *Psychiatric intensive care*. Cambridge: Cambridge University Press.

Bharani, N., & Snowden, M. (2005). Evidence-based interventions for nursing home residents with dementia-related behavioral symptoms. *Psychiatric Clinics of North America, 28,* 985–1005.

Bijou, S. W., Peterson, R. F., & Ault, M. H. (1968). A method to integrate descriptive and experimental field studies at the level of data and empirical concepts. *Journal of Applied Behavior Analysis, 1,* 175–191.

Blatt, B., & Kaplan, F. (1966). *Christmas in purgatory*. Syracuse: Human Policy Press.

Bodfish, J. W., Crawford, T. W., Powell, S. B., & Parker, D. E. (1995). Compulsions in adults with mental retardation: Prevalence, phenomenology, and comorbidity with stereotypy and self-injury. *American Journal on Mental Retardation, 100,* 183–192.

Bodfish, J. W., Symons, F. J., Parker, D. E., & Lewis, M. H. (2000). Varieties of repetitive behavior in autism: Comparisons to mental retardation. *Journal of autism and developmental disorders, 30,* 237–243.

Boo, K. (1999). Forest Haven is gone, but the agony remains. *Washington Post*, Sunday, March 14, 1999. http://www.washingtonpost.com/wp-srv/local/daily/march99/grouphome14.htm, downloaded 12/20/14.

Borckardt, J. J., Madan, A., Grubaugh, A. L., Danielson, C. K., Pelic, C. G., Hardesty, S. J., et al. (2011). Systematic investigation of initiatives to reduce seclusion and restraint in a state psychiatric hospital. *Psychiatric Services, 62,* 477–483.

Branford, D. (1996). Factors associated with the successful or unsuccessful withdrawal of antipsychotic drug therapy prescribed for people with learning disabilities. *Journal of Intellectual Disability Research, 40,* 322–329.

Brend, M. (2008). *First and last. Closing learning disabilities hospital*. London: Choice Press.

Briggs, R. (1989). Monitoring and evaluating psychotropic drug use for persons with mental retardation: A follow-up report. *American Journal on Mental Retardation, 93,* 633–639.

British Institute of Learning Disabilities. (2002)

British Institute of Learning Disabilities. (2014). *BILD Code of Practice for minimising the use of restrictive physical interventions: Planning, developing and delivering training*. Kidderminster: BILD.

Brooker, J. E., Webber, L., Julian, J., Shawyer, F., Graham, A. L., Chan, J., & Meadows, G. (2014). Mindfulness-based training shows promise in assisting staff to reduce their use of restrictive interventions in residential services. *Mindfulness*, 1–6.

Bull, M., & LaVecchio, F. (1978). Behavior therapy for a child with Lesch-Nyhan syndrome. *Developmental Medicine and Child Neurology, 20,* 368–375.

Burgio, L., & Burgio, K. (1986). Behavioral gerontology: Application of behavioral methods to the problems of older adults. *Journal of Applied Behavior Analysis, 19,* 321–328.

Campbell, A. J., Robertson, M. C., Gardner, M. M., et al. (1999). Psychotropic medication withdrawal and a home-based exercise program to prevent falls: A randomized, controlled trial. *Journal of the American Geriatric Society, 47*, 850–853.

Capezuti, E., Maislin, G., Strumpf, N., & Evans, L. K. (2002). Side rail use and bed-related fall outcomes among nursing home residents. *Journal of the American Geriatrics Society, 50,* 90–96.

Capezuti, E., Strumpf, N. E., Evans, L. K., Grisso, J. A., & Maislin, G. (1998). The relationship between physical restraint removal and falls and injuries among nursing home residents. *The Journals of Gerontology Series A: Biological Sciences and Medical Sciences, 53,* M47–M52.

Capezuti, E., Talerico, K. A., Cochran, I., Becker, H., Strumpf, N., Evans, L. (1999). Individualized interventions to prevent bed-related falls and reduced siderail use. *Journal of Gerontological Nursing, 25,* 26–34.

Care Quality Commission. (2011). Review of compliance. Castelbeck Care Ltd. (Tyneside). http://www.cqc.org.uk/sites/default/files/documents/1-116865865_castlebeck_care_teesdale_ltd_1-138702193_winterbourne_view_roc_20110517_201107183026.pdf, downloaded 12/20/14.

Care Quality Commission. (2012). *What we think about St Lukes.* Easy read report. (http://www.cqc.org.uk/sites/default/files/old_reports/1-102643354_Mild_Professional_Homes_Limited_1-138212443_St_Lukes_Hospital_LDR_20120405_Easy_Read.pdf), downloaded 12/20/14.

Castle, N. G. (1998). Physical restraints in nursing homes: A review of the literature since the Nursing Home Reform Act of 1987. *Medical Care Research and Review, 55,* 139–170.

Castle, N. G. (2008). Nursing home caregiver staffing levels and quality of care. A literature review. *Journal of Applied Gerontology, 27,* 375–405.
Centers for Medicare and Medicaid Services. (2008). Freedom from unnecessary physical restraints: Two Decades of National Progress in Nursing Home Care". http://www.cms.gov/Medicare/Provider-Enrollment-and-Certification/SurveyCertificationGenInfo/downloads/SCLetter09-11.pdf, downloaded 12/17/14.
Centers for Medicare and Medicaid Services. (2008b). Nursing home data compendium 2013 Edition. https://www.cms.gov/Medicare/Provider-Enrollment-andCertification/CertificationandComplianc/downloads/nursinghomedatacompendium_508.pdf, downloaded 12/14/14.
Chan, J., LeBel, J., & Webber, L. (2013). The dollars and sense of restraints and seclusion. *Journal of Law and Medicine, 20,* 73–81.
Chaplin, E., Tsakanikos, E., Wright, S., & Bouras, N. (2009). Clinical psychopathology, untoward incidents and the use of restrictive procedures in adults with intellectual disability. *Journal of Applied Research in Intellectual Disabilities, 22,* 169–178.
Chapman, M. J., Hare, D. J., Caton, S., Donalds, D., McInnis, E., & Mitchell, D. (2013). The use of mindfulness with people with intellectual disabilities: A systematic review and narrative analysis. *Mindfulness, 4,* 179–189.
Christensen, L. W. (2006). *Extreme joint locking and breaking: Restraint and submission techniques for the street.* Boulder: Paladin.
Coalition Against Institutionalized Child Abuse. (2011). List of restraint deaths. http://www.leg.state.co.us/CLICS/CLICS2011A/commsumm.nsf/b4a3962433b52fa787256e5f00670a71/43604896fe25c9bb87257856006a0516/$FILE/110317AttachI.pdf, downloaded 12/17/14.
Colaizzi, J. (2005). Seclusion and restraint: A historical perspective. *Journal of Psychosocial Mental Health Service, 43,* 31–37.
Colonial Times. New York: Columbia University Press
Conolly, J. (1856/1973). *Treatment of the insane without mechanical restraints.* London: Dawson of Pall Mall.
Conor Ward, O. (1999). John Langdon Down 1828-1896: A caring pioneer. *Journal of the Royal Society of Medicine, 92,* 322–323.
Consumer Product Safety Commission. (2012). Adult portable bed rail-related deaths, injuries, and potential injuries: January 2003 to September 2012. http://www.cpsc.gov//PageFiles/133466/adultbedrail.pdf, downloaded 12/28/14.
Cooper, J. O., Heron, T. E., & Heward, W. L. (2007). *Applied behavior analysis* (2nd ed.). Upper Saddle River: Pearson.
Cotter, V. T. (2005). Restraint free care in older adults with dementia. *The Keio Journal of Medicine, 54,* 80–84.
Council of Parent Attorneys and Advocates. (2009). Unsafe in the schoolhouse. Abuse of children with disabilities. http://c.ymcdn.com/sites/www.copaa.org/resource/collection/662B1866-952D-41FA-B7F3-D3CF68639918/UnsafeCOPAAMay_27_2009.pdf, downloaded 12/17/14.
Curran, C., Adnett, C., & Zigmond, T. (2005). Seclusion: Factors to consider when designing and using a seclusion suite in a mental health hospital. Downloaded from http://www.sykehusplan.no/data/seclusion.pdf, 12/15/14.
Currier, G. W. (2003). The controversy over chemical restraint in acute care psychiatry. *Journal of Psychiatric Practice, 9,* 59–70.
Currier, G. W., & Farley-Toombs, C. (2002). Datapoints: Use of restraint before and after implementation of the new HCFA rules. *Psychiatric Services, 53,* 138–138.
Damen, I. M. (2009). *The effectiveness of a restraint reduction policy implemented to reduce the use of physical restraint with children and adolescents in a residential care facility.* Doctoral dissertations, 30. http://trace.tennessee.edu/cgi/viewcontent.cgi?article=1062&context=utk_graddiss&sei-redir=1&referer=http%3A%2F%2Fscholar.google.com%2Fscholar%3Fq%3DRestraint%2BAND%2BDamen%2B%25282009%2529%26btnG%3D%26hl%3Den%26as_sdt%3D0%252C33#search=%22Restraint%20Damen%20%282009%29%22, downloaded 12/31/14.
Davidson, N. A., Hemmingway, M. J., & Wysocki, T. (1984). Reducing the use of restrictive procedures in a residential facility. Psychiatric Services, 35, 164–167.

Day, P. (2002). What evidence exists about the safety of physical restraint when used by law enforcement and medical staff to control individuals with acute behavioural disturbance? *NZHTA TECH BRIEF SERIES*, 1, downloaded from http://www.otago.ac.nz/christchurch/otago014012.pdf 12/15/14.

De Hert, M., Dirix, N., Demunter, H., & Correll, C. U. (2009). Prevalence and correlates of seclusion and restraint use in children and adolescents: A systematic review. *European Child and Adolescent Psychiatry, 20,* 221–230.

De Hert, M., Dirix, N., Demunter, H., & Correll, C. U. (2011). Prevalence and correlates of seclusion and restraint use in children and adolescents: A systematic review. *European Child and Adolescent Psychiatry, 20,* 221–230.

Dean, S. (2014). EXCLUSIVE: Strapped in and locked up: Shocking photos reveal how autistic children are treated in Australian schools. http://www.dailymail.co.uk/news/article-2744571/Strapped-locked-Shocking-photos-reveal-disabled-children-treated-Australian-schools.html#ixzz3NJ6DHaLL, downloaded 12/28/14.

Dean, A. J., Duke, S. G., George, M., & Scott, J. (2007). Behavioral management leads to reduction in aggression in a child and adolescent psychiatric inpatient unit. *Journal of the American Academy of Child and Adolescent Psychiatry, 46,* 711–720.

Dean, A. J., McDermott, B. M., & Scott, J. (2009). Changing utilization of pro re nata ('as needed') sedation in a child and adolescent psychiatric inpatient unit. *Australian and New Zealand Journal of Psychiatry, 43,* 360–365.

Delafon, V., Kiani, R., Barrett, M., Vahabzadeh, A., Vaidya, H., Walker, G., et al. (2010). Use of PRN medication in people with intellectual disabilities. *Advances in Mental Health and Intellectual Disabilities, 7,* 346–355.

Delaney, K. R. (2001). Developing a restraint-reduction program for child/adolescent inpatient treatment. *Journal of Child and Adolescent Psychiatric Nursing, 14,* 128–140.

Delaney, K. R. (2006). Evidence base for practice: Reduction of restraint and seclusion use during child and adolescent psychiatric inpatient treatment. *Worldviews on Evidence-Based Nursing, 3,* 19–30.

Denunzio, M. M., & Hogan, J. D. (2012). Chiarugi, Vincenzo. In *Encyclopedia of the History of Psychological Theories* (pp. 174–175). US: Springer.

Department for Children, Schools and Families. (2013). Use of reasonable force in schools. https://www.gov.uk/government/publications/use-of-reasonable-force-in-schools, downloaded 12/28/14.

Department of Health. (2012). *Transforming care: A national response to Winterbourne View Hospital. Department of* Health Review: Final Report. https://www.gov.uk/government/uploads/system/uploads/attachment_data/file/213215/final-report.pdf, downloaded 12/20/14.

Deutsch, A. (1946). *The mentally ill in American. A history of their care and treatment from colonial times*. New York: Columbia University Press.

Deveau, R., & McGill, P. (2009). Physical interventions for adults with intellectual disabilities: Survey of use, policy, training and monitoring. *Journal of Applied Research in Intellectual Disabilities, 22,* 145–151.

Didden, R., Duker, P. C., & Korzilius, H. (1997). Meta-analytic study on treatment effectiveness for problem behaviors with individuals who have mental retardation. *AJMR—American Journal on Mental Retardation, 101,* 387–399.

Didden, R., Korzilius, H., van Oorsouw, W., & Sturmey, P. (2006). Behavioral treatment of challenging behaviors in individuals with mild mental retardation: Meta-analysis of single-subject research. *American Journal on Mental Retardation, 111,* 290–298.

Dix, R., & Betteridge, C. (2001). Seclusion. In M. D. Beer, S. M. Pereira, & C. Patton (Eds.), *Psychiatric intensive care* (pp. 133–156). Cambridge: Cambridge University Press.

Donat, D. C. (1998). Impact of a mandatory behavioral consultation on seclusion/restraint utilization in a psychiatric hospital. *Journal of Behavior Therapy and Experimental Psychiatry, 29,* 13–19.

Donat, D. C. (2002). Impact of improved staffing on seclusion/restraint reliance in a public psychiatric hospital. *Psychiatric Rehabilitation Journal, 25,* 413–416.

Donat, D. C. (2003). An analysis of successful efforts to reduce the use of seclusion and restraint at a public psychiatric hospital. *Psychiatric Services, 54,* 1119–1123.

Donat, D. C. (2006). Impact of a clinical-administrative review procedure on reducing reliance on psychotropic PRN medication. *Psychiatric Rehabilitation Journal, 29,* 215–218.

Dube, A. H., & Mitchell, E. K. (1986). Accidental strangulation from vest restraints. *Journal of the American Medical Association, 256,* 2725–2726.

Duker, P. C., & Seys, D. M. (1997). An inventory method for assessing the degree of restraint imposed by others. *Journal of Behavior Therapy and Experimental Psychiatry, 28,* 113–121.

Duker, P. C., & Seys, D. M. (2000). A quasi-experimental study on the effect of electrical aversion treatment on imposed mechanical restraint for severe self-injurious behavior. *Research in Developmental Disabilities, 21,* 235–242.

Dunbar, J. M., Neufeld, R. R., White, H. C., & Libow, L. S. (1996). Retrain, don't restrain: The educational intervention of the National Nursing Home Restraint Removal Project. *The Gerontologist, 36,* 539–542.

Dykens, E. M., & Kasari, C. (1997). Maladaptive behavior in children with Prader–Willi syndrome, Down syndrome, and nonspecific mental retardation. *American Journal on Mental Retardation, 102,* 228–237.

Education Act. (1996). http://www.legislation.gov.uk/ukpga/1996/56/contents, downloaded 12/28/14.

Ekdawi, M. Y. (1987). Asylum of Leros. *Psychiatric Bulletin, 11,* 275–275.

Ellenor, G. L., & Frisk, P. A. (1977). Pharmacist impact on drug use in an institution for the mentally retarded. *American Journal of Health-System Pharmacy, 34,* 604–608.

Emerson, E. (2002). The prevalence of use of reactive management strategies in community of community-based strategies in the UK. In D. Allen (Ed.), *Ethical approaches to physical interventions Volume I: Responding to challenging behaviour in people with intellectual disabilities* (pp. 15-30). Kidderminster: BILD.

Emerson, E., Robertson, J., Gregory, N., Hatton, C., Kessissoglou, S., Hallam, A., & Hillery, J. (2000). *Journal of Applied Research in Intellectual Disabilities, 13,* 197–215.

Equip for Equality. (2011). Equip for equality national review of restraint, restraint related deaths of children and adults with disabilities. The Lethal Consequences of Restraint. http://www.equipforequality.org/wp-content/uploads/2014/04/National-Review-of-Restraint-Related-Deaths-of-Adults-and-Children-with-Disabilities-The-Lethal-Consequences-of-Restraint.pdf, downloaded 12/17/14.

Esther, R. J. (1997). Use of physical restraints in a nineteenth-century state hospital. *History of Psychiatry, 8,* 83–93.

Evans, D., Wood, J., & Lambert, L. (2002). A review of physical restraint minimization in the acute and residential care settings. *Journal of Advanced Nursing, 40,* 616–625.

Evans, E., Strumpf, L. K., Allen, N. E., Taylor, S. L., et al. (1997). A clinical trial to reduce restraints in nursing homes. *Journal of the American Geriatrics Society, 45,* 675–681.

Everston. (1994–2004). Greek mental care failures exposed. June 30, 2009. http://news.bbc.co.uk/2/hi/europe/8124976.stm, downloaded 12/20/14.

Favell, J. E., McGimsey, J. F., & Jones, M. L. (1978). The use of physical restraint in the treatment of self-injury and as positive reinforcement. *Journal of Applied Behavior Analysis, 11,* 225–241.

Favell, J. E., McGimsey, J. F., Jones, M. L., & Cannon, P. R. (1981). Physical restraint as positive reinforcement. *American Journal of Mental Deficiency, 85,* 425–432.

Feldman, M. A., Atkinson, L., Foti-Gervais, L., & Condillac, R. (2004). Formal versus informal interventions for challenging behaviour in persons with intellectual disabilities. *Journal of Intellectual Disability Research, 48,* 60–68.

Fielding, L. T., Murphy, R. J., Reagan, M. W., & Peterson, J. L. (1980). An assessment programme to reduce drug use with the mentally retarded. *Hospital and Community Psychiatry, 31,* 771–773.

Finn, L. L., & Sturmey, P. (2009). Analysis of the distribution and social antecedents of restrictive behavioural practices in a community day service for adults with intellectual disabilities. *Journal of Applied Research in Intellectual Disabilities, 22,* 179–186.

Fisher, W. A. (1994). Restraint and seclusion: A review of the literature. *American Journal of Psychiatry, 151,* 1584–1591.

Fisher, W. A. (2003). Elements of successful restraint and seclusion reduction programs and their application in a large, urban, state psychiatric hospital. *Journal of Psychiatric Practice, 9,* 7–15.

Fisher, W. W., Grace, N. C., & Murphy, C. (1996). Further analysis of the relationship between self-injury and self-restraint. *Journal of Applied Behavior Analysis, 29,* 103–106.

Fisher, W. W., & Iwata, B. A. (1996). On the function of self-injurious behavior and its relationship to self-injury. *Journal of Applied Behavior Analysis, 29,* 93–98.

Fisher, W. W., Piazza, C. C., Bowman, L. G., Hanley, G. P., & Adelinis, J. D. (1997). Direct and collateral effects of restraints and restraint fading. *Journal of Applied Behavior Analysis, 30,* 105–120.

Forman, D., Hall, S., & Oliver, C. (2002). Descriptive analysis of self-injurious behaviour and self-restraint. *Journal of Applied Research in Intellectual Disabilities, 15,* 1–7.

Foxx, R. M. (1977). Attention training: The use of overcorrection avoidance to increase the eye contact of autistic and retarded children. *Journal of Applied Behavior Analysis, 10,* 489–499.

Foxx, R. M. (1980). *Harry. Behavioral treatment of self-abuse.* Champaign Illinois: Research Press.

Foxx, R. M. (2005). The National Institutes of Health Consensus development conference on treatment of destructive behaviors: A study in professional politics. In J. W. Jacobson, R. M. Foxx, & J. A. Mulick (Eds.), *Controversial therapies for developmental disabilities* (pp. 461–477). Mahwah: Lawrence Erlbaum.

Foxx, R. M., & Dufrense, D. (1984). "Harry": The use of physical restraint as a reinforcer, timeout from restraint, and fading restraint in treating a self-injurious man. *Analysis and Intervention in Developmental Disabilities, 4,* 1–13.

Foxx, R. M., & Shapiro, S. T. (1978). The timeout ribbon: A nonexclusionary timeout procedure. *Journal of Applied Behavior Analysis, 11,* 125–136.

G4S guards cleared over Jimmy Mubenga death. (2014). http://www.bbc.com/news/uk-england-30494548, downloaded 12/28/14.

Gardner-Hill. (1838/1976). *Total abolition of personal restraint in the treatment of the insane.* New York: Arno Press.

Gaskin, C. J., Elsom, S. J., & Happell, B. (2007). Interventions for reducing the use of seclusion in psychiatric facilities review of the literature. *The British Journal of Psychiatry, 191,* 298–303.

Gaskin, C. J., McVilly, K. R., & McGillivray, J. A. (2013). Initiatives to reduce the use of seclusion and restraints on people with developmental disabilities: A systematic review and quantitative synthesis. *Research in Developmental Disabilities, 34,* 3946–3961.

General Accounting Officer. (1999a). Mental health. Improper restraint or seclusion use places people at risk. http://www.gao.gov/archive/1999/he99176.pdf, downloaded 12/17/14.

General Accounting Officer. (1999b). Mental health. Extent of risk from improper restraint or seclusion is unknown. http://www.gao.gov/archive/2000/he00026t.pdf, downloaded 12/17/14.

General Accounting Officer. (2008a). Residential facilities. State and Federal oversight gaps may increase risk to youth well-being. http://www.gao.gov/new.items/d08696t.pdf, downloaded 12/17/14.

General Accounting Officer. (2009). Seclusions and restraints. Selected cases of death and abuse at public and private schools and treatment centers. http://www.gao.gov/new.items/d09719t.pdf, downloaded 12/15/14.

Gerard, D. L. (1997). Chiarugi and Pinel considered: Soul's brain/person's mind. *Journal of the History of the Behavioral Sciences, 33,* 381–403.

Gillies, J., Moriarty, H., Short, T., Pesnell, P., Fox, C., & Cooney, A. (2005). An innovative model for restraint use at the Philadelphia Veterans Affairs Medical Center. *Nursing Administration Quarterly, 29,* 45–56.

Gilligan, J., & Lee, B. (2013). Report to the New York City Board of Correction. http://solitary-watch.com/wp-content/uploads/2013/11/Gilligan-Report.-Final.pdf, downloaded 12/28/14.

Gillis, J. (1996). *Bad habits and pernicious results: Thumb sucking and the discipline of late-*

Gianoumis, T., & Sturmey, P. (2012). Generalization procedures in training interventionists for individuals with developmental disabilities. *Behavior Modification, 36,* 619–629.

Glover, G., Brown, I. J., & Hatton, C. (2014). How psychiatric in-patient care for people with learning disabilities is transforming after Winterbourne View. *Tizard Learning Disability Review, 19,* 8–8.

Godfrey, J. L., McGill, A. C., Jones, N. T., Oxley, S. L., & Carr, R. M. (2014). Anatomy of a transformation: A systematic effort to reduce mechanical restraints at a state psychiatric hospital. *Psychiatric Services, 65,* 1277–1280.

Government Accountability Office. (2008a). Residential programs: Selected cases of death, abuse, and deceptive marketing. Testimony Before the Committee of Education and Labor, U.S. House of Representatives. Washington, D.C.

Greene, R., Ablon, J. S., & Martin, A. (2006). Innovations: Child & adolescent psychiatry: Use of collaborative problem solving to reduce seclusion and restraint in child and adolescent inpatient units. *Psychiatric Services, 57,* 610–612

Grove, E. (2010). Plainfield school accused of food denial, using 'jail cell'. *Medical history, 40,* 55–73. http://www.norwichbulletin.com/article/20100307/News/303079 960, downloaded 12/28/14.

Gulpers, M. J. M., Bleijlevens, M. H. C., Ambergen, T., Capezuti, E., van Rossum, E., & Hamers, J. P. H. (2011). Belt restraint reduction in nursing homes: Effects of a multicomponent intervention program. *Journal of the American Geriatrics Society, 59,* 2029–2036.

Gulpers, M. J., Bleijlevens, M. H. C., Ambergen, T., Capezuti, E., Rossum, E., & Hamers, J. P. (2013). Reduction of belt restraint use: Long-term effects of the EXBELT intervention. *Journal of the American Geriatrics Society, 61,* 107–112.

Hadjimatheou, C. (2009). Greek mental care failures exposed. June 30, 2009. http://news.bbc.co.uk/2/hi/europe/8124976.stm, downloaded 12/20/14.

Hakim. (2011a). $5 million payment to end suits over death of 13-year-old boy in State Care. http://www.nytimes.com/2011/09/22/nyregion/ny-state-settles-jonathan-carey-wrongful-death-lawsuits.html, downloaded 12/20/14.

Hakim. (2011b). Abused and used. http://www.nytimes.com/interactive/nyregion/abused-and-used-series-page.html?module=Search&mabReward=relbias%3As, downloaded 12/20/14.

Harper, S. K., Webb, T. L., & Rayner, K. (2013). The effectiveness of mindfulness-based interventions for supporting people with intellectual disabilities: A narrative review. *Behavior modification,* 0145445513476085.

Harris, J. (1996). Physical restraint procedures for managing challenging behaviours presented by mentally retarded adults and children. *Research in Developmental Disabilities, 17,* 99–134.

Haw, C., & Wolstencroft, L. (2014). A study of the use of sedative PRN medication in patients at a secure hospital. *Journal of Forensic Psychiatry and Psychology, 25,* 307–320.

Haw, C., & Yawston, G. (2004). Thomas Prichard and the non-restraint movement at the Northampton asylum. *Psychiatric Bulletin, 28,* 140–142.

Hawes, C. H., Morris, J. N., Phillips, C. D., Fries, B. E., Murphy, K., & Mor, B. E. (1997). Development of the nursing home Resident Assessment Instrument in the USA. *Age Ageing, 26*(suppl 2), 19–25.

Healthcare Commission. (2006). Joint investigation into the provision of services for provision of services for people with learning disability at Cornwall Partnership NHS trust. http://webarchive.nationalarchives.gov.uk/20060502043818/http:/healthcarecommission.org.uk/_db/_documents/cornwall_investigation_report.pdf, downloaded 12/20/14.

Healthcare Commission. (2007). Investigation into the services for people with learning disabilityies provided by Sutton and MertonPrimary Care Trust. http://webarchive.nationalarchives.gov.uk/20060502043818/ http://healthcarecommission.org.uk/_db/_documents/Sutton_and_Merton_inv_Main_Tag.pdf, downloaded 12/20/14.

Held, K. S. (2013). Couple charged with keeping autistic child in cage. http://www.ksdk.com/story/news/2013/10/20/3107709/ downloaded 12/20/14.

Hellerstein, D. J., Staub, A. B., & Lequesne, E. (2007). Decreasing the use of restraint and seclusion among psychiatric inpatients. *Journal of Psychiatric Practice, 13,* 308–317.

Heyveart, M., Saenen, L. M., Baes, J. M., & Onghena, P. (2014). Efficacy of behavioral interventions for reducing problem behavior in persons with autism: An updated quantitative synthesis of single-subject research. *Research in Developmental Disabilities, 35,* 2463–2476.

Hofmann, H., & Hahn, S. (2013). Characteristics of nursing home residents and physical restraint: A systematic literature review. *Journal of Clinical Nursing, 23,* 3012–3024.

Hollins, L. P., & Paterson, B. Physical intervention trainers: The case for greater accountability. *Journal of Psychiatric and Mental Health Nursing, 16,* 376–381.

Holmes & Simmons. (2008). *Rapid tranquillisation.* In M. D. Beer & S. M. Pereira (Eds.), *Psychiatric intensive care* (pp. 32–49). Cambridge: Cambridge University Press.

Holt, E. (2004). Rest and restraint. *Lancet, 364*(9437), 829–830.

Holt, G., Costello, H., Bouras, N., Diareme, S., Hillery, J., Moss, S., Dimitrakaki, C., et al. (2000). BIOMED-MEROPE project: Service provision for adults with intellectual disability: A European comparison. *Journal of Intellectual Disability Research, 44,* 685–696.

Houten, R., & Rolider, A. (1984). The use of response prevention to eliminate nocturnal thumbsucking. *Journal of Applied Behavior Analysis, 17,* 509–520.

Huang, L. (2011). Alternatives to seclusion and restraint in behavioral health care. http://www.integration.samhsa.gov/clinical-practice/promoting_alternatives_to_seclusion_and_restraint.pdf), downloaded 12/17/14.

Huefner, J. C., Griffith, A. K., Smith, G. L., Vollmer, D. G., & Leslie, L. K. (2014). Reducing psychotropic medications in an intensive residential treatment center. *Journal of Child and Family Studies, 23,* 675–685.

Hughes, R. (2009). *Rights, risk and restraint-free care of older people: Person-centred approaches in health and social care.* London: Jessica Kingsley.

Huizing, A. R., Hamers, J. P., Gulpers, M. J., & Berger, M. P. (2006). Short-term effects of an educational intervention on physical restraint use: A cluster randomized trial. *BMC Geriatrics, 6,* 17.

Huizing, A. R., Hamers, J. P., Gulpers, M. J., & Berger, M. P. (2009). A cluster-randomized trial of an educational intervention to reduce the use of physical restraints with psychogeriatric nursing home residents. *Journal of the American Geriatrics Society, 57,* 1139–1148.

Humza Bin Saeed, M., Daly, B., & Newton, J. T. (2012). Knowledge and practice of behavioral management principles among dentists treating adults with learning disabilities. *Special Care in Dentistry, 32,* 190–195.

Hwang, Y. S., & Kearney, P. (2013). A systematic review of mindfulness intervention for individuals with developmental disabilities: Long-term practice and long lasting effects. *Research in Developmental Disabilities, 34,* 314–326.

Hyman, P., Oliver, C., & Hall, S. (2002). Self-injurious behavior, self-restraint, and compulsive behaviors in Cornelia de Lange syndrome. *American Journal on Mental Retardation, 107,* 146–154.

Isley, E. M., Kartsonis, C., McCurley, C. M., Eager Weisz, K., & Roberts, M. S. (1991). Self-restraint: A review of etiology and applications in mentally retarded adults with self-injury. *Research in Developmental Disabilities, 12,* 87–95.

Iwata, B. A., Dorsey, M. F., Slifer, K. J., Bauman, K. E., & Richman, G. S. (1982). Toward a functional analysis of self-injury. *Analysis and Intervention in Developmental Disabilities, 2,* 3–20.

Iwata, B. A., Rolider, N. U., & Dozier, C. L. (2009). Evaluation of timeout programs through phased withdrawal. *Journal of Applied Research in Intellectual Disabilities, 22,* 203–209.

Jacobsen, P. B., Manne, S. L., Gorfinkle, K., Schorr, O., Rapkin, B., & Redd, W. H. (1990). Analysis of child and parent behavior during painful medical procedures. *Health Psychology, 9,* 559–576.

Jacoby, M. G., Babikian, H., McLamb, E., & Hohlbein, B. (1958). A study in non-restraint. *American Journal of Psychiatry, 115,* 114–120.

James, J. E. (1981). Behavioral self-control of stuttering using time-out from speaking. *Journal of Applied Behavior Analysis, 14,* 25–37.

Jancar, J. (1970). Gradual withdrawal of tranquillizers with the help of ascorbic acid. *The British Journal of Psychiatry, 117,* 238–239.

Jarvis, E., & Clark, J. (1869/2013). *A memoir of John Conolly M. D. D. C. L. comprising a sketch of the treatment of the insane in Europe and America.* Cambridge: Cambridge University Press.

Jay, S. M., Elliot, C. H., Ozolins, M., Olson, R. A., & Pruitt, S. D. (1985). Behavioral management of children's distress during painful medical procedures. *Behaviour, Research and Therapy, 23,* 513–520.

Jensen, C. C., Lydersen, T., Johnson, P. R., Weiss, S. R., Marconi, M. R., Cleave, M. L., & Weber, P. (2012). Choosing staff members reduces time in mechanical restraint due to self-injurious behaviour and requesting restraint. *Journal of Applied Research in Intellectual Disabilities, 25,* 282–287.

Jerome, J., & Sturmey, P. (2008). Reinforcing efficacy of interactions with preferred and non-preferred staff under progressive-ratio schedules. *Journal of Applied Behavior Analysis, 41,* 221–225.

Jerome, J., & Sturmey, P. (2014). The effects of pairing non-preferred staff with preferred stimuli on increasing the reinforcing value of non-preferred staff attention. *Research in Developmental Disabilities, 35,* 849–860.

Johnson, S. F. (2010). *Preventing physical restraints in schools.* Warner: Education Law Resource Center, LLC.

Johnson, S. (n.d.). *Preventing physical restraints in schools: A guide for parents, educators & professionals.* Warner: The Education Resource Center.

Joint Commission on Accreditation of Healthcare. (2002). *Restraint and seclusion: Complying with Joint Commission Standards.* Joint Commission on Accreditation of Healthcare.

Jonikas, J. A., Cook, J. A., Rosen, C., Laris, A., & Kim, J. B. (2004). Brief reports: A program to reduce use of physical restraint in psychiatric inpatient facilities. *Psychiatric Services, 55,* 818–820.

Kalhan, A. (2010). Rethinking immigration detention. *Colombia Law Review, 110,* 42–58.

Karim, S. (2014). *A human rights perspective on reducing restrictive practices in intellectual disability and autism.* Birmingham: BILD.

Kearns, R. R., & Spencer, R. L. (2013). An unexpected increase in restraint duration alters the expression of stress response habituation. *Physiology and Behavior*, 2013.03.029

Kerth, D. M., Progar, P. R., & Morales, S. (2009). The effects of non-contingent self-restraint on self-injury. *Journal of Applied Research in Intellectual Disabilities, 22,* 187–193.

King, B. H. (1993). Self-injury by people with mental retardation: A compulsive behavior hypothesis. *American Journal of Mental Retardation, 98,* 93–112.

Knutzen, M., Bjørkly, S., Eidhammer, G., Lorentzen, S., Mjøsund, N. H., Opjordsmoen, S., & Friis, S., et al. (2014). Characteristics of patients frequently subjected to pharmacological and mechanical restraint—A register study in three Norwegian acute psychiatric wards. *Psychiatry Research, 215,* 127–133.

Kojima, T., Akishita, M., Nakamura, T., Nomura, K., Ogawa, S., Iijima, K., & Ouchi, Y., et al. (2012). Polypharmacy as a risk for fall occurrence in geriatric outpatients. *Geriatrics and Gerontology International, 12,* 425–430.

Konetzka, R. T., Brauner, D. J., Shega, J., & Werner, R. M. (2014). The effects of public reporting on physical restraints and antipsychotic use in nursing home residents with severe cognitive impairment. *Journal of the American Geriatrics Society, 62,* 454–461.

Kotynia-English, R., McGowan, H., & Almeida, O. P. (2005). A randomized trial of early psychiatric intervention in residential care: Impact on health outcomes. *International Psychogeriatrics, 17,* 475–485.

Kumar. (2007). *The CMS restraint training requirements handbook paperback.* Danvers: HCPro Inc.

Kupfersmid, J., & Monkman, R. (Eds.). (1988). *Assaultive youth: Responding to physical assaultiveness in residential, community and health care settings.* New York: Haworth Press.

Kuske, B., Luck, T., Hanns, S., Matschinger, H., Angermeyer, M. C., Behrens, J., & Riedel-Heller, S. G. (2009). Training in dementia care: A cluster-randomized controlled trial of a training program for nursing home staff in Germany. *International Psychogeriatrics, 21,* 295–308.

Lambeth, L. G. J. (2013). Chemical restraint. Chief Forensic Psychiatrist. Clinical guideline 10. Downloaded from 10 http://www.dhhs.tas.gov.au/__data/assets/pdf_file/0004/148261/24_CFP_Clinical_Guideline_10_-_Chemical_Restraint.pdf on 12/15/14.

Lane, K. L., Kalberg, J. R., & Menzies, H. M. (2009). *Developing schoolwide programs to prevent and manage problem behaviors: A step-by-step approach.* London: Guilford.

Lay, B., Nord, C., & Russler, W. (2007). Mental hospital admission rates of immigrants in Switzerland. *Social Psychiatry and Psychiatric Epidemiology, 42,* 229–236.

LeBel, J., & Goldstein, R. (2005). The economic cost of using restraint and the value added by restraint reduction or elimination. *Psychiatric Services, 56,* 1109–1114.

LeBel, J., Stromberg, N., Duckworth, K., Kerzner, J., Goldstein, R., Weeks, M., & Sudders, M., et al. (2004). Child and adolescent inpatient restraint reduction: A state initiative to promote strength-based care. *Journal of the American Academy of Child and Adolescent Psychiatry, 43,* 37–45.

LeBel, J., Huckshorn, K. A., & Jacobs, H. E. (2014). An organizational approach to reducing and preventing restraint and seclusion use with people with acquired brain injury. *Neuro Rehabilitation,* 671–680.

LeBlanc, L. A., Piazza, C. C., & Krug, M. A. (1997). Comparing methods for maintaining the safety of a child with pica. *Research in Developmental Disabilities, 18,* 215–220.

Lee, S., Gray, R., & Gournay, K. (2012). Comparing the outcomes of the application of C & R (general service) and SCIP in the management of disturbed behaviour in mental health care. *Journal of Mental Health, 21,* 307–317.

Leitenberg, H. (1965). Is time-out from positive reinforcement an aversive event? A review of the experimental evidence. *Psychological Bulletin, 64,* 428–441.

Leoni, M., Corti, S., Chiodelli, G., Fioriti, F., Cavagnola, R. (June, 2012). *Deinstitutionalization process for persons with IDD. An Italian experience.* Presented to the 136th annual meeting of the American Association on Intellectual and Developmental Disabilities, Charlotte, North Carolina, US.

Lepler, S., Hodas, A., & Cotter-Mack, A. (1994). What input do community-based psychiatrists need from staff and families of our consumers? *Mental Retardation, 32,* 245–247.

Lerman, D. C., & Iwata, B. A. (1996). A methodology for distinguishing between extinction and punishment effects associated with response blocking. *Journal of Applied Behavior Analysis, 29,* 231–233.

Lerman, D. C., Iwata, B. A., Smith, R. G., & Vollmer, T. R. (1994). Restraint fading and the development of alternative behaviour in the treatment of self-restraint and self-injury. *Journal of Intellectual Disability Research, 38,* 135–148.

Levering, N. J., & Wellie, J. V. M. (2011). Current status of nitrous oxide as a behavior management practice routine in pediatric dentistry. *Journal of Dentistry for Children, 78,* 24–30.

Levine, J. M., Marchello, V., & Totolos, E. (1995). Progress toward a restraint-free environment in a large academic nursing facility. *Journal of the American Geriatrics Society, 43,* 914–918.

Lewis, M., Shilton, P., & Fuqua, W. R. (1981). Parental control of nocturnal thumbsucking. *Journal of Behavior Therapy and Experimental Psychiatry, 12,* 87–90.

Lipson, J. V., & Braun, S. (1993). *Toward a restraint-free environment: Reducing the use of physical and chemical restraints in long-term and acute care settings.* Baltimore: Health Professions Press.

Luchins, D. J., Dojka, D., & Hanrahan, P. (1993). Factors associated with reduction in antipsychotic medication dosage in adults with mental retardation. *American Journal of Mental Retardation, 98,* 165–175.

Luiselli, J. K. (2009). Physical restraint of people with intellectual disability: A review of implementation reduction and elimination procedures. *Journal of Applied Research in Intellectual Disabilities, 22,* 126–134.

Luiselli, J. K., Kane, A., Treml, T., & Young, N. (2000). Behavioral intervention to reduce physical restraint of adolescents with developmental disabilities. *Behavioral Interventions, 15,* 317–330.

Luiselli, J. K., Pace, G., & Dunn, E. K. (2003). Antecedent analysis of therapeutic restraint in children and adolescents with acquired brain injury: A descriptive study of four cases. *Brain Injury, 17,* 255–264.

Luiselli, J., Dunn, E. K., & Pace, G. M. (2005). Antecedent assessment and intervention to reduce physical restraint (protective holding) of children and adolescents with acquired brain injury. *Behavioral Interventions, 20,* 51–65.

Lyon, C., & Pimor, A. (2004). *Physical interventions and the law*. Kidderminster: BILD.

Maas, A. P., Didden, R., Bouts, L., Smits, M. G., & Curfs, L. M. (2009). Scatter plot analysis of excessive daytime sleepiness and severe disruptive behavior in adults with Prader–Willi syndrome: A pilot study. *Research in Developmental Disabilities, 30,* 529–537.

MacPherson, R., Dix, R., & Morgan, S. (2005). A growing evidence base for management guidelines Revisiting … Guidelines for the management of acutely disturbed psychiatric patients. *Advances in Psychiatric Treatment, 11,* 404–415.

Madan, A., Borckardt, J. J., Grubaugh, A. L., Danielson, C. K., McLeod-Bryant, S., Cooney, H., Hardesty, S. H., & Frueh, B. C. (2014). Efforts to reduce seclusion and restraint use in a state psychiatric hospital: A ten-year perspective. *Psychiatric Services, 65,* 1273–1276.

Mador, J. E., Giles, L., Whitehead, C., & Crotty, M. (2004). A randomized controlled trial of a behavior advisory service for hospitalized older patients with confusion. *International Journal of Geriatric Psychiatry, 19,* 858–863.

Magee, S. K., & Ellis, J. (2001). The detrimental effects of physical restraint as a consequence for inappropriate classroom behavior. *Journal of Applied Behavior Analysis, 34,* 501–504.

Manne, S. L., Redd, W. H., Jacobsen, P. B., Gorfinkle, K., Schorr, O., & Rapkin, B. (1990). Behavioral intervention to reduce child and parent distress during venipuncture. *Journal of Consulting and Clinical Psychology, 58,* 565–572.

Marlatt, G. A., & Kristeller, J. L. (1999). Mindfulness and meditation. In W. R. Miller (Ed.), *Integrating spirituality into treatment: Resources for practitioners* (pp. 67–84). Washington, DC: American Psychological Association.

Martin, B. (2002). Restraint use in acute and critical care settings: Changing practice. *AACN Advanced Critical Care, 13,* 294–306.

Mason, T. (1992). Seclusion: Definitional interpretations. *The Journal of Forensic Psychiatry, 3,* 261–270.

Mayhew, P. A., Kimbera, C., Berkebile, J., Miller, C., & Farrish, A. (1999). Restraint reduction: Research utilization and case study with cognitive impairment. *Geriatric Nursing, 20,* 305–308.

McClelland, R. J. (1988). The madhouses and mad doctors of Ulster. *The Ulster Medical Journal, 57,* 101–120.

McCue, R. E., Urcuyo, L., Lilu, Y., Tobias, T., & Chambers, M. J. (2004). Reducing restraint use in a public psychiatric inpatient service. *The Journal of Behavioral Health Services and Research, 31,* 217–224.

McDonnell, A., Sturmey, P., Oliver, C., Cunningham, A., Hayes, S., & Galvin, M., Walshe, M., & Cunningham, C. (2008). The effects of staff training on staff confidence and challenging behavior in services for people with autism spectrum disorders. *Research in Autism Spectrum Disorders, 2,* 311–319.

McGaughey, J., & Bell, J. (2013). Report of the office of protection and advocacy for persons with disabilities and the office of the child advocate. No more "scream rooms" in Connecticut schools: An investigation into seclusion practices at Farm Hill Elementary School, including analysis of the responses of the state departments of education and children and families, and recommendations for reform July 2013. http://www.ct.gov/oca/lib/oca/No_More_Scream_Rooms_OPA-OCA_REPORT_7-13_FINAL.pdf), downloaded 12/17/15.

McGaw, S., & Sturmey, P. (1989). The effects of text readability and summary exercises on parent knowledge of behaviour therapy: The Portage parent readings. *Educational Psychology, 9,* 127–132.

McGill, P., Murphy, G., & Kelly-Pike, A. (2009). Frequency of use and characteristics of people with intellectual disabilities subject to physical interventions. *Journal of Applied Research in Intellectual Disabilities, 22,* 152–158.

McNett, M., Sarver, W., & Wilczewski, P. (2012). The prevalence, treatment and outcomes of agitation among patients with brain injury admitted to acute care units. *Brain Injury, 26,* 1155–1162.

Medley, N. S., Little, S. G., & Akin-Little, A. (2008). Comparing individual behavior plans from schools with and without schoolwide positive behavior support: A preliminary study. *Journal of Behavioral Education, 17,* 93–110.

Mental Disability Advocacy Center. (2012). European court finds use of restraints constitutes inhuman and degrading treatment. http://www.mdac.info/en/19/10/2012/european-court-finds-use-restraints-constitutes-inhuman-and-degrading-treatment, downloaded 12/28/14.

Mental Disability Advocacy Center. (2014). Cage beds and coercion in Czech psychiatric Institutions. http://www.mdac.org/sites/mdac.info/files/cagebed_web_en_20140624.pdf, downloaded 12/20/14.

Mental Health Act. (1983). London: HMSO.

Merineau-Cote, J., & Morin, D. (2013). Correlates of restraint and seclusion for adults with intellectual disabilities in community services. *Journal of Intellectual Disability Research, 57,* 182–190.

Mercer, J. (2001). "Attachment therapy" using deliberate restraint: An object lesson on the identification of unvalidated treatments. *Journal of Child and Adolescent Psychiatric Nursing, 14,* 105–111.

Mercer, J. (2002). Child psychotherapy involving physical restraint: Techniques used in four approaches. *Child and Adolescent Social Work Journal, 19,* 303–314.

Mercer, J. (2007). *Unconventional therapies evaluating unconventional mental health treatments.* London: Rowman & Littlefield.

Meyer, G., Köpke, S., Haastert, B., & Mühlhauser, I. (2008). Restraint use among nursing home residents: Cross-sectional study and prospective cohort study. *Journal of Clinical Nursing, 18,* 981–990.

Miles, S. H., & Irvine, P. (1992). Deaths caused by physical restraints. *The Gerontologist, 32,* 762–766.

Miller, J. A., Hunt, D. P., & Megan, G. A. (2006). Reduction of physical restraints in residential treatment facilities. *Journal of Disability Policy Studies, 16,* 202–208.

Mohler, R., Richter, T., Sascha, S., & Meyer, G. (2012). Interventions for preventing and reducing the use of physical restraints in long-term geriatric care. The Cochrane library downloaded from http://onlinelibrary.wiley.com/doi/10.1002/14651858.CD007546.pub2/abstract 12/15/14.

Morris, C. (2011). Tethered teenage psychiatric patient shocks Netherlands. http://www.bbc.co.uk/news/world-europe-12256811, downloaded 12/20/14.

Morris, S. (2014). Teacher 'put sticky tape over children's mouths'. http://www.theguardian.com/uk-news/2014/mar/04/teacher-put-sticky-tape-childrens-mouths, downloaded 12/28/14.

Murphy, G. H., Oliver, C., Corbett, J. A., Crayton, L., Hales, J., Head, D., & Hall, S. (1993). Epidemiology of self injury, characteristics of people with severe self-injury and initial treatment outcome. In C. Kiernan (Ed.), *Research to Practice?: Implications of research on the challenging behaviour of people with learning disability* (pp. 1–35). Clevedon: BILD.

Murphy, G., Kelly-Pike, A., & McGill, P. (2001). Physical interventions for people with intellectual disabilities: Initial survey of training and evaluation of a policy framework. *Journal of Applied Research in Intellectual Disabilities, 14,* 401–411.

Murphy, G., Kelly-Pike, A., McGill, P., Jones, S., & Byatt, J. (2003). Physical interventions with people with Intellectual Disabilities: Staff training and policy frameworks. *Journal of Applied Research in Intellectual Disabilities, 16,* 115–125.

National Association of State Mental Health Program Directors Research Institute. (n.d.). National Public Rates. Behavioral Healthcare Performance Measurement System. http://media.wix.com/ugd/186708_fa2f69a9194844c4815755ef8b2544b4.pdf, downloaded 12/17/14.

National Disability Rights Network. (2009). School is not supposed to hurt. Update on progress in 2009 to prevent and reduce restraint and seclusion in schools. http://www.ndrn.org/images/Documents/Resources/Publications/Reports/School-is-Not-Supposed-to-Hurt-NDRN.pdf. downloaded 12/17/15.

National Disability Rights Network. (2012). School is not supposed to hurt: The U.S. Department of Education must do more to protect school children from restraint and seclusion. http://www.ndrn.org/images/Documents/Resources/Publications/Reports/School_is_Not_Supposed_to_Hurt_3_v7.pdf, downloaded 12/17/14.

National Institute of Clinical Excellence. (2005). Violence: The short-term management of disturbed/violent behaviour in in-patient psychiatric settings and emergency departments. Downloaded from https://www.nice.org.uk/guidance/cg25/chapter/about-this-guideline, 12/16/2014.

National Institute of Clinical Excellence. (2014). Rapid tranquillisation in mental health settings: Promethazine hydrochloride. Downloaded from http://www.nice.org.uk/advice/esuom28, 12/15/14.

National Mental Health Consumer and Career Forum. (2009). *Ending seclusion and restraint in Australian Mental Health Services*. Dowloaded from http://www.nmhccf.org.au/documents/Seclusion%20&%20Restraint.pdf, 12/15/14.

National Union of Teachers. (2012). NUT Notes 2-12-2013. Education the law and you. http://www.teachers.org.uk/files/the-law-and-you-8251-.pdf, downloaded 12/28/14.

Nazir, A., Unroe, K., Tegeler, M., Khan, B., Azar, J., & Boustani, M. (2013). Systematic review of interdisciplinary interventions in nursing homes. *Journal of the American Medical Directors Association, 14,* 471–478.

Nelson, E. A. S., Schiefenhoevel, W., & Felizitas, H. (2000). Child care practices in nonindustrialized societies. *Pediatrics, 105,* S. e75.

Nelstrop, L., Chandler-Oatts, J., Bingley, W., Bleetman, T., Corr, F., Cronin-Davis, J., et al. (2006). A systematic review of the safety and effectiveness of restraint and seclusion as interventions for the short-term management of violence in adult psychiatric inpatient settings and emergency departments. *Worldviews Evidence-Based Nursing, 3,* 8–18.

Neufeld, R. R., Libow, L. S., Foley, W. J., Dunbar, J. M., Cohen, C., & Breuer, B. (1999). Restraint reduction reduces serious injuries among nursing home residents. *Journal of the American Geriatrics Society, 47,* 1202–1207.

Newton, J. T. (2009). Restrictive behaviour management procedures with people with Intellectual disabilities who require dental treatment. *Journal of Applied Research in Intellectual Disabilities, 22,* 118–125.

Newton, T., & Sturmey, P. (2002) Acceptability of methods of behaviour control for dentally anxious children. *Journal of Dental Research, 81,* A–32.

Newton, J. T., Naidu, R., & Sturmey, P. (2003). The acceptability of the use of sedation in the management of dental anxiety in children: Views of dental students. *European Journal of Dental Education, 7,* 72–76.

Newton, J. T., Patel, H., Shah, S., & Sturmey, P. (2004). Attitudes towards the use of hand over mouth (HOM) and physical restraint amongst paediatric specialist practitioners in the UK. *International Journal of Paediatric Dentistry, 14,* 111–117.

Newton, J. T., Patel, H., Shah, S., & Sturmey, P. (2005). Perceptions of detention in treatment of people with eating disorders. *Psychological Reports, 96,* 701–706.

Njus, E. (2011). Parents accused of caging autistic children in Vancouver plead not guilty. http://www.oregonlive.com/clark-county/index.ssf/2011/04/parents_accused_of_caging_autistic_children_in_vancouver_plead_not_guilty.html, downloaded 12/28/14.

Nurses and Midwives Board of Western Australia. (2009) Guidelines for the use of restraints in WA. Downloaded from http://www.acas.edu.au/the_house/guideline_for_use_of_restraint.pdf on 12/15/14.

Nyman, S., & Oliver, D. (2010). Preventing falls and avoiding restraint. In R. Hughes (Ed.), *Rights, risk and restraint-free care of older people: Person-centred approaches in health and social care* (pp. 167–177). London: Jessica Kingsley.

O'Brien, F., Azrin, N. H., & Bugle, C. (1972). Training profoundly retarded children to stop crawling. *Journal of Applied Behavior Analysis, 5,* 131–137.

O'Callaghan, P. M., Allen, K. D., Powell, S., & Salama, F. (2006). The efficacy of noncontingent escape for decreasing children's disruptive behavior during restorative dental treatment. *Journal of Applied Behavior Analysis, 39,* 161–171.

O'Neill, D. (2006). Lea cross review. http://www.hse.ie/eng/services/publications/olderpeople/Leas_Cross_Report_.pdf, downloaded 12/28/14.

Office for Civil Rights. (2012). Civil rights data collection. Data snapshot: School Discipline. http://www2.ed.gov/about/offices/list/ocr/docs/crdc-discipline-snapshot.pdf, downloaded 12//15/114.

Oliver, C., Hall, S., Hales, J., Murphy, G., & Watts, D. (1998). The treatment of severe self-injurious behavior by the systematic fading of restraints: Effects on self-injury, self-restraint, adaptive behavior, and behavioral correlates of affect. *Research in Developmental Disabilities, 19,* 143–165.

Oliver, C., Murphy, G., & Hall, S., Arron, K., & Leggett, J. (2003). Phenomenology of self-restraint. *American Journal on Mental Retardation, 108,* 71–81.

Oliver, D., Connelly, J. B., Victor, C. R., Shaw, F. E., Whitehead, A., Genc, Y., Vanoli, A., Martin, F. C., & Gosney, M. A. (2007). Strategies to prevent falls and fractures in hospitals and care homes and effect of cognitive impairment: Systematic review and meta-analyses. *The British Medical Journal, 33,* 82.

Oueis, H. S., Ralstrom, E., Miriyala, V., Molinari, G. E., & Casamassimo, P. (2010). Alternatives for hand over mouth exercise after its elimination from the clinical guidelines of the American Academy of Pediatric Dentistry. *Pediatric Dentistry, 32,* 223–228.

Pace, G. M., Iwata, B. A., Edwards, G. L., & McCosh, K. C. (1986). Stimulus fading and transfer in the treatment of self-restraint and self-injurious behavior. *Journal of Applied Behavior Analysis, 19,* 381–389.

Parkes, J. (2000). Sudden death during restraint: A study to measure the effect of restraint positions on the rate of recovery from exercise. *Medicine, Science and the Law, 40,* 39–44.

Parry-Jones, W. L. (1972). *The trade in lunacy: A study of private madhouses in England in the 18th and 19th centuries*. London: Routledge & Kegan Paul.

Paterson, B., Bradley, P., Stark, C., Saddler, D., Leadbetter, D., & Allen, D. (2003). Deaths associated with restraint use in health and social care in the UK. The results of a preliminary survey. *Journal of Psychiatric and Mental Health Nursing, 10,* 3–15.

Paton, C., Barnes, T. R., Cavanagh, M. R., Taylor, D., & Lelliott, P. (2008). High-dose and combination antipsychotic prescribing in acute adult wards in the UK: The challenges posed by PRN prescribing. *The British Journal of Psychiatry, 192,* 435–439.

Pellfolk, T. J. E., Gustafson, Y., Bucht, G., & Karlsson, S. (2010). Effects of a restraint minimization program on staff knowledge, attitudes, and practice: A cluster randomized trial. *Journal of the American Geriatrics Society, 58,* 62–69.

Persel, C. S., Persel, C. H., Ashley, M. J., & Krych, D. K. (1997). The use of noncontingent reinforcement and contingent restraint to reduce physical aggression and self injurious behaviour in a traumatically brain injured adult. *Brain Injury, 11,* 751–760.

Peterson, R. F., & Peterson, L. R. (1968). The use of positive reinforcement in the control of self-destructive behavior in a retarded boy. *Journal of Experimental Child Psychology, 6,* 351–360.

Peterson, R. C., Ryan, J. B., & Rozalski, M. (2013). *Physical restraint and seclusion in schools*. Arlington: Council for Exceptional Children.

Pilowsky, L. S., Ring, H., Shine, P. J., Battesby, M., & Lader, M. (1992). Rapid tranquilization. A survey of emergency prescribing in a general psychiatric hospital. *British Journal of Psychiatry, 161,* 831–835.

Pogge, D. L., Pappalardo, S., Buccolo, M., & Harvey, P. D. (2011). Prevalence and precursors of the use of restraint and seclusion in a private psychiatric hospital: Comparison of child and adolescent patients. *Administration and Policy in Mental Health and Mental Health Services Research, 40,* 224–231.

Police Injured due to 'Horseplay'. (2009). Downloaded from http://news.bbc.co.uk/2/hi/uk_news/england/london/7967985.stm on 12/15/14.

Powell, S. B., Bodfish, J. W., Parker, D., Crawford, T. W., & Lewis, M. H. (1996). Self-restraint and self-injury: Occurrence and motivational significance. *American Journal of Mental Retardation, 101,* 41–48.

Powers, K. V., Roane, H. S., & Kelley, M. E. (2007). Treatment of self-restraint associated with the application of protective equipment. *Journal of Applied Behavior Analysis, 40,* 577–581.

Premack, D. (1963). Prediction of the comparative reinforcement values of running and drinking. *Science, 139*(3559), 1062–1063.

Propublica. (2014). Restraint. http://www.propublica.org/series/restraints, downloaded 12/16/14.

Pudelski, S. (2012). Keeping schools safe: Ensuring federal policy supports school safety. http://www.aasa.org/uploadedFiles/Policy_and_Advocacy/AASA-July-2012-Keeping-Schools-Safe.pdf, downloaded 12/17/14.

Quinn, C. A. (1994). The four A's of restraint reduction: Attitude, assessment, anticipation, avoidance. *Orthopaedic Nursing, 13,* 11–19.

Rainier, N. C. (2014). Reducing physical restraint use in alcohol withdrawal patients: A literature review. *Dimensions of Critical Care Nursing, 33,* 201–206.

Ray, W. A., Taylor, J. A., Meador, K. G., Lichtenstein, M. J., Griffin, M. R., Fought, R., & Blazer, D. G., et al. (1993). Reducing antipsychotic drug use in nursing homes: A controlled trial of provider education. *Archives of Internal Medicine, 153,* 713–721.

Reed, J. (2010). Bar and club bouncers to get restraint training. http://www.bbc.co.uk/newsbeat/10186122, downloaded 12/17/14.

Rezendes, M. (2014a). A death in restraints after 'standard procedure'. http://www.bostonglobe.com/metro/2014/02/16/homicide-bridgewater-state-hospital-raises-profound-questions-about-care-for-mentally-ill/TqgMJdNZ8SPjLcFQ6hRkTN/story.html?p1=Article_Related_Box_Article_More, downloaded 12/28/14.

Rezendes, M. (2014b). Bridgewater restraints use rose, even after patient's death. http://www.bostonglobe.com/metro/2014/04/05/bridgewater-restraints-use-rose-even-after-patient-death/iVt77HVAplzKD5Eh3vaF4M/story.html, downloaded 12/28/14.

Rezendes, M. (2014c). Restraints cited in three deaths at Bridgewater. http://www.bostonglobe.com/metro/2014/10/11/doubts-about-quality-massachusetts-prison-health-care-after-three-deaths-bridgewater-state-hospital/1oRBH0×7JHJxzU2kbm2AlL/story.html, downloaded 12/28/14.

Richter, T., Meyer, G., Möhler, R., & Köpke, S. (2012). Psychosocial interventions for reducing antipsychotic medication in care home residents. *Cochrane Database of Systematic Reviews* 2012, (12). Art. No.: CD008634. doi:10.1002/14651858.CD008634.pub2.

Roberts, Y. (2013). Trauma of autistic boy shackled by police. http://www.theguardian.com/uk/2013/feb/17/police-restraint-autistic-boy, downloaded 12/28/14.

Robertson, J., Emerson, E., Pinkney, L., Caesar, E., Felce, D., Meek, A., & Hallam, A., et al. (2005). Treatment and management of challenging behaviours in congregate and noncongregate community-based supported accommodation. *Journal of Intellectual Disability Research, 49,* 63–72.

Rojahn, J., Schroeder, S. R., & Mulick, J. A. (1980). Ecological assessment of self-protective devices in three profoundly retarded adults. *Journal of Autism and Developmental Disorders, 10,* 59–66.

Romijn, A., & Frederiks, B. J. (2012). Restriction on restraints in the care for people with intellectual disabilities in the Netherlands: Lessons learned from Australia, UK, and United States. *Journal of Policy and Practice in Intellectual Disabilities, 9,* 127–133.

Rooker, G. W., & Roscoe, E. M. (2005). Functional analysis of self-injurious behavior and its relation to self-restraint. *Journal of Applied Behavior Analysis, 38,* 537–542.

Rovner, B. W., Steele, C. D., Shmuely, Y., & Folstein, M. F. (1996). A randomized trial of dementia care in nursing homes. *Journal of the American Geriatrics Society, 44,* 7–13.

Royal College of Psychiatrists. (2005). *Violence: The short-term management of disturbed/violent behaviour in psychiatric in-patient and emergency departments guideline NCC-NSC 22/02/05.* London: Royal College of Psychiatrists.

Ryan, C. (2010). *Manual restraints in psychiatric settings: Empirical realities: A rare insight from patients' and nurses' perspectives.* Saarbruken: VDM.

Ryan, J. B., Peterson, R., Tetreault, G., & Vander Hagen, E. (2007). Reducing seclusion timeout and restraint procedures with at-risk youth. *The Journal of at Risk Issues, 13,* 7-–12.

Sailas, E., & Fenton, M. (2000). Seclusion and restraint for people with serious mental illness (Cochrane Review) (2):CD001163.

Sambrook, C. (2013). G4S guard fatally restrains 15 year old—gets promoted. http://www.opendemocracy.net/ourkingdom/clare-sambrook/g4s-guard-fatally-restrains-15-year-old-gets-promoted, downloaded 12/28/14.

Sanders, K. (2009). The effects of an action plan, staff training, management support and monitoring on restraint use and costs of work-related injuries. *Journal of Applied Research in Intellectual Disabilities, 22,* 216–220.

Santini, S., & Ness S. (2011). *The catalog of cruelty: An illustrated collection of ancient restraints and medieval instruments of torture and execution.* Scotts Valley: Steven Santini.

Scanlan, J. N. (2010). Interventions to reduce the use of seclusion and restraint in inpatient psychiatric settings: What we know so far a review of the literature. *International Journal of Social Psychiatry, 56,* 412–423.

Scheuermann, R., Peterson, R. L., & Billingsley, G. (2013). Ethical issues in the use of restraint and seclusion. In R. L. Peterson, J. B. Ryan, & M. Rozalski (Eds.). *Physical restraint and seclusion in schools* (pp. 31–50). Arlington: Council for Exceptional Children.

Schieb, D. A., Protas, E. J., & Hasson, S. M. (1996). Special feature: Implications of physical restraint and restraint reduction of older persons. *Topics in Geriatric Rehabilitation, 12,* 70–83.

School staff get 1,700 complaints. (2010). http://www.bbc.co.uk/news/education-10918940, downloaded 12/28/14.

Schussler, S., Dassen, T., & Lohrmann, C. (2014). Comparison of care dependency and related nursing care problems between Austrian nursing home residents with and without dementia. *European Geriatric Medicine, in press.*

Shaw. (2014). Report of the independent advisory panel on non-compliance management. https://www.gov.uk/government/uploads/system/uploads/attachment_data/file/324130/report-iap-ncm-mar-14.pdf, downloaded 12/28/14.

Siegler, E. L., Capezuti, E., Maislin, G., Baumgarten, M., Evans, L., & Strumpf, N. (1997). Effects of a restraint reduction intervention and OBRA '87 regulations on psychoactive drug use in nursing homes. *Journal of the American Geriatrics Society, 45,* 791–796

Silverman, K., Watanabe, K., Marshall, A. M., & Baer, D. M. (1984). Reducing self-injury and corresponding self-restraint through the strategic use of protective clothing. *Journal of Applied Behavior Analysis, 17,* 545–552.

Simoni-Wastila, L., Wei, Y.-J., Luong, M., Franey, C., Huang, T.-Y., Rattinger, G. B., Zuckerman, I. H., et al. (2014). Quality of psychopharmacological medication use in nursing home residents. *Research in Social and Administrative Pharmacy, 10,* 494–507.

Singh, N. N., Lancioni, G. E., Wahler, R. G., Winton, A. S., & Singh, J. (2008). Mindfulness approaches in cognitive behavior therapy. *Behavioural and Cognitive Psychotherapy, 36,* 659–666.

Singh, N. N., Lancioni, G. E., Winton, A. S., Adkins, A. D., Wahler, R. G., Sabaawi, M., & Singh, J. (2007). Individuals with mental illness can control their aggressive behavior through mindfulness training. *Behavior Modification, 31,* 313–328.

Singh, N. N., Lancioni, G. E., Winton, A. S., Curtis, W. J., Wahler, R. G., Sabaawi, M., & McAleavey, K., et al. (2006). Mindful staff increase learning and reduce aggression in adults with developmental disabilities. *Research in Developmental Disabilities, 27,* 545–558.

Singh, N. N., Lancioni, G. E., Winton, A. S., Singh, A. N., Adkins, A. D., & Singh, J. (2009a). Mindful staff can reduce the use of physical restraints when providing care to individuals with intellectual disabilities. *Journal of Applied Research in Intellectual Disabilities, 22,* 194–202.

Singh, A. N., Matson, J. L., Cooper, C. L., & Adkins, A. D. (2009b). Readability and reading level of behavior treatment plans in intellectual disabilities. *Journal of Developmental and Physical Disabilities, 21,* 185–194.

Singh, N. N., Wahler, R. G., Adkins, A. D., & Myers, R. E. (2003). Soles of the feet: A mindfulness-based self-control intervention for aggression by an individual with mild mental retardation and mental illness. *Research in Developmental Disabilities, 24,* 158–169.

Skinner, B. F. (1953). *Science and human behavior.* New York: Free Press.

Smallridge, P., & Williamson, A. (2011). Report on implementing the independent review of restraint in juvenile settings. https://www.gov.uk/government/uploads/system/uploads/attachment_data/file/217362/report-implement-review-restraint-juvenile-secure-settings.pdf, downloaded 12/28/14.

Smalls, Y. (2004). *Utility of the implementation of programmatic systems to reduce and eliminate restraint use for the treatment of problem behaviors with individuals with mental retardation.* Doctoral dissertation, Louisiana State University.

Smith, G. M., Davis, R. H., Bixler, E. O., Lin, H.-M., Altenor, A., Altenor, R. J., et al. (2005). Special section on seclusion and restraint: Pennsylvania state hospital system's seclusion and restraint reduction program. *Psychiatric Services, 56,* 1115–1122.

Smith, R. G., Iwata, B. A., Vollmer, T. R., & Pace, G. M. (1992). On the relationship between self-injurious behavior and self-restraint. *Journal of Applied Behavior Analysis, 25,* 433–445.

Smith, R. G., Lerman, D. C., & Iwata, B. A. (1996). Self-restraint as a positive reinforcement for self-injurious behavior. *Journal of Applied Behavior Analysis, 29,* 99–102.

Smith, R. G., Russo, L., & Le, D. D. (1999). Distinguishing between extinction and punishment effects of response blocking: A replication. *Journal of Applied Behavior Analysis, 32,* 367–370.

Sourander, A., Ellilä, H., Välimäki, M., & Piha, J. (2002). Use of holding, restraints, seclusion and time-out in child and adolescent psychiatric in-patient treatment. *European Child and Adolescent Psychiatry, 11,* 162–167.

Spinney, L. (2007). Therapy for autistic children causes outcry in France. *Lancet, 370,* 645–646.

Spreat, S., Lipinski, D., Hill, J., & Halpin, M. E. (1986). Safety indices associated with the use of contingent restraint procedures. *Applied Research in Mental Retardation, 7,* 465–481.

Steinert, T., Lepping, P., Bernhardsgrütter, R., Conca, A., Hatling, T., Janssen, W., et al. (2010). Incidence of seclusion and restraint in psychiatric hospitals: A literature review and survey of international trends. *Social Psychiatry and Psychiatric Epidemiology, 9,* 889–897.

Stewart, D., Van der Merwe, M., Bowers, L., Simpson, A., & Jones, J. (2010). A review of interventions to reduce mechanical restraint and seclusion among adult psychiatric inpatients. *Issues in Mental Health Nursing, 31,* 413–424.

Stickney, S. B. (1974). Problems in implementing the right to treatment in Alabama: The Wyatt v. Stickney case. *Psychiatric Services, 4,* 32–45.

Stojanovic, D. (2007). *Report. Disabled people abused in Serbia.* http://www.nbcnews.com/id/21790870-nbc_nightly_news_with_brian_williams/#.VJXrF_8w4Q, downloaded 12/20/14.

Stokes, T. F., & Baer, D. M. (1977). An implicit technology of generalization. *Journal of Applied Behavior Analysis, 10,* 349–367.

Stone, K. (2009). Gatehouse school. *An Independent Management Review.* January, 2009.

Strickland, T. (2009). Executive order 2009–13-s. *Establishing restraint policies including ban on prone restraint.* https://education.ohio.gov/getattachment/Topics/Other-Resources/School-Safety/Building-Better-Learning-Environments/Policy-Positive-Behavior-Interventions-and-Support/Seclusion-and-Restraint-EO-09-13S.pdf.aspx, downloaded 12/17/14.

Strumpf, N., Robinson, J., Wagner, J., & Evans, L. K. (1998). *Restraint-free care: Individualized approaches for frail elders.* New York: Springer.

Stubbs, B., & Alderman, N. (2008). Physical interventions in the management of aggression arising from brain injury: Frequency of use and injuries associated with implementation. *Brain Injury, 22,* 691–696.

Sturmey, P. (1990). Goal planning manuals: Their readability, human interest and content. *Mental Handicap Research, 3,* 70–80.
Sturmey, P. (1993). The reliability and human interest of information leaflets from major British charities: An unintelligible, boring replication? *Mental Handicap Research, 6,* 174–182.
Sturmey, P. (1996). *Functional analysis in clinical psychology*. Chichester: Wiley.
Sturmey, P. (1999). Correlates of restraint use in an institutional population. *Research in Developmental Disabilities, 20,* 339–346.
Sturmey, P. (2003). Aging-related behavioral interventions. In P. W. Davidson, V. Prasher, & M. P. Janicki (Eds.), *Mental health, intellectual disabilities, and the aging process.* London: Blackwell.
Sturmey, P. (2007). *Functional analysis in clinical treatment.* Chichester: Wiley.
Sturmey, P. (2009). Restraint, seclusion and PRN medication in English services for people with learning disabilities: An analysis of the 2007 National Audit Survey. *Journal of Applied Research in Intellectual Disabilities, 22,* 140–144.
Sturmey, P. (2014a). Evidence-based practice: An overview. In P. Sturmey & R. Didden (Eds.), *Evidence-based practice in intellectual disabilities* (pp. 3–28). Chichester: Wiley.
Sturmey, P. (2014b). Adaptive behavior. In P. Sturmey & R. Didden (Eds.), *Evidence-based practice in intellectual disabilities* (pp. 29–61). Chichester: Wiley.
Sturmey, P. (2014c). Maladaptive behavior. In P. Sturmey & R. Didden (Eds.), *Evidence-based practice in intellectual disabilities* (pp. 62–84). Chichester: Wiley.
Sturmey, P. (2014d). But is it worth it? In P. Sturmey & R. Didden (Eds), *Evidence-based practice in intellectual disabilities* (pp. 85–100). Chichester: Wiley.
Sturmey, P., & Didden, R. (Eds.). (2014). *Evidence-based practice in intellectual disabilities.* Chichester: Wiley.
Sturmey, P., Lee, R., Reyer, H., & Robek, A. (2003a). Assessing preferences for staff: Some pilot data. *Behavioural and Cognitive Psychotherapy, 31,* 99–102.
Sturmey, P., & McGlynn, A. P. (2003). Restraint reduction. In D. Allen (Ed.), *Responding to challenging behaviour in persons with intellectual disabilities: Ethical approaches to physical intervention* (pp. 203–218). Kidderminster: BILD.
Sturmey, P., Thomsett, M., Sundaram, J., & Newton, J. T. (2003b). The effects of method of behaviour management client characteristics, and outcome on public perceptions of intervention acceptability in paediatric dentistry. *Behavioural and Cognitive Psychotherapy, 31,* 169–176.
Sullivan-Marx, E. M., & Strumpf, N. E. (1996). Restraint-free care for acutely ill patients in the hospital. *AACN Advanced Critical Care, 7,* 572–578.
Sullivan-Marx, E. M., Strumpf, N. E., Evans, L. K., Baumgarten, M., & Maislin, G. (1999). Predictors of continued physical restraint use in nursing home residents following restraint reduction efforts. *Journal of the American Geriatrics Society, 47,* 342–348.
Sundel, M., Garrett, R. M., & Horn, R. D. (1994). Restraint reduction in a nursing home and its impact on employee attitudes. *Journal of the American Geriatrics Society, 42,* 381–387.
Sundram, C. J. (2011). The measure of a society. Protection of vulnerable persons in residential facilities against abuse and neglect. https://archive.org/stream/327142-ny-abuse-report#page/n0/mode/2up, downloaded 12/20/14.
Tardiff, K. (1984). *The psychiatric uses of seclusion and restraint.* Washington, DC: American Psychiatric Publishing.
TASH. (2000). Positive behavior supports. http://tash.org/about/resolutions/tash-resolution-positive-behavioral-supports/, downloaded 12/17/14.
Taub, E. (2012). The behavior-analytic origins of constraint-induced movement therapy: An example of behavioral neurorehabilitation. *The Behavior Analyst, 35,* 155–178.
Taylor, S. J. (2009). *Acts of conscience: World War II, mental institutions, and religious objectors.* Syracuse: Syracuse University Press.
Testad, I., Aasland, A. M., & Aarsland, D. (2005). The effect of staff training on the use of restraint in dementia: A single-blind randomised controlled trial. *International Journal of Geriatric Psychiatry, 20,* 587–590.

Texas Education Agency. (2009). Restraint report. 2007–2009. http://www.txbehaviorsupport.org/docs/9Final%20Restraint%20Report%20%28Feb%202011%29.pdf, downloaded 12/15/14.

Thompson, R. H., Iwata, B. A., Conners, J., & Roscoe, E. M. (1999). Effects of reinforcement for alternate behavior during punishment of self-injury. *Journal of Applied Behavior Analysis, 32,* 317–328.

Thompson, T., & Grabowski, J. (1972). *Behavior modification of the mentally retarded.* Oxford: Oxford University Press.

Tiffany, F. (1890). *Life of Dorothea Dix.* New York: Houghton Mifflin.

Timeline: Winterbourne View abuse scandal. (2012). http://www.bbc.com/news/uk-england-bristol-20078999, downloaded 12/20/14.

Tinetti, M. E., Liu, W. L., & Ginter, S. L., (1992). Mechanical restraint use and fall-related injuries among residents of skilled nursing facilities. *Annals of Internal Medicine, 116,* 369–374.

Toledo News Now. (n.d.). Authorities find 11 children locked in cages. *Toledo News Now.* http://www.toledonewsnow.com/story/3841482/authorities-find-11-children-locked-in-cages), downloaded 12/28/14.

Touchette, P. E., MacDonald, R. F., & Langer, S. N. (1985). A scatter plot for identifying stimulus control of problem behavior. *Journal of Applied Behavior Analysis, 18,* 343–351.

Trahan, M. A., Kahng, S., Fisher, A. B., & Hausman, N. L. (2011). Behavior-analytic research on dementia in older adults. *Journal of Applied Behavior Analysis, 44,* 687–691.

Travis, R., & Sturmey, P. (2010). Functional analysis and treatment of the delusional statements of a man with multiple disabilities. Four year follow-up. *Journal of Applied Behavior Analysis, 43,* 745–749.

Tsakanikos, E., Costello, H., Holt, G., Sturmey, P., & Bouras, N. (2007). Behaviour management problems as predictors of psychotropic medication and use of psychiatric services in adults with autism. *Journal of Autism and Developmental Disorders, 37,* 1080–1085.

Tuke, S. (1813/2009). *Description of the retreat: An institution Near York, for the insane persons of the society of friends.* Charleston: Bibliolife.

United Nations. (2006). Convention on the rights of persons with disabilities. (http://www.un.org/disabilities/convention/conventionfull.shtml, downloaded 12/17/14.

Unsted Park 'self-harm blades' head teacher cleared. (2014). BBC News May 16, 2014, downloaded from http://www.bbc.com/news/uk-england-surrey-27443496, 12/28/14.

US Department of Justice. (2014). CRIPA Investigation of the New York City Department of Correction Jails on Rikers Island. http://www.justice.gov/usao/nys/pressreleases/August14/RikersReportPR/SDNY%20Rikers%20Report.pdf, downloaded 12/28/14.

van Houten, R. (1998). Unpublished paper.

Van Houten, R., Axelrod, S., Bailey, J. S., Favell, J. E., Foxx, R. M., Iwata, B. A., & Lovaas, O. I. (1988). The right to effective behavioral treatment. *The Behavior Analyst, 11,* 111–114.

van der Schaaf, P. S., Dusseldorp, E., Keuning, F. M., Janssen, W. A., & Noorthoorn, E. O. (2014). Impact of the physical environment of psychiatric wards on the use of seclusion. *British Journal of Psychiatry, 202,* 142–149.

Vogel, H. (2014). Violent and legal: The shocking ways school kids are being pinned down, isolated against their will. http://www.propublica.org/article/schools-restraints-seclusions/, downloaded 12/16/14.

Vollmer, T. R., Iwata, B. A., Zarcone, J. R., & Rodgers, T. A. (1992). A content analysis of written behavior management programs. *Research in Developmental Disabilities, 13,* 429-–441.

Wagner, M. (2014). California couple locked 11-year-old autistic son in dog cage to control tantrums: Cops. http://www.nydailynews.com/news/crime/calif-couple-locked-autistic-son-dog-cage-cops-article-1.1851973, downloaded 12/16/14.

Wainwright, M. (2011). Unlawful restraint contributed to death of boy in custody. http://www.theguardian.com/society/2011/jan/27/unlawful-restraint-inquest-adam-rickwood, downloaded 12/28/14.

Walk, A. (1970). Lincoln and non-restraint. *British Journal of Psychiatry, 117,* 481–495.

Wallace, M. D., Iwata, B. A., Zhou, L., & Goff, G. A. (1999). Rapid assessment of the effects of restraint on self-injury and adaptive behavior. *Journal of Applied Behavior Analysis, 32,* 525–528.
Wang, W. W., & Moyle, W. (2005). Physical restraint use on people with dementia: A review of the literature. *Australian Journal of Advanced Nursing, 22,* 46–52.
Webber, L. S. (2013). *Senior practitioner report. 2012–2013.* Melbourne: Department of Human services.
Webber, L. S., Lambrick, F., Donley, M., Buchholtz, M., Chan, J. B., Carracher, R., & Patel, G. (2010). Restraint and seclusion of people on compulsory treatment orders in Victoria, Australia in 2008–2009. *Psychiatry, Psychology and Law, 17,* 562–573.
Webber, L., Richardson, B., Lambrick, F., & Fester, T. (2012). The impact of the quality of behaviour support plans on the use of restraint and seclusion in disability services. *International Journal of Positive Behavioural Support, 2,* 3–11.
Weintraub, D., & Spurlock, M. (2002). Change in the rate of restraint use and falls on a psychogeriatric inpatient unit: Impact of the health care financing administration's new restraint and seclusion standards for hospitals. *Journal of Geriatric Psychiatry and Neurology, 15,* 91–94.
Welch. (1989). *Holding time.* New York: Fireside.
Wieman, D. A., Camacho-Gonsalves, T., Huckshorn, K. A., & Leff, S. (2014). Multisite study of an evidence-based practice to reduce seclusion and restraint in psychiatric inpatient facilities. *Psychiatric Services, 65,* 345–351.
Wilder, D. A., Masuda, A., O'Connor, C., & Baham, M. (2001). Brief functional analysis of bizarre vocalizations in an adult with schizophrenia. *Journal of Applied Behavior Analysis, 34,* 65–68.
Williams, D. (1998). Those who've come across the seas. https://www.humanrights.gov.au/funnelback/search?query=restraint&start=81, downloaded 12/28/14.
Williams, D. E. (2009). Restraint safety: An analysis of injuries related to restraint of people with intellectual disabilities. *Journal of Applied Research in Intellectual Disabilities, 22,* 135–139.
Williams, D. E., & Grossett, D. L. (2011). Reduction of restraint of people with intellectual disabilities: An organizational behavior management (OBM) approach. *Research in Developmental Disabilities, 32,* 2336–2339.
Williams, D. E., Kirkpatrick-Sanchez, S., Enzinna, C., Dunn, J., & Borden-Karasack, D. (2009). The clinical management and prevention of Pica: A retrospective follow-up of 41 individuals with intellectual disabilities and Pica. *Journal of Applied Research in Intellectual Disabilities, 22,* 210–215.
Williams, D. E., Kirkpatrick-Sanchez, S., & Iwata, B. A. (1993). A comparison of shock intensity in the treatment of longstanding and severe self-injurious behavior. *Research in Developmental Disabilities, 14,* 207–219.
Wilson, E. B. (1996). Physical restraint of elderly patients in critical care: Historical perspectives and new directions. *Critical Care Nursing Clinics of North America, 8,* 61–70.
Winterbourne View: Earlier abuse at hospital. (2012). http://www.bbc.com/news/uk-england-bristol-19990628, downloaded 12/20/14.
Wressell, S. E., Tyrer, S. P., & Berney, T. P. (1990). Reduction in antipsychotic drug dosage in mentally handicapped patients. A hospital study. *The British Journal of Psychiatry, 157,* 101–106.
Wurtele, S. K., King, A. C., & Drabman, R. S. (1984). Treatment package to reduce SIB in a Lesch-Nyhan patient. *Journal of Mental Deficiency Research, 28,* 227–234.
Yeh, S. H., Lee, L. N., Ho, T. H., Chiang, M. C., & Lin, L. W. (2004). Implications of nursing care in the occurrence and consequences of unplanned extubation in adult intensive care units. *International Journal of Nursing Studies, 41,* 255–262.
Zusman, J. (1997). *Restraint and seclusion: Improving practice and conquering the JCAHO standards.* New York: Opus Communications.
Zusman, J. (1999). *Restraint and seclusion: Improving practice and maintaining JCAHO compliance.* New York: Opus Communications.

Index

P. Sturmey, *Reducing Restraint and Restrictive Behavior Management Practices*,
Autism and Child Psychopathology Series, DOI 10.1007/978-3-319-17569-0

MIX
Papier aus verantwortungsvollen Quellen
Paper from responsible sources
FSC® C105338

If you have any concerns about our products,
you can contact us on
ProductSafety@springernature.com

In case Publisher is established outside the EU,
the EU authorized representative is:
Springer Nature Customer Service Center GmbH
Europaplatz 3, 69115 Heidelberg, Germany

Printed by Libri Plureos GmbH
in Hamburg, Germany